FOURTH EDITION

LPN *to* RN
TRANSITIONS

Lora Claywell, PhD, MSN, RN, CNE

Professor
Affiliate Faculty Coordinator and RN-BSN Coordinator
Department of Graduate and Post-Licensure Nursing
Loretto Heights School of Nursing
Rueckert-Hartman College for Health Professions
Regis University
Denver, Colorado

ELSEVIER

ELSEVIER

3251 Riverport Lane
St. Louis, Missouri 63043

LPN TO RN TRANSITIONS, FOURTH EDITION   ISBN: 978-0-323-40151-7

Notices

Knowledge and best practice in this field are constantly changing. As new research and experience broaden our understanding, changes in research methods, professional practices, or medical treatment may become necessary. Practitioners and researchers must always rely on their own experience and knowledge in evaluating and using any information, methods, compounds, or experiments described herein. In using such information or methods they should be mindful of their own safety and the safety of others, including parties for whom they have a professional responsibility. With respect to any drug or pharmaceutical products identified, readers are advised to check the most current information provided (i) on procedures featured or (ii) by the manufacturer of each product to be administered, to verify the recommended dose or formula, the method and duration of administration, and contraindications. It is the responsibility of practitioners, relying on their own experience and knowledge of their patients, to make diagnoses, to determine dosages and the best treatment for each individual patient, and to take all appropriate safety precautions. To the fullest extent of the law, neither the Publisher nor the authors, contributors, or editors, assume any liability for any injury and/or damage to persons or property as a matter of products liability, negligence or otherwise, or from any use or operation of any methods, products, instructions, or ideas contained in the material herein.

Library of Congress Cataloging-in-Publication Data

Names: Claywell, Lora, author.
Title: LPN to RN transitions / Lora Claywell.
Description: Fourth edition. | St. Louis, Missouri : Elsevier, Inc., [2018] |
    Includes bibliographical references and index.
Identifiers: LCCN 2017028515 (print) | LCCN 2017029384 (ebook) | ISBN
    9780323474122 (Ebook) | ISBN 9780323401517 (pbk. : alk. paper)
Subjects: | MESH: Education, Nursing | Nurse's Role | Nursing Process |
    Career Mobility | Vocational Guidance | Nursing, Practical
Classification: LCC RT82 (ebook) | LCC RT82 (print) | NLM WY 18 | DDC
    610.7306/9--dc23
LC record available at https://lccn.loc.gov/2017028515

Senior Content Strategist: Sandra Clark
Senior Content Development Manager: Laurie Gower
Associate Content Development Specialist: Madison Autry
Publishing Services Manager: Deepthi Unni
Project Manager: Radhika Sivalingam
Design Direction: Ryan Cook

Printed in the United States of America

Last digit is the print number: 9   8   7   6   5   4   3   2

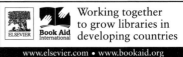

Working together
to grow libraries in
developing countries

www.elsevier.com • www.bookaid.org

Linda S. Barren, EdD, RNC, MS
Associate Professor
Nurse Science
Oklahoma State University—Oklahoma City
Oklahoma City, Oklahoma

Kelly W. Butler, MSN, RN, PHN
Professor of Nursing
Assistant Program Director,
ADN Program
Modesto Junior College
Nursing – Allied Health
Modesto, California

Jo-Ann B. Dean, MSN, MS, RN
National Dean of Nursing
National Dean of Nursing Education
West Orange, New Jersey

Carolyn Gersch, PhD (Candidate), MSN, RN, CNE
Associate Professor of Nursing
Kettering College
Kettering, Ohio

Sharon D. Henderson, MSN, RN
Associate Professor
Hillsborough Community College
Adjunct Faculty
The University of Tampa
Tampa, Florida

Barbara A. Lodge, BSN, RN
Assistant Professor
Nursing Department
Jefferson College
Hillsboro, Missouri

Pamela S. Sealover, RN, MSN, CNE
Associate Professor of Nursing,
Associate Director of Nursing
Ohio University-Zanesville
Zanesville, Ohio

Instructor and Student Ancillary Writers
Amber Ballard, MSN, RN
Sparrow Health System
Michigan State University
Lansing, Michigan

Lora Claywell, PhD, MSN, RN, CNE
Professor
Affiliate Faculty Coordinator and
RN-BSN Coordinator
Department of Graduate and
Post-Licensure Nursing
Loretto Heights School of Nursing
Rueckert-Hartman College for Health Professions
Regis University
Denver, Colorado

Laura Bevlok Kanavy, MSN, RN
Director of Practical Nursing
Career Technology Center of
Lackawanna County
Scranton, Pennsylvania

PREFACE

This edition of *LPN to RN Transitions* builds on the solid work of the first three editions, expanding as nursing knowledge and roles have expanded. The topics in the new and improved text were carefully selected in the hope of fully supporting the practical/vocational nurse in the early stage of transition to become a registered nurse.

This book is divided into five major parts, addressing not only the move back into the role of student but also progressing through each of the roles of the RN, and ultimately transitioning to the new role.

Unit 1 was created for the practical/vocational nurse who is once again becoming a student and taking that leap of faith back into nursing education. It addresses content that students need to have the best opportunity for success in educational endeavors. Time management, study skills, test-taking strategies, and learning as an adult.

Unit 2 honors and clarifies the unique perspective of the student who is already in a nursing role so that the new role can come into focus as distinctly different. Concepts and principles that are foundational to **members of the discipline** of nursing are presented as the cornerstone upon which to shape your professional nursing practice.

Unit 3 completes the essential foundational information for the role of **Provider of Care** with improved chapters on nursing theory and nursing process, critical thinking, and evidence-based practice. Professional nursing today—from the bedside to the community and university settings—requires that we diligently bridge the gap from theory and research to practice. This unit will help you form a clear understanding of how your Provider of Care role is guided through theory and evidence.

Unit 4 takes you through the professional nursing role of **Manager of Care**, where leading, delegating, and collaborating are hallmarks of contemporary nursing practice.

Unit 5 prepares you to make the transition and to socialize into the role of **Registered Nurse**, particularly focusing on preparing to take the NCLEX-RN®.

Finally, this new edition brings with it several online resources within Elsevier's awesome website, Evolve at http://evolve.elsevier.com/Claywell/transitions. NCLEX Review Questions broken down by chapter, a searchable online Glossary, and Résumé and Cover Letter Templates are all designed to further enhance your opportunity for learning. In addition, you will find an updated chapter on writing professionally to help you advance your writing skills. You are encouraged to make use of all of these resources as you go along your way.

ACKNOWLEDGMENTS

It has been nearly two decades now since I first began the process of researching and writing about the transition of practical/vocational nurses to registered nurses., So much has changed in health care and nursing education, but much has also stayed the same. Clearly, nursing is more critical to the health of the people of the world than ever. Nurses at every level are called upon to practice to the very limits of their preparation and licensure. Nursing education is challenged with providing more education for and engendering more competencies in students within an environment where time and clinical experiences are at a premium. LPNs/LVNs are uniquely positioned to enter professional nursing at a whole new level, and their previous experience can be a fine place from which to build the bridge. I am honored to be allowed to create a small part of that connection through this text. I believe that this new edition will go farther to support you as you take those steps to assume your new role.

In creating this new and improved work, many are to be acknowledged for their careful and considered input. First, I would like to thank Bradley Corbin, the co-author of the original edition of this text. His work remains relevant and appreciated. I also wish to recognize Kathy Ham, whose original work both informed and contributed to the development of this text. There are several other superb nurses whose contributions to, and focused review of, both the text and ancillary materials added brilliantly to both the breadth and depth of this edition. For those past and present, thank you!

To the staff at Elsevier, both those working behind the scenes and those who are known to me and with whom I have enjoyed working over the years, I am forever grateful. Yvonne Alexopoulos had the first conversation with me that ignited the fire in the belly for creating the first edition of the text. Thank you for listening and for making it happen! Sandy Clark, Lisa Newton, Laurie Gower, and Madison Autry, over the years, have been an invaluable resource and support; what a pleasure it is to work with such superb professionals! Your talent, competence, and patience are all beyond measure. I thank you. Writing this fourth edition has extended my dream come true!

To Jim, my husband, best friend, and the love of my life, I simply cannot imagine life or even my purpose in it without you! Thank you for your love, for always believing in me, for supporting me, and for your gentle understanding, caring, and devotion! To my children Cameron and Kaitlin, the lights of my life, you were so young when I wrote the first edition, and now in the blink of an eye you are grown and off on your own adventures. I am so proud of you and how you have pursued your dreams. Thank you for just being you, my precious loves. To my wonderful mom and dad, you have always supported me and cheered me on, always providing your unfailing strength and support. I have always admired you both and hope I have made you proud. I love you all more than words can say!

Last but not least, I wish to thank God. For I know that all good things come only from Him. I have been blessed with purpose and opportunity, with love and joy, and with family who support me and who mean everything to me. I pray that all that I do is acceptable to Him and will be to His purpose and glory.

Lora G. Claywell

CONTENTS

UNIT THREE   THE RN AS A PROVIDER OF CARE, 120

UNIT FOUR   THE RN AS MANAGER OF CARE, 236

UNIT FIVE   PUTTING IT ALL TOGETHER, 284

UNIT 1

Essential Skills to Begin Your Transition

CHAPTER

1

Honoring Your Past, Planning Your Future

evolve WEBSITE

Additional resources are available online at:
http://evolve.elsevier.com/Claywell/transitions

OBJECTIVES

After completing this chapter, the student will be prepared to:
1. Identify how experiences influence learning in adults.
2. Create an experiential résumé.
3. Delineate both positive and negative impact experiences.
4. Examine personal and professional selves.
5. Identify motivations and personal outcome priorities for returning to school.
6. Identify both short- and long-term personal and professional goals.
7. Understand change theory and how it applies to becoming an RN.

KEY TERMS

adult learning	long-term goal	scheme
cohort	moving	short-term goal
driving force	outcome priority	transition
experiential résumé	refreezing	unfreezing
lifelong learning	restraining force	

OVERVIEW

In this chapter you will begin to assess yourself closely and prepare for your nursing education experience. In doing so you will consider why you believe you want to be a registered nurse (RN). You will review the positive and negative aspects of your past. You will look closely at the present, set goals, and chart your course into your future as an RN.

UNDERSTANDING TRANSITION

As the title of this text implies, you are about to undergo a series of transitions and the experience of **transition** might be best prepared for by taking a look at a nursing theory regarding human transition. Afaf Meleis (2010) created and refined Transitions Theory over several decades, and it has become a foundational theory for nursing practice. Not only can it be applied to our patients and serve as a basis for understanding how they move, for example, from health to illness and back again, but it can be applied to any individual and his or her family who is experiencing change. Meleis (2010) says that change is the catalyst that causes a person to begin to move, "from one fairly stable state to another fairly stable state…" (p. 11). It is during these transitional times that nurses can influence the experience for the individual and their families. In this same way, if you are aware that you are embarking on a period of transition, there are things you can do to facilitate a smoother experience for both you and your family.

According to Transitions Theory, it is important to understand the type of transition at hand as well as its complexity with regard to timing and whether it influences other elements of a person's life. Transition does not happen in a vacuum, and, therefore, a wide-angle view of the conditions associated with the transition is key. Consider those things that will influence the transition such as economics, family situation, cultural beliefs, personal health, confidence, education, previous experience, and so on (Meleis, 2010). With these things in mind, you can take action to prepare yourself and your family for the transitions to come as you enter nursing school.

Just as our interventions are those things we do to facilitate the transitions in our patients, we can plan interventions for ourselves as well. This book, and in particular the first few chapters, will help you prepare for your transition, gain confidence, and plan ways to cope with the inevitable challenges that come with going back to school as an adult with a full and complex life.

LEARNING AS AN ADULT

As you will see as you go along in this text, there are a number of references to Adult Learning Theory, also known as andragogy. Malcolm Knowles, one of the earliest and most popular theorists to study *adult learning* (as opposed to learning in children), identified adult learning as a process that can be understood and supported. There are six underlying assumptions associated with the way adults learn. First, as adults, we need to understand why we need to know what is being taught and how it is important to our future. Second, as adults, we want to be in control of what we learn; this is also known as self-direction. This means we like to have a say in what and how we learn, and teaching us as if we were children will not work. Third, as adults, we have lived full and complex lives that accumulate experience that cannot be ignored. Your experience as an LPN/LVN should be incorporated and celebrated rather than ignored. Your experience has value, and it will come to bear on new material you will learn, one way or the other. Fourth, we like to solve problems, and we draw upon the whole of our lives and experience when it comes to being ready to learn something new or change what we learned in the past. Fifth, we like to be able to apply what we are learning immediately and in a practical way. Gaining as much learning by doing as possible will help us remember. Finally, we are motivated to learn by being faced with a problem (Knowles, Holton, & Swanson, 2015). Our maturity has led us to recognize that we can and must problem-solve to get to the next level. This goes right along with Transitions Theory…basically hand in hand. If we understand these things about ourselves as adult learners, we can better prepare ourselves and our families for the transitions to come. More about adult learning theory is woven into later segments of this chapter. See Box 1.1 for a brief list of the principles of adult learning.

WHERE IT ALL BEGINS

As an LPN/LVN returning to nursing school, you have universal and individual needs that must be addressed in order to make the transition meaningful, productive, and positive. Having been to LPN/LVN school, you have some idea of what likely lies ahead, and returning to nursing school might be a daunting challenge. Very likely you are experiencing a degree of fear or even guilt associated with your decision, and it is important to recognize it. You may be asking yourself these questions:

- Will I fit in?
- Will it be too expensive and cause my family to have to scrimp to get by?
- Will it take up too much of my time and cause problems with my family and friends?
- Will it really be worth it; after all, I already have a career?
- Will my co-workers understand my need for flexibility in my scheduling now?

Admitting fear and guilt is a good first step in dealing with these feelings, and this book will give you practical tools for doing just that. There are times when the journey to becoming an RN might seem too steep, with treacherous footing. Take a deep breath and pat yourself on the back, for you have already accomplished a great deal.

BOX 1.1 KNOWLES' SIX PRINCIPLES OF ADULT EDUCATION

- Adults **need to know** the why, what, and how of what is to be learned
- Adults prefer to be in control of their learning; are **self-directed**
- Adults have **life experiences** that influence the learning
- Adult **readiness to learn** is associated with need or change
- Adult **orientation to learning** is practical and for immediate application
- Adults are **motivated to learn** when there will be a personal gain or problem solved

(Knowles, Holton, & Swanson, 2015)

You believe you can do it! Believing in yourself is the cornerstone of success. Very few people reach their goals without persistence and overcoming adversity. As you begin your journey, remember that a challenge is lost only if one ceases to try. Any effort is an accomplishment, and sometimes we have to measure our progress in small steps.

If asked why you decided to resume nursing education, your answers might vary from needing to improve your financial prospects to hoping to fulfill a lifelong dream. Students who are already LPN/LVNs have reported that one reason they decided to return to school was the inability to find the often higher-paying jobs in acute care nursing. Acute care facilities are moving toward an all-RN primary care provider model, and this makes the LPN/LVN position in hospitals more difficult to find. Other students report that their organizations required returning to school to earn the RN designation in order to advance and, in some cases, to remain employed (Cook et al., 2010). In any case, most adults seek to continue their education due to particular life circumstances, having identified needs in their lives. The desire to return to college may have been present for some years, but the lack of time or money made returning to school an impossibility. However, once certain conditions prevail, resuming nursing education becomes the priority.

Both internal factors, such as your personal desire or aspirations, and external factors, like the need to increase your income potential, may definitively make becoming an RN the most important outcome in your life. When you enrolled in nursing school, you were acting on your **outcome priority,** the essential issue or need to be addressed at any given time within a set of conditions or circumstances. This term, which is threaded throughout this book, may be applied to virtually any situation. In the first several chapters of this book we will address your individual outcome priorities as related to making the transition back into school and from LPN/LVN to RN.

REVIEWING THE PAST

One of the greatest strengths a person has is the realization that experiences and accomplishments are key tools when working toward a new goal. Knowles, Holton, and Swanson (2015) describe four ways that experience influences learning. First, it develops and accentuates differences among learners. Experience is also a source for insight and motivation, but it can also be a barrier or a rigid mold into which new learning may have a hard time fitting. Finally, experience is the foundation upon which you define yourself.

As a learner, you will become part of a **cohort,** a group of people engaging in a common experience at the same time. You will gravitate toward those in your cohort whose experiences have shaped their habits, attitudes, and other traits such that you become compatible with or complementary to them. The experiences you and your cohort share are valuable tools in gaining understanding and perspective. The more you engage with your classmates, the better your experience will be.

Experience can also make some learning difficult. An old concept or detail may seem clear in your mind, but it can be challenged or modified with new information. Often adults must be able to make sense of new material in the presence of previously established beliefs or knowledge. Finding critical links between what you already know and integrating new information will be a key to learning as an adult. This can be especially challenging as a student who may be considered an expert in the LPN/ LVN role but who is reentering nursing school at the novice or advanced beginner level as a student in a new role. As an adult, making this transition may prove to be a significant challenge. Keeping an open mind toward new or modified information (even if it contradicts what you have known in the past) is key.

Experience adds layers of description to definition of the self. You may consider yourself "good" or "bad" at starting IVs based on patient reaction in the past. Such self-definition may influence your actions. You may either avoid having to start IVs or seek additional practice and instruction so that your skills improve. Use good or bad experience as a link to new learning, and be open to the possibility of accommodating something new.

Relate each new piece of information to your daily practice. You can likely recall examples of patients or experiences in the past that will make the critical connection not only for you but also for those in your cohort group with whom you share your experience. Life stories are an important element in integrating new learning. These and your experiences, as well as prior learning, make up the **scheme,** or web of connections, to which all new learning must be related so that it makes sense. Work with each new concept and detail until it feels comfortable in your already well-developed scheme. Your faculty will expect you, as an adult learner, to be able to critically assess both your strengths and your weaknesses related to knowledge, skills, and attitudes regarding both previously and newly learned didactic content, psychomotor skills, and the values associated with the whole of the experience of becoming an RN.

To move forward, you need to determine where you have been. You must closely and critically examine the path you have traveled to this point. In Exercise 1.1, briefly sketch your *experiential résumé,* a concise list of your experiences and prior learning. Begin at the point of completion of your LPN/LVN program. Make a timeline, including events, accomplishments, and setbacks that stand out in your mind, detailing the surrounding circumstances and other aspects as much as possible. Looking at your experiential résumé, what are some of the lessons you learned along the way? What will you do similarly or differently as you embark upon the next leg of your journey?

Let's look at experiences more critically now. Research in adult education has determined that experiences may either help or hinder both present and future educational endeavors (Knowles et al., 2015). Experience may serve as a chain to which new learning may be linked, making concepts understandable within your personal context. Conversely, some experiences make learning more difficult in that new information may contradict previously accepted information and make it necessary to unlearn it. The process of unlearning is more difficult than initial learning.

In Exercise 1.2, separate the items you wrote in your experiential résumé into either the positive-impact or negative-impact category. Determine the impact based on your beliefs at this time (you may always switch them later). For instance, perhaps after high school, you entered nursing school but were in an accident and had to withdraw. Maybe you were unsuccessful in your first nursing science class and dropped out. How did this influence subsequent decisions and actions? You might have decided that the nursing program was just not appropriate, or you might have tried to determine what needed to be done to ensure success the next time.

❓ EXERCISE 1.1

Experiential Résumé
Secondary education completed _____ (date).

Entrance to RN school _____ (date).

❓ EXERCISE 1.2

POSITIVE-IMPACT EXPERIENCES	NEGATIVE-IMPACT EXPERIENCES

We leave the past for now. As we move into the present, keep your experiential résumé in mind. Along the way, it may be necessary to revisit the list in Exercise 1.2 to determine the roots of problem situations that may arise. Having noted both positive and negative experiences, you have armed yourself with a portion of a key tool to success: self-awareness.

❓ EXERCISE 1.3

I define my personal self as:

I define my professional self as:

❓ EXERCISE 1.4

PERCEPTION OF CURRENT LPN/LVN ROLE	PERCEPTION OF NEW RN ROLE

EXAMINING WHERE YOU ARE NOW

"The most difficult of all perspectives is to see oneself as one really is."

(Wilson & Porter-O'Grady, 1999, p. 230)

Montgomery and O'Grady (2010) state, "Self-perception and expectations are parts of the critical learning infrastructure" (p. 45). Now that you have reviewed your experiences and accomplishments, it is time to examine your current personal and professional statuses. To grow beyond the status quo, you must be fully able to assess who you are; your motivations; and the conditions, environment, or role that you currently occupy. How would you describe your personal self? The personal realm includes the areas of your life before and after work and those that relate to your private goals rather than company goals. What are your roles and your traits? What can be said about you professionally? That is, regarding the business in which you earn your living, how would you describe your roles and traits? In Exercise 1.3, define who you are by completing the phrases.

Now that you have defined who you are, what do you want to change about yourself? What motivates you to return to nursing school, to spend the next few years preparing yourself to become an RN?

Too many times, LPN/LVNs resuming their nursing education have misjudged their current levels of knowledge, experience, and even their licensure when planning how they will go about successfully negotiating a professional nursing program. LPN/LVN school is a challenge, and you have met that challenge effectively and passed the NCLEX-PN examination. Your current licensure is evidence of your ability to succeed. In Exercise 1.4, write what it currently means to you to practice in the role of an LPN/LVN. Then speculate about how your practice will change as you take on the role of an RN.

Knowles, Holton, and Swanson (2015) apply Vroom's Expectancy Theory to explain that adults are motivated to learn when they believe that the outcome of that learning will be useful and important to themselves or others. In the struggle to continue, it can be easy to forget why the journey began. Understanding your individual motivation for resuming your education will be helpful for keeping you on the right, albeit winding and occasionally uphill, path. In Exercise 1.5, explain your motivations or most important reasons for returning to school.

SETTING YOUR GOALS

"By taking the time to create a vision and a purpose for your life, you will approach your work with a broader, more critical, and more strategic outlook."

(Wilson & Porter-O'Grady, 1999, p. 222)

A map can be helpful when planning a journey if you understand where you have been and where you are now. Now is the time to define where you are going. To avoid drifting in the sea of education, your destination must be clearly defined. It is not often that airplane tickets are bought for just any airport in a large region. The itinerary is more precise. Charting a course does not necessarily mean plotting the shortest distance between two points, however. Rather, the route should accommodate individual needs and desires. The key is to keep moving in a purposeful manner.

Determining the path begins with defining both short- and long-term goals. A **short-term goal** may be something that could be attained in 6 months or fewer. A **long-term goal,** then, would take longer than 6 months. Being true to your inner self, the examination of personal goals occurs first.

In Exercise 1.6, write your personal goals. The personal realm encompasses everything outside of your professional life. Such goals might include getting married, having children, and moving into a new home. Write the goals first, then label them "ST" (short-term) or "LT" (long-term). Finally, prioritize them, placing the number 1 next to the most important or most immediate, the number 2 for the next most important, and so on.

In Exercise 1.7, using your professional goals, complete the same process as in Exercise 1.6.

Prioritizing

Now that you have determined both your personal and professional goals, choose the number-one short-term goal of each type and write the associated outcome priority.

⁇ EXERCISE 1.5

My outcome priorities and most important reasons prompting my return to nursing school are:

⁇ EXERCISE 1.6

PERSONAL GOALS

Goal	ST or LT	Priority

Remember, the outcome priority is the need or situation that must be addressed above all others for you to reach the goal. For example, consider what you have to do to accomplish the goal of going to the "rush-hour" show with your family on Friday. Several things must be planned from before the time you leave for work to the time the feature begins. Maybe you purchase theater tickets early in the week. Friday morning you take hamburger out of the freezer for dinner. You leave for work early enough to fill the gas tank. You complete your banking during lunch. These are all priorities that will make it possible to enjoy the Friday feature.

This is just an example for one family outing, but much the same process of prioritizing and planning can move you steadily toward your larger life goals. Wilson and Porter-O'Grady (1999) ask an important question: "Do you set daily priorities that move you forward toward your dreams?" (p. 221).

In Exercise 1.8, complete the statements.

The final exercise in plotting your course is the development of a timeline to gauge your progress. In Exercise 1.9, arrange your short- and long-term goals along the time continuum. Be sure to write down where you imagine yourself 5 and 10 years from now.

Change Theory

Similar to Vroom's Expectancy Theory, the Empirical-Rational Change Theory suggests that adults will make a change if they can foresee the benefits that may result (Marquis & Huston, 2015; Tomey, 2008). That is, adult students who perceive the

---

? EXERCISE 1.7

PROFESSIONAL GOALS

Goal	ST or LT	Priority

? EXERCISE 1.8

The outcome priority related to my number-one short-term personal goal is:

The outcome priority related to my number-one short-term professional goal is:

? EXERCISE 1.9

Present _____ (date)

5 years

10 years

---

change as important to their self-interests will seek what is needed in order to make the change on their own. Students may need help in visualizing or reconceptualizing what the future may hold, but once the vision is in place, adults will go about the activities required to achieve the goal (Shapiro, 2005). Keeping this in mind, let's explore the process of change and how it will help move you toward achieving your goals. In 1951, Kurt Lewin described three phases of change as well as what he termed **driving forces** and **restraining forces,** pushing toward and away from change, respectively (Tomey, 2008). A driving force is a facilitator toward change; it helps to move the situation toward the desired outcome. A restraining force shifts the momentum away from the desired outcome, hindering progress toward the change (Nursing Theoris, 2011). Those descriptions still apply today. According to Lewin's theory, one goes through unfreezing, moving, and refreezing during the change process (Fig. 1.1).

You have engaged in the process of change while working through this chapter. You have examined your needs or motivations for change as well as those forces that make change easier or more difficult. You have identified why you want to change your current life routine to include going back to college, going to clinical experiences, and the rest of what a nursing program brings. This is known as **unfreezing.** The more reasons you find that compel you to take action (in this case, to resume your education), the more unfrozen you become. As an ice cube must be melted to water before assuming a new state, so must your current life state unfreeze for you to move toward your dreams.

You have also engaged in the second phase of change: you are **moving**—actively planning changes and taking action on them. Moving also means you are dealing with both positive and negative forces as they ebb and flow, and you are modifying your plan as needed (Marquis & Huston, 2015).

Refreezing happens when a change becomes an integral part of who you are and what you do. This is not to imply that the change is permanent. Any change you desire must be continually renewed in order to maintain stability. Once a positive change has been integrated, a person often begins the unfreezing process again to begin working toward another dream or goal. Let's say that after you become an RN, you find that you especially enjoy teaching and decide that you would like to become a nursing faculty member. The new goal requires that you have an advanced or even terminal degree (MSN or doctorate) to achieve success.

Tomey (2008) defines eight types of change that you may experience: coercive, emulative, indoctrinizing, interactive, natural, social, technocratic, and planned. The meanings of each are embedded in the terms. The type of change

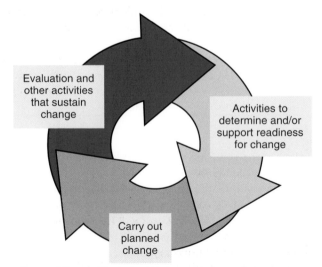

FIG. 1.1 According to Change Theory, the three phases of change are activities to determine and/or support readiness for change, carrying out planned change, and evaluation and other activities that sustain change (unfreezing, moving, and refreezing).

in which you are currently engaged is likely the last listed: planned change. You have identified your needs, have made a plan, are implementing the plan, and will experience the integration of the change into your life as a part of this planned process.

LIFELONG LEARNING

What goes hand in hand with change besides learning? As adults we have come to know that we learn constantly. We are very aware that there is always more to learn, new discoveries to be made, and new ways of doing and thinking. In your role as an LPN/LVN you were subject to constant updates of your knowledge of policies and procedures, new medications, new equipment, and new technologies. There is no escape from the requirement to constantly learn and adapt. Likewise, crucial to transitioning to the role of RN and then moving through the stages (again) from novice to expert and being able to maintain our knowledge and skill is lifelong learning. Our patients manage their health and illness through learning, and you will manage your transitions in a similar manner. The key to lifelong learning is knowing how to find the information, knowledge, and experience you need, when you need it. The fact that you have returned to nursing school is an indicator that you recognize the value in continued education. Lifelong learning is rarely accomplished alone; it is active and often self-directed; it is more than knowing, as it applies and includes our values and attitudes; it increases confidence and competence and is pervasive in that every aspect of our lives requires learning for growth and development (Collins, 2009). The profession of nursing depends on the development of a culture of curiosity within each of us as professionals whereby we seek evidence in support of better outcomes for our patients and ourselves.

The American Nurses Association (2010) identifies education as a standard of professional performance, stating, "The registered nurse attains knowledge and competence that reflects current nursing practice" (p. 11). Inherent in this standard is the requirement that we constantly seek the knowledge and experiences required to maintain our competence. "Registered nurses must continually reassess their competencies and identify needs for additional knowledge, skills, personal growth, and integrative learning experiences" (ANA, 2010, p. 13).

KEY POINTS

After completion of this chapter, you have:
- Learned about the outcome priority theme of this textbook.
- Applied the outcome priority concept to your past, present, and future.
- Realized that what you learned in the past can both help and hinder new learning.
- Defined yourself both personally and professionally.
- Established both short- and long-term goals.
- Developed a timeline with identified milestones related to your development.
- Applied change theory to your LPN to RN transition.

CRITICAL THINKING QUESTIONS

1. Name an RN whom you admire. What characteristics help you define him or her as an expert nurse? How would you envision your practice as an expert nurse?
2. You are attempting to balance your job, family, and work, and you are not satisfied with your grades in school.
   a. How would you describe your problem?
   b. What is your outcome priority related to this situation?
   c. What measures could you take to help with the balance and meet the goal of getting better grades?
3. How is your current practice as an LPN/LVN legally differentiated from that of an RN in your state?
4. In what ways do you already engage in lifelong learning, and how do you see yourself continuing in this practice as an RN?

REFERENCES

American Nurses Association. (2010). *Nursing: scope and standards of practice* (2nd ed.). Silver Spring, Maryland: American Nurses Association.

Collins, J. (2009). Education techniques for lifelong learning: lifelong learning in the 21st century and beyond. *RadioGraphics, 29*(2), 613–622.

Cook, L., Dover, C., Dickson, M., & Engh, B. (2010). Returning to school: the challenges of the licensed practical nurse-to-registered nurse transition student. *Teaching and Learning in Nursing, 5,* 125–128.

Knowles, M. S., Holton, E. F., & Swanson, R. A. (2015). *The adult learner: the definitive classic in adult education and human resource development* (8th ed.). New York, NY: Routledge.

Marquis, B. L., & Huston, C. J. (2015). *Leadership roles and management functions in nursing: theory and application* (7th ed.). Philadelphia, PA: Wolters Kluwer Health/Lippincott Williams & Wilkins.

Meleis, A. I. (2010). *Transitions theory: middle range and situation specific theories in nursing research and practice.* New York: Springer.

Montgomery, K. K., & Porter-O'Grady, T. (2010). Innovation and learning: creating the DNP nurse leader. *Nurse Leader, 8*(4), 44–47.

Nursing theories. (2011). Retrieved from http://currentnursing.com/nursing_theory/change_theory.html.

Shapiro, I. (2005). *Theories of change.* Retrieved from. http://beyondintractability.org/bi-essay/theories-of-change.

Tomey, A. M. (2008). *Guide to nursing management and leadership* (8th ed.). St. Louis, MO: Mosby.

Wilson, C. K., & Porter-O'Grady, T. (1999). *Leading the revolution in healthcare: advancing systems, igniting performance* (2nd ed.). Gaithersburg, MD: Aspen.

Assessing Yourself and Designing Success

⊖volve WEBSITE

Additional resources are available online at:
http://evolve.elsevier.com/Claywell/transitions

OBJECTIVES

After completing this chapter, the student will be prepared to:
1. Identify personal gifts and barriers.
2. Identify outcome priorities related to both gifts and barriers.
3. Create an action plan to address outcome priorities.
4. Describe how learning style affects the learning process.
5. Identify the impact of self-directedness on learning.
6. Define personal empowerment.
7. Interpret the role of locus of control on personal empowerment.
8. Explain the impact of positive self-talk.
9. Describe how self-defeating behavior negatively affects personal empowerment.
10. Describe self-defeating behaviors.
11. Explain four key work habits that contribute to success.
12. Explain the impact of health on personal empowerment.
13. Identify steps that aid in stress reduction.

KEY TERMS

empowerment	self-awareness
learning styles	self-defeating behaviors
locus of control	self-directedness
personal empowerment	self-talk

OVERVIEW

In this chapter you will identify your individual learning tools. In doing so, you will examine your gifts and barriers and consider your learning style and how they affect your study habits. In addition, you will learn about personal empowerment. **Empowerment** means providing a way of doing something, setting free the ability to move forward, and enabling. **Personal empowerment** means giving yourself the opportunity to succeed, or enabling your own success. Being empowered can also be thought of as having a positive attitude, feeling in control of your own destiny, and believing that you are important (Nugent & Vitale, 2016).

One can improve his or her personal empowerment skills by assuming an internal locus of control, practicing positive self-talk, eliminating self-defeating behaviors, managing the work of success, and managing health. At the end of this chapter, you should feel more competent in identifying individual tools that will enable you to be more successful.

GIFTS AND BARRIERS

Many people are uncomfortable with the idea of listing their individual gifts (strengths) and barriers (weaknesses). Etiquette has taught us to be modestly self-deprecating about positive attributes to avoid seeming arrogant or pompous. We may also try to ignore characteristics within us that are less positive. The effects of understanding and addressing your gifts and barriers are twofold. Being aware of the traits that make you unique will both keep you from repeating mistakes and give you the ability to internally support yourself, providing the best opportunity for success.

In Exercise 2.1, list, in as much detail as you wish (the more, the better), all of your gifts and barriers. Self-awareness, being conscious of and understanding yourself, is your ongoing self-portrait. It is not a measure of what others may think of you or your performance but of what you understand about yourself. This exercise will heighten your sense of yourself. Studying the self-portrait can be a very healthy experience if you are then motivated to support the strengths and work to lessen the impact of the weaknesses you've identified. You may or may not choose to share such insights.

Once you have several items listed, you can prioritize them, which is necessary to keep you from becoming overwhelmed and to focus your energy on where it can make the most difference. Prioritize the items you've listed by numbering them, placing a number 1 next to what you consider your greatest gift and another 1 by your most troublesome barrier. Give a number 2 to your next best and next worst traits. Go down both lists, numbering each item.

? EXERCISE 2.1

GIFTS   BARRIERS

Develop a statement regarding the outcome priority for both the number-one gift and the number-one barrier. Write the statements in Exercise 2.2. Here, the outcome priority is related to the first or most important gift or barrier issue to be dealt with. For example, if you wrote "good listener" as your greatest gift, an outcome priority might be "Apply listening skills at each class session." Similarly, if "procrastination" is your greatest barrier, then an outcome priority might be "Seek guidance from an advisor regarding techniques and behaviors to avoid procrastinating."

Self-awareness is essential but will not give its full benefit unless you take action to correct or minimize your weaknesses and capitalize on or maximize your gifts. Make a plan of action, a self-care plan, to specify how to go about addressing the outcome priorities you have established. When writing the plan of action, be as specific as possible. Include target dates or time periods for reassessment. Reevaluate your plan of action periodically to determine whether changes are necessary.

Note your plan's similarities to how you plan patient care. Patients are assessed for needs that require intervention as well as for strengths that require support. Patients are periodically reassessed, and interventions are continued, discontinued, or modified to meet their changing health status. This process may be visualized as a succession of phases that are circular and in motion (Fig. 2.1).

In Exercise 2.3, write a care plan (self-care plan) to support the outcome priorities for the gifts and barriers you determined earlier. An example is provided. Return to your self-care plan from time to time, at least at each target date, to assess your progress with

---

? EXERCISE 2.2

The outcome priority related to my greatest gift is:

The outcome priority related to my most troublesome barrier is:

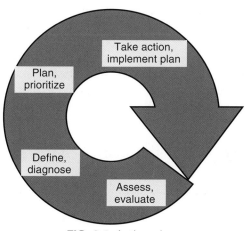

FIG. 2.1 Action plan.

💡 EXERCISE 2.3

INTERVENTIONS TO CORRECT OUTCOME PRIORITY	INTERVENTIONS TO SUPPORT OUTCOME PRIORITY	EXPECTATIONS AND TARGET DATES FOR REASSESSMENT
Decrease procrastination behaviors.	1. Make a list of all assignments. 2. Prioritize list items according to due dates and difficulty. 3. Assign work dates and time needed; place on calendar.	1. By the end of the first week of class (add specific date here), I will have created a complete list of all assignments including due dates, with level of difficulty/complexity identified. 2. By the end of the first week of class (add specific date here), I will have all work dates and times on the calendar for the term and will have scheduled time to work on all assignments. 3. Every week thereafter (include specific dates here), I will reassess and make adjustments to the schedule and plan of priorities.

---

each outcome priority. When you revisit your self-care plan, ask yourself the following questions: "Am I making progress toward the outcomes I've established?" If not: "What can I do differently?" "Are my target dates realistic?" "Do I need more help?" If you are consistently mastering your specified outcome: "Is it time to focus on a new area?" Writing about your experiences along the way will help. Keeping a journal is a great way to reflect on what you learn about yourself. Use your journal to evaluate your progress and to examine the questions that arise.

Now that you have determined gifts and barriers that influence your personal and professional identities and performance, point out other characteristics you possess that influence abilities and behaviors.

LEARNING STYLE

Many instruments are designed to help you better understand your learning styles, or the manners in which you prefer to learn. Many studies have attempted to correlate learning styles and the methods of teaching and studying that best suit each style category. In general, although it remains inconclusive how predictive most instruments and inventories are, they are still considered excellent tools for gaining personal insight.

Numerous studies have applied Kolb's Learning Styles Inventory to various types of nursing students. The studies came up with different results, all of which were significant. The greatest impact, however, is likely within the individual student, as insight is gained into how to apply one's strengths. Knowing your preferred style of learning is important, but you must adapt your preferred style to the learning context (Fig. 2.2).

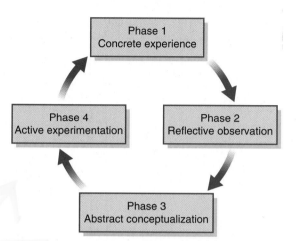

FIG. 2.2 Kolb's LSI (From Brooker C & Waugh A: Foundations of nursing practice: fundamentals of holistic care, ed 1, Edinburgh, 2008, Mosby Ltd.)

All learning preferences are valuable, and none is considered better than the others. Kolb (1984) developed a Theory of Experiential Learning as a cycle composed of four phases: concrete experience, reflective observation, abstract conceptualization, and active experimentation. The cycle begins with an experience that the learner reflectively observes and conceptualizes. This leads to participating in an experiment or experience, which then begins the cycle anew. Based on this theory, Kolb developed the Learning Styles Inventory to determine individual learning style preferences. The responses to a 12-item questionnaire place the learner into one of four categories, each having unique characteristics and preferences related to the four phases of the learning cycle. Kolb believes that as a learner matures, the preferred style integrates the traits of all four categories, not just the initially dominant one; thus, the learner effectively moves among all of the styles as needed.

People who prefer learning through concrete experiences relish being directly involved in new experiences in a hands-on fashion. These learners are likely to solve problems as they go and are good at adapting to new situations. Others prefer what Kolb calls reflective observation: watching events or experiences without having to be directly involved. These learners are usually good listeners and prefer to bring problems to harmonious solutions. Those predisposed to abstract conceptualization are considered data organizers. These learners order and arrange information in meaningful ways and are often happier in a lecture-type format, where they will write and arrange notes to their liking. People who prefer the active experimentation learning style seem to learn best by doing, by "trying it out." Such learners may try many different solutions to a problem before settling on one (Kolb, 1984).

Your preferred style of learning is not restricted to the school setting. Learning takes place every day in all the situations you encounter. You likely participate in learning along the lines of each of Kolb's categories in a wide variety of activities. In Exercise 2.4, identify learning situations that would be examples of Kolb's four theoretical categories.

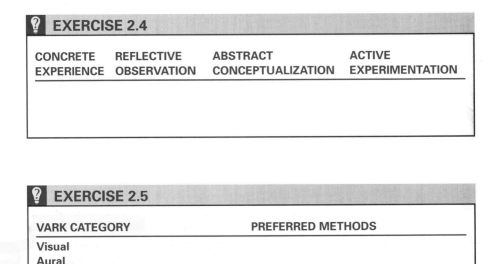

EXERCISE 2.4

CONCRETE EXPERIENCE	REFLECTIVE OBSERVATION	ABSTRACT CONCEPTUALIZATION	ACTIVE EXPERIMENTATION

EXERCISE 2.5

VARK CATEGORY	PREFERRED METHODS
Visual	
Aural	
Read/Write	
Kinesthetic	

Another very helpful tool for understanding how you best learn is called the VARK guide to learning styles. If you go online to http://vark-learn.com/the-vark-questionnaire/ you will be able to take this free, very quick, 16-question survey that will help you determine the way in which you prefer to learn. After completing the VARK questionnaire online, fill in Exercise 2.5, writing in examples of what you might do or what types of methods of learning you might seek to adjust to your preferred learning style. In the acronym VARK, V is for visual, A is for aural, R is for read/write, and K is for kinesthetic. Each of us has a preferred way to interact with information, and for those who have a higher preference in the visual category learning is likely promoted through the use of diagrams, maps, charts, shapes, lines, and other symbols that could have been described in words. Interestingly, this group does not include a preference for movies or photographs or PowerPoint, which is so popular in nursing education these days. For those with a higher preference in the aural category, the best way to promote learning is through hearing, such as in discussions, listening to the radio or taped lectures, talking to others or to oneself, and even through email. One might think email belongs in the read/write group, but interestingly it does not. Those in the read/write group often prefer reading and writing in all manners, such as reading and writing papers, rewriting notes, reading manuals, searching the Internet, and anything that is displayed in words. Finally, those with a preference in the kinesthetic category prefer doing, hands-on practice, simulation, and other personal physical or concrete experiences. Most often each learner is a combination of all of these categories, but understanding your preferences can help you to seek out ways of learning and manipulating the content that is presented such that it makes the most sense to you (VARK Learn Limited, 2016).

BEHAVIORS	HOW TO TRANSFER BEHAVIORS INTO LEARNING SITUATION

SELF-DIRECTEDNESS

Self-directedness has been described in numerous ways. Knowles, Holton, and Swanson (2015) identify two perspectives of self-directed learning. Learners seen as teaching themselves engage in the learning environment and determine the pace and methodology of study, such as in-home or independent study. The other perspective is one of autonomy, or the learner takes control of the learning, which causes the learner to feel compelled to question what is learned. These two perspectives are considered independent and may be present in a learner either alone or together.

The ability to engage in self-directed learning may be considered a requirement for the nontraditional student. More programs are attempting to meet the needs of adults returning to school by increasing the amount and complexity of material provided in a learner-paced, learner-directed manner. Therefore, the learner must be prepared to exercise initiative, independence, and persistence, along with the discipline and determination to meet goals and solve problems when challenges arise. Being self-directed is not necessarily inherent but may be viewed instead as a process that requires practice, time, and experience (Merriam, Caffarella, & Baumgartner, 2007). Like most adults managing multifaceted lives, you may have come to understand that success in life outside the classroom requires behaviors similar to those identified as self-directedness. As you transition back to the role of student, it is expected that you assume responsibility for your educational experiences and opportunities, thus transferring those adult, self-directed behaviors into your role as a student.

Consider for a moment how you exhibit behaviors consistent with self-directedness in your daily life outside of school. List the behaviors in Exercise 2.6, and then write about how you might transfer those behaviors into the learning situation.

If you understand your individual learning style as a student as well as your personality traits and preferences, then you and your instructors will be able to plan learning experiences that better suit your needs. In addition, understanding your needs as a learner, particularly related to becoming more self-directed, will empower you to take control of your learning. Capitalize on your strengths, and build upon areas that require nurturing for growth. Gone are the days when faculty were the pitcher and students the empty vessel waiting to be filled with knowledge. Today students are responsible for their own learning, and faculty serve as guides and facilitators.

Personal empowerment skills are behaviors that you practice to improve your ability to accomplish goals or that motivate you to engage in your education and other life activities from a position of strength and control. Most personal empowerment skills are learned skills that most people do not already possess or regularly practice, such as assuming an internal locus of control, practicing positive self-talk, eliminating self-defeating behaviors, managing the work of success, and managing your health.

Cattaneo and Chapman (2010) developed a model for empowerment. They define *empowerment* as "an iterative process in which a person who lacks power sets a personally meaningful goal oriented toward increasing power, takes action toward that goal, and observes and reflects on the impact of this action, drawing on his or her evolving self-efficacy, knowledge, and competence related to the goal" (p. 647). Briefly, their stepwise approach to the process of attaining personal empowerment involves identifying a goal, knowledge, self-efficacy, competence, action, and impact.

First, identifying personally meaningful and power-oriented goals is the key step. A personally meaningful goal is self-explanatory, but a power-oriented goal requires more explanation. Cattaneo and Chapman define a power-oriented goal as "an aim to increase one's influence in social relations at any level of human interaction" (p. 652). You could wish to improve your own interest (becoming an RN) or the interests of a group. Second, self-efficacy (or belief that you can reach your goal) is needed for personal empowerment. Next, knowledge is the understanding of the paths to get to the goal, what is needed to get there, and how to get the means necessary for fulfilling the goal. Fourth, competence is knowing how to accomplish your goal within your skill set. Fifth, action is the actual execution of your plan. Finally, impact is the personal evaluation of your actions. If the entire process of empowerment was successful, you may have increased feelings of efficacy. If you had a negative experience, you might not believe that you are the master of your destiny (Exercise 2.7).

ASSUMING AN INTERNAL LOCUS OF CONTROL

Internal or external locus of control describes where you believe the power in your life resides. If you have an external locus of control, you believe that the responsibility for your action or inaction lies outside of yourself. For example, in the case of a less-than-satisfactory grade on a test, the student may externalize the locus of control by saying, "The test was too hard" or "The instructor gave me a B." If your locus of control is internal, you take responsibility for what happens to you, for your mistakes as well as your accomplishments. Using the same example, the student with an internal locus of control might say, "I need to study harder next time to improve my grade" or "I earned a B on my paper."

? EXERCISE 2.7

Think about a goal.
1. Why is the goal personally meaningful to you? (Personally meaningful and power-oriented goal)
2. Do you believe you can accomplish this goal? (Self-efficacy)
3. What do you need to know about how to achieve the goal? (Knowledge)
4. Do you have the skills necessary to reach the goal? (Competence) If not, how do you obtain these skills?
5. What steps will you take to carry out your goal? (Action)
6. What happened as you followed through on your plan? How did it make you feel? Will you try the same steps next time? (Impact)

In the left column of Exercise 2.8, write statements that you have made in the past that represent an external locus of control. In the right column rewrite the statement so it reflects an internal locus of control. Discuss how this process might aid in your transition from LPN/LVN to RN.

POSITIVE SELF-TALK

People who are empowered often think good thoughts about themselves and engage in positive self-talk, defined as talking to themselves kindly and with encouraging words, in a manner that would support and affirm. Consider the child faced with trying to ride a bike and repeatedly wobbling and weaving, with a near-fall here or there. A parent might relate the story of *The Little Engine That Could,* a powerful story for all ages. If you think you can and you tell yourself that you can, then you can. It feels great when someone we love, trust, or admire tells us "Great job!" or "I am so proud of you for working so hard!"

An affirmation from yourself is also very valuable. Only you really know how much work and sacrifice went into doing something well by "giving it your all." Be as kind, understanding, forgiving, and encouraging to yourself as you would be to a fellow student, a child, or a friend who is doing the best possible. Learning is a process of forward motion but also steps back, with reflection and inner contemplation.

Tell yourself, "What I am doing is important to me and to the world. I will make a difference in my own life as well as in those of others." The affirmation that is in order at this point in your education is "I can do this." When life in nursing school gets a little hectic, as it inevitably will, repeat to yourself silently or out loud, "I can do this."

Nothing is more counterproductive than convincing yourself, "I don't get it" or "I can't do this." Negative self-talk is a damaging coping mechanism that may seem to lift the stress of a situation temporarily by claiming that what is before you is insurmountable, out of your league, or over your head. The pressure is off for a moment if you excuse yourself from facing and conquering the fear of doing what a situation requires. The pressure will only be replaced with shame, guilt, or regret; however, do not allow your mind to begin to chatter such untruths.

You can do this. You have what it takes. You can will yourself to work through every situation. Be positive and empower yourself to succeed.

Exercise 2.9 will enable you to turn negative self-talk into positive affirmations. We have all experienced self-doubt and self-defeating behaviors. Think back to a time when you recall having said to yourself, "I cannot do this" or "I'll never get this right." Any statements about yourself that were less than positive will work here.

? EXERCISE 2.8

EXTERNAL LOCUS OF CONTROL	INTERNAL LOCUS OF CONTROL

⚑ EXERCISE 2.9

Scenario:

NEGATIVE STATEMENTS	POSITIVE AFFIRMATIONS

In Exercise 2.9, write a short but meaningful scenario. Below the scenario in the left column, list the negative phrases that likely occurred to you at that time. Then think of an affirming statement that counters each negative phrase and write it in the right column. If you are comfortable doing so, say your affirmations out loud. At first, you may feel odd doing this, but this is one way to ensure that you will not experience the same negativity should the same or a similar scenario arise again.

ELIMINATION OF SELF-DEFEATING BEHAVIORS

Another crucial skill of personal empowerment is the recognition and elimination of self-defeating behaviors, which put us at risk of failure. These behaviors, when routinely permitted, can lead us to fulfill the prophecies that our positive affirmations seek to counter. Chenevert (2010) describes several behaviors that directly impede our ability to succeed. These include pessimism, nit-picking, worrying, and perfectionism. Blaming is another prevalent form of negative conduct. The remedy for such self-defeating behavior, as suggested by Chenevert, may be in continually recognizing their presence in ourselves.

Pessimism

A pessimist is the type of person who views current situations and anticipates outcomes from a negative perspective, viewing a glass of milk as half empty rather than half full. Pessimism creates the negative self-talk we seek to eliminate. The choice between pessimism and optimism in an otherwise healthy person is simply that: a choice. Choose to be optimistic.

Validating that little voice inside that says, "Be careful" or "Don't do it" is not the same as being pessimistic. Pessimism is expecting that success is not possible, no matter what the situation. Pessimism removes our power and makes us give up any control we may have over the events in our lives.

A note of caution here: chronic pessimistic behaviors and perceptions can be symptoms of a serious illness or disorder. If you find that you experience frequent pessimistic feelings, it is best to seek the advice of your primary health care provider.

Nit-Picking

Nit-picking is one way of rationalizing a decision that otherwise could not be supported. Nit-picking is a damaging compensatory mechanism that seems to release the nit-picker from the responsibility for getting the job done. A person with a nit-picking attitude seems to look for the tiniest fault. If the nit-picker chips away at small details, sooner or later the sum of all the imperfections will lead to a reason not to move forward. This may be simply a sign of uneasiness or perhaps of some undisclosed concern.

Worrying

In a similar way, worrywarts often immobilize themselves with fear. Worry wastes time and uses energy better placed into planning and proactivity. When you've done your best, listened to your internal voice of reason, and made your decisions based on all the evidence at hand, you can stop worrying. Worrying about what might happen will change nothing, but it robs you of the energy you will need to plan for, or cope with, the outcome either way. Worrying is not action, and only action provides any hope of changing the outcome.

Perfectionism

Perhaps one of the most discreetly cloaked self-defeating behaviors of all is perfectionism. How old were you when your parent first told you, "Nobody's perfect"? What is it, then, that makes us believe that we must be perfect? To strive for perfection is to be perpetually unhappy, as we fall short. This is not to say that trying to improve ourselves is futile but rather that we should set goals that are humanly possible and go for them. Each time we try, we learn, and we are therefore closer than before. Perfection is out of the question, but continuous improvement is not.

Blaming

Shifting blame to others is one of the most destructive self-defeating behaviors. To blame is to reject the responsibility of control over outcomes, saying if something goes wrong, it is someone else's fault. If we are unable to accept the responsibility for our actions or inactions, we are not going to benefit from reflecting about what we could have done differently that might have changed the outcome.

Accountability is a major creed for professional nursing. Being a nurse means accepting responsibility not only for the care you personally give but also for the care given by those under your supervision. If you are constantly looking to blame someone else, then you are not accepting responsibility for your actions and therefore not learning from them.

MANAGING THE WORK OF SUCCESS

Success at home, at work, and at school is directly related to your ability to manage the work of success. Having completed a practical nursing program, you are well aware that success takes work. The four key work habits that need to be developed and maintained in order to manage your success are decision making, planning, commitment, and time management.

Decision Making

A strong decision-making ability shows that you are in control. You have settled on what you want. Stick to your decision unless you are strongly compelled to change your mind. This applies to all decisions. One decision you might make is to earn a B or better in a particular course. This is your decision. The teacher does not give you a grade; you earn it. As you read earlier, this keeps your locus of control internal.

Planning

There is no more powerful builder of self-esteem than to have accomplished all you had planned by the end of the day. Planning is essential to the smooth functioning of the busy life of an adult in school. Planning requires close assessment of every aspect of the task at hand and its context. What are the conditions and requirements? What instructions, parameters, or guidelines do you have?

To plan means making sure you have all the necessary resources to complete an assignment as well as a backup plan. What are you going to do if your car breaks down on the way to the library and you lose all the time you had set aside for study that day?

Planning includes breaking down a goal into its individual parts and prioritizing them so you first complete the most urgent or otherwise logically first tasks. Doing well in a course involves a series of small tasks that, once summed, equal the whole. Divide your course into separate testing periods or projects. Make each of them a separate goal, and then break it down further into even smaller steps that will lead to successful completion.

We can often be immobilized by the sheer size of an entire project or task that lies ahead. Breaking down a project or study session into more manageable pieces is a strong motivator for continuing the work until it is finished. Just looking at one small part of the whole brings back your motivation. Completing one part at a time and concentrating on only that one part will eventually lead you to completion of the entire task. Before you know it, you are at the end of the semester, you've completed all the assignments, and the grade you had set out to earn is yours.

Think for a moment what it feels like after you've said goodnight to your last dinner guest, only to come to the kitchen doorway and see piles of messy dishes, a greasy stove, and an otherwise perfectly shiny floor (which you had spent 2 hours scrubbing) dribbled with drips and spills of various foods and beverages. It is all just too much to deal with. Or is it? If you separate the cleanup into its individual tasks, the job won't seem so big.

Likewise, if you have a 70-page reading assignment to be prepared for the next class, the time to plan is as soon as you are aware of the assignment. Examine your schedule. Determine the study time you have to devote to this assignment, and then divide it up. Read and take notes on all that you had planned—and more, if your energy level and time permit. When the next class rolls around, you should be ready if you have stuck to the plan.

Commitment

The third habit for managing your success is commitment, or total dedication, to your plan (Watford, 1996). Commitment requires discipline. You have carefully dissected a goal into its parts and then each of those parts into its individual pieces. You have made the necessary assessments to prioritize, and you have all the necessary resources to see it through. Dedicate yourself to the plan.

Initial dedication to your plan will be wholehearted and vigorous. The challenge comes later, when you are required to maintain the plan in the face of other mounting responsibilities and waning resolve. You must have the discipline to turn away from a more attractive proposal of how to spend your evening when you know you have a test the next morning. For example, instead of going out to a midnight movie that would interfere with a full night's rest, opt for a quiet evening of study and reflection that ends early so that you can take the test the next morning fully rested and ready to do your best.

To further bolster your commitment, try to remember your original inspiration for going to nursing school. What can keep you going? Perhaps you have a picture, poem, or phrase that sums up your motivation. Keep a tangible reminder near you. Take time to reflect, take stock of your accomplishments, and praise yourself for working toward your goal.

Time Management

Unfortunately, poor time management skills can get in the way of carefully made plans by the most committed individuals. Learning effective time management skills is crucial to success. Effective time management applied consistently can be a great asset and may be considered the box that organizes and carries all the essential study skills and other tools that you use to build your education. Planning and completing a task without your toolbox can be difficult.

Before we investigate the contents of the box, let's examine the box itself. As an LPN/LVN, you are most likely returning to school with a busy, well-established life. You no longer have the luxury of hanging out at the library every day, like you did when you first went off to school. Your home life, work life, and school life must be well orchestrated. To manage time effectively, you must learn to set and prioritize goals (Meltzer & Palau, 1997). The importance of these skills cannot be overemphasized.

Assessment

Assessment is the first task to help you develop effective time management. Exercise 2.10 will help you begin to address the management of the time you spend on how your life is structured. This is a personal assessment that could be very beneficial, so take your time and make it count. Be certain to include even the smallest activities and be realistic with the time each will take. Consider this example: In a recent faculty

---

? EXERCISE 2.10

On a separate sheet of paper, write out every activity that you do during your average day. For example, choose a Monday and complete the following:
1. List everything you do on a typical Monday, from waking up your children to brushing your teeth, making coffee, and showering. Include relaxation and personal time.
2. Next to each item, write how much time you spend on each task. Be realistic, and do not leave anything out. At this point, you are not deciding what to change, just assessing your usual day.

Now add up all the time spent. The idea of time management is not to stuff 20 hours of work into 16 hours but to determine what needs to be done, what can be delegated to others, and what can be done differently to maximize the quality of the time you spend on each activity.

? EXERCISE 2.11

SEMESTER GOALS	ORDER OF PRIORITY

---

meeting a complaint was mentioned that meetings are often scheduled back to back without thought to the need to actually walk to and from different meeting rooms or buildings or the need to stop off at the restroom or drinking fountain or to glance at the cell phone to check for important messages. Remember that there must be time allotted for these necessary moments. It may seem silly, but many times, our days can be thrown off because we did not schedule a few moments to eat lunch or return calls.

Setting Goals and Prioritizing

Setting goals is the next necessary step. The goals here are different from those you developed in Chapter 2. Here we examine one semester.

In Exercise 2.11, list the activities and events you need or want to participate in this semester. This list should include things such as attending school part- or full-time, working part- or full-time, serving as den parent or room parent, volunteering, having your family over for Thanksgiving, or hosting a birthday party. Place the number 1 next to the most important thing that you must accomplish, a 2 by the second most important, and so on.

Meltzer and Palau (1997) point out that every activity cannot be the top priority. Some activities require that you change or limit others. Even during a nursing program, you must balance your goals so that you do not ignore what makes you happy.

Now that you have listed and prioritized your semester goals or activities, place them on your calendar. Most advisors agree that a key to success in college is the ritual use of this essential organizational tool. A calendar that shows days, weeks, and months is an absolute necessity. Keep it with you at all times.

Go back now to your semester goals. Note your number-one priority. What do you need to do to accomplish this? For example, if working full- or part-time is your first priority, include in your schedule not only your work hours but also the time it takes to get ready, pack your lunch, and drive or catch the bus to and from work. (Remember the daily assessment you completed in Exercise 2.4.) Repeat this process for your second priority and so on down the list.

The syllabus given out during course orientation is the key to accomplishing your school goals. Go through the syllabus and transfer class dates, times, and locations to your calendar. Block off time for travel and walking to and from the parking lot. Some other things you will want to mark on your calendar are exam dates, paper due dates, project due dates, group work sessions, study sessions, anticipated library and computer lab time, and advising and registration for next semester. Most schools expect you to study or prepare at least 2 to 3 hours for every hour you spend in class or clinical. Do not scrimp on this time. The time you spend engrossed in study will pay off when you prepare to take the NCLEX-RN.

❓ EXERCISE 2.12

TIME WASTERS	SOLUTION

Write on your calendar all of your personal or family responsibilities of which you are aware. These may be things such as doctor and dentist appointments; exercise class or going to the gym; taking out the garbage, doing laundry, and paying bills; family birthdays, movies, concerts, and going out to dinner; church and choir practice; doing your nails and going to the salon; and getting the car inspected and the oil changed. The personal list is endless. Refer to your average daily assessment. Can you delegate some activities on the list to another family member? While you are in school, allow others to help you. The point of time management is not to enable you to cram everything into a day but to help you choose the few most important priorities and apply quality time to those activities.

Time Wasters

This is the difficult part: identifying the ways you waste time. Be aware of the time you spend that is not productive. This is not to say that resting and relaxing are not productive; they are essential to keeping your body and mind functioning at their best.

In Exercise 2.12, list the time wasters that interfere with your daily productivity. After you've listed the things that steal your time, write what you believe you could do to solve each problem. For instance, if you get caught up in watching TV, talking on the telephone, surfing the Internet, visiting with friends, or reading for recreation, then set limits on the amount of time you will spend in such activities and stick to them.

Chenevert (2010) points out that procrastination may be recognized as a self-defeating behavior. Procrastination seems to accompany tasks that are difficult, complex, or do not have immediate apparent application. Procrastination can be harmless, or it can be devastating. Procrastination is defined as, for any number of reasons (excuses), delaying or putting off an activity or responsibility until one is at or past the deadline. If you recognize that you are putting off a task, take a closer look. What about the task specifically causes you discomfort? Separate the whole into its parts and work with the individual pieces. If you've been unable to find the time to go enroll in that next class, then you probably dread a specific part of the class or the enrollment procedure. Work toward resolution of the situation one issue at a time.

Time wasters are often procrastination in disguise. Not everyone procrastinates for the same reasons. Experts say that procrastination comes in many disguises. Do you recognize any of these?

- Paralysis by planning. You plan and plan to perfection but never implement. You spend so much time planning that you run out of either time or motivation to complete the task.

- Perfection. Often perfection is not required, and usually it is out of reach. Some students turn in assignments late, claiming they just weren't happy with them. Work your best within a limited amount of time.
- Boredom. If the task is not interesting to you, you must discipline yourself to get it done. Strive to find significance and personal purpose in every assignment.
- Hostility. Perhaps you have negative feelings toward the person assigning the task, you are required to work within a group that has historically been a less-than-optimal match for you, or you are angry or upset regarding the characteristics of the assignment, such as its complexity, amount of work, or due date ("too hard, too much, too soon"). Try to remove emotion from the action needed for completing the assignment.
- Adrenaline rush. Working against a deadline can provide an intense, satisfying adrenaline rush. Unfortunately, while this may serve as a positive influence for some, adrenaline junkies may find that their work does not get finished when an unforeseen last-minute complication happens. If you're likely to say, "I work better with a deadline," consider that this may mean that you need external pressure to create the urgency to force you into action. If you do your best work at the eleventh hour, then consider doing most of the work early, saving only the polishing or finishing touches for near-deadline time. In any case, the first time you miss a deadline or have to ask for an extension for an assignment that is due, you have crossed the line from a late starter–strong finisher to a full-fledged procrastinator, and behaviors must change for you to preserve both your sanity and your grade. FYI 2.1 on page 29 lists 10 ways to help you avoid procrastinating.

MANAGING YOUR HEALTH

Living a healthy life and paying attention to your personal health needs are critical to achieving self-empowerment. Students often sabotage otherwise gallant efforts by ignoring their basic needs for adequate rest, relaxation, exercise, and nutrition. As a practical/vocational nurse, you are well aware of the labor-intensive nature of the nursing profession. If you are to be able to concentrate fully on the task at hand and help those in need, you must meet your own needs first. A brain that is well nourished and well rested is a more powerful brain.

In nursing school you will learn (if you haven't already) that people who are ill or injured or lacking nutrients, hydration, rest, or shelter often feel powerless. The saying is true: "If you do not have your health, nothing else matters." In today's society, more than ever before, health equals power. At the very least, those who are trying to maintain or regain their health are considered powerful consumers and are the target of much product marketing. Think about how you feel when you are making smart choices about eating, drinking, exercise, and lifestyle in general. How do you feel when you achieve balance between work and play? You feel in control. This is how it feels to be self-empowered.

Stress and Stress Reduction

One of the most disabling experiences of nursing school is a high level of stress, which seems to affect every nursing student at some point. To some, mild stress is a motivator, but to others, even mild stress on top of an already complicated life is nearly lethal.

> ## 🏃 FYI 2.1   10 WAYS TO AVOID PROCRASTINATING
>
> 1. Be rational. Understand that many people can justify almost any action or inaction through faulty reasoning. Examine your reasoning and separate what is true rationalization from what is false rationalization. Do this by writing down your rationale, or scheme of reasons, for believing the way you do. Beside each reason identify the source of the information. If you further identify actual fact rather than hearsay and what conditions you know to exist rather than what you or others speculate, then you are thinking carefully through your decisions.
> 2. Maintain positive self-motivation. Always speak in positives. Tell yourself, "The sooner, the better" and "I can do this."
> 3. Do not predict the worst. If you expect the worst, the worst may happen as you paralyze yourself with fear and self-doubt.
> 4. Set goals. Be realistic and stick to the plan.
> 5. Prioritize. Begin each day by dealing with the number-one priority. Remind yourself of what must be accomplished.
> 6. Break it down. Large tasks will often overwhelm you into immobility. Take the project apart and assign each part, in order of priority, to a different block of time or date.
> 7. Organize your life. Nothing wastes more time than disorganization. The time invested in getting organized will be rewarded exponentially.
> 8. Commit. Publicly committing yourself to a task or project by sharing with a friend, relative, or classmate often keeps you on track. You will have more trouble wasting time if you know others are expecting you to complete the job.
> 9. Employ reminders. Often we forget that we "were going to do something." Whether this was a conscious or subconscious act is not really important. What is important is that we remember. To improve your chances of remembering, put obvious notes around your house, at the office, or in your car.
> 10. Celebrate. There is nothing like positive reinforcement to keep a good thing going. Give yourself a pat on the back.

Stress

Sources of stress are many and varied. While research has identified common causes and manifestations of stress, every person experiences stress and the stress response differently. Commonly reported stressors for student nurses include significant others, finances, and grades (Twiname & Boyd, 2002).

Your significant others will experience their own stresses as you progress through college. They may feel neglected or burdened when school responsibilities require you to give up time with family and friends. You in turn will feel the result of that stress. Children, spouses, and other family members and friends will vie for your attention in ways that are positive and not so positive. To help relieve the tension, be sure to block out time throughout every week just to be with your significant other, and keep it sanctified. Let nothing interfere with that time so that each minute is quality time. Hold family meetings to discuss what it means for you and for them that you are back in college and working hard. Do the same with friends. Keep everyone up to date on your progress and let them know how they are helping to make your success possible.

Finances and work responsibilities are among the most worrisome stressors for adult students returning to school. As an adult, you have a well-established life and, as such, one that is already full of responsibilities that require you to manage a delicate balance between work and home, which school only complicates. Furthermore, returning to school is an expensive endeavor. Not only does it involve added costs for tuition, fees, books, and uniforms but nursing students also find that they must cut back the number of hours they normally work to have time for classes, clinical, projects, and study. Financial assistance is available in the form of grants, scholarships, and loans; however, to receive assistance, you must ask for it. You must often complete interviews and paperwork to qualify. Ask your advisor or school financial counselor about how to access the many types of financial assistance available.

Grades seem to be a major source of stress for many students. The minimum acceptable grade in nursing school is higher than that in many other programs of learning, and earning a D is not acceptable. Many students must maintain a certain grade point average to keep a scholarship. This puts a great deal of pressure on the student. In addition, some students are not happy with anything below an A, which is just not reasonable for many. Give yourself a break. Be happy, but not complacent, when you have done everything you know how to do, have given your all, and still received a B or a C.

If you do not have command of a topic, study it until you do, even after the test. Nursing education is designed to build on prior learning, documented or not. Some people among the world's top nurses earned grades lower than As in nursing school, likely because they did their best when in school and continued to work at it until they fully understood what they needed to know.

Stress Reduction

Just as the manifestations of stress are individual, so too are the techniques that aid in stress reduction. What works beautifully for one person may serve to add stress for another. The literature generously reports coping mechanisms and techniques to reduce stress. Holistic cognitive therapy, however, engages a process that may lead an individual to optimum stress reduction. Four steps are involved in cognitive therapy (Dossey, & Keegan 2016):

1. Achieve awareness. You achieve awareness through understanding how you feel under stress. How does your body physically feel? Does your head ache or your shoulder feel tight? Maybe your stomach gets queasy or you lose your appetite. Maybe your appetite increases. Become aware of the early signs of stress, and take steps to reduce or neutralize the symptoms.

2. Identify automatic thoughts. These are usually immediate responses made without reflection. They have formed before we even realize the entirety of a situation. They are almost always negative in nature, with hard or blaming words like *should* and *never* correlating the discomfort directly to an outside source, real or imagined. Automatic thoughts are usually distorted and irrational, with little or no basis in reality. The only way to deal with automatic thoughts is to acknowledge the possibility of their existence and to identify them as what they are.

3. Identify cognitive distortions. These are illogical, irrational thoughts. Look carefully at the following list of 10 cognitive distortions, and try to identify any of these in yourself during a past (or present) time of stress:
   - All-or-nothing thinking. This includes thoughts such as "If I cannot be the best, then I won't play at all" or "Anything less than perfect equals failure."
   - Overgeneralization. This involves lumping all similar situations, events, or people into broad (usually negative) categories.
   - Mental filtering. This is manifested by identifying one negative detail and then characterizing the whole by that one part.
   - Disqualifying the positive. This is characterized by the inability to see positive experiences as important or by refusing to accept compliments on a job well done.
   - Jumping to conclusions. This is identified as "mind reading" or acting or making decisions without evidence.
   - Magnification. This involves making a problem seem worse than it actually is. The converse—failure to see the importance of what went well—is also a cognitive distortion.
   - Emotional reasoning. Just because you believe or feel a certain way does not make it so. A distorted way of thinking is confusing feelings with fact.
   - "Should" statements. Although statements that contain the word *should* are meant to bring about action, they seldom do.
   - Labeling. When a person, situation, or event is labeled, it is automatically characterized and burdened inappropriately with the characteristics of others within the category.
   - Personalizations. These are manifested by placing yourself at the center of everything. If you are personalizing, you feel that everything negative that happens in your world is all because of you.

   Scary, isn't it? Facing the reality behind the façade of cognitive distortions is neither easy nor painless. Accept yourself as you are without the façade and work from there. There is no right or wrong or judgment to be passed, only an opportunity to get to know yourself so that you can empower yourself to succeed in a world that is unpredictable and imperfect.

4. Choose coping mechanisms that work. To come up with an appropriate response to a stressor, you must identify both the practical side of the issue (the factual information surrounding the situation) and the emotional side (how you feel about it). They will likely each need a different method for effective coping. Following is a list of mechanisms that may help you cope:
   - Distraction. Deciding to lay aside the stress until it is necessary to deal with it is not a means to avoid the situation but to reserve the angst until such time as the situation can be dealt with directly.
   - Direct action. There is something you can do to resolve the problem.
   - Relaxation. Employ techniques or activities that bring about relaxation at the initial awareness of stress. This can help change your physical and psychological responses as well as the action taken either proactively or in response.

- Reframing. *Looking* at the situation from another perspective often sheds a different light on it and can alter your behavior within the moment. This may also be referred to as "looking for the silver lining."
- Affirmation. A positive thought is an affirmation. As you learned previously, thinking positively can benefit the outcome. People who think they can, can!
- Spirituality. One very powerful means of coping is to think deeply about what feeds you spiritually. Turning to your faith may help you put life back into perspective.
- Catharsis. Crying and laughter are both often helpful as emotional releases.
- Journal writing. One safe way to bring out thoughts and feelings and to work through them is on paper. Writing can be an effective means of processing stressful situations.
- Social support. Sharing with family members or friends is an effective means of dealing with stress for many people. Talking about stressors often leads to learning not only new ways to cope but also ways to avoid stress, where possible, by changing behavior.
- Assertive communication. Your ability to communicate needs and desires clearly is important for others to be able to respond appropriately.
- Empathy. Being able to put yourself in the place of another helps you understand him or her.
- Acceptance. Forgiveness and letting go of those things that are beyond your control help you maintain balance when you are unable to alter or avoid the situation.

This list is not an all-inclusive grouping of techniques but a place to begin the process of cognitive therapy, a most personal voyage toward self-empowerment.

To take a quiz that will help to measure your current level of stress and anxiety, go online to http://greatergood.berkeley.edu/quizzes/take_quiz/8 and complete the 16-item questionnaire. After you receive your results, you will also find suggestions for how to manage stress. For an additional stress quiz, Go online to http://www.medicine net.com/stress_quiz/quiz.htm and take the Stress Quiz, being certain to read the rationale under the correct answers, and then click on http://www.medicinenet.com/stress _management_techniques/article.htm to learn more about how to manage your stress.

KEY POINTS

After completion of this chapter, you have:
- Analyzed your gifts and barriers for returning to nursing school and assuming the student role.
- Developed a self-care plan to reduce your weaknesses and capitalize on your strengths.
- Gained self-awareness.
- Learned about Kolb's stages of the learning cycle: concrete experience, reflective observation, abstract conceptualization, and active experimentation.
- Come to know that self-directedness is associated with the most successful learners.
- Learned that becoming self-empowered is an active process and that it cannot be bestowed upon you; rather, you achieve it.

- Realized that five basic skills are required for success:
  - Assuming an internal locus of control
  - Engaging in positive self-talk
  - Eliminating self-defeating behaviors
  - Managing the work of success
  - Managing your health
- Learned that the moment you begin to engage in self-empowering behavior, you will feel the surge.

CRITICAL THINKING QUESTIONS

1. The concept of professionalism is a thread throughout the history of nursing. Working in a group of at least three or four student nurses, each of you chooses a time in the history of nursing and composes a single report comparing the significance of the past events with present nursing conditions.
2. You have identified your learning style preference. As you work in the group on question 1, note the differences in learning styles among the team members.
   a. What aspects of your learning style will be challenged?
   b. What aspects will be enhanced?
3. Goals help to create the map, or step-by-step guide, by which you can plan your personal and professional life and then evaluate your progress. Consider this, and then respond to each of the following:
   a. What are the potential consequences of not setting personal and professional goals?
   b. What would it look like, feel like, and seem like if you fail to reach the goals you set for yourself?
   c. What measure can you implement to ensure that you will feel good about your successes even if you do not meet all of your goals?
4. All reasoning begins with basic assumptions. You started this chapter with a basic assumption that your gifts and barriers will potentially help or hinder your progress toward professional development.
   a. What assumptions can you make about how each of your gifts will assist you in completing your mobility program?
   b. How would you test your hypothesis that this gift will help you?
   c. What measure will you take to ensure that your barriers do not hinder your progress?
5. Your patient needs an IV started for antibiotic therapy. During report you learn that the patient is a difficult IV start and that the RN leaving the shift, one of the most skilled IV starters, tried to start the IV two times without success. You walk into the room and introduce yourself and are introduced to the patient's son and daughter, a nurse, and a physician. Write a brief but honest narration as to how you feel about this situation.
   a. What will be the consequences if you do not have positive self-talk going into this situation?
   b. From the patient's point of view, what are the main concerns related to the IV?
   c. What could you do to put a positive and supportive spin on this event?

6. You have clinical on Tuesdays and Wednesdays, with clinical paperwork due Thursday morning at the beginning of class. This paperwork generally takes you 2 hours to complete. Although you have been keeping up with the daily class assignments, you would like to schedule some study time. This week you have a unit exam scheduled on Thursday at 0900. Your study group wants to meet Wednesday evening before the unit exam.
   a. What decisions must you make?
   b. What will your action plan need to look like for you to complete the work as well as study for the exam and meet with your study group?
   c. What will be your top priority and lowest priority? List potential consequences to your selections (remember, *consequence* is a neutral term, so list both positive and negative consequences to your prioritized items).
7. Reframe the following statements or concepts to be positive:
   a. The glass is half empty.
   b. This door is closed to me.
   c. The cardiovascular unit is too hard to understand.
   d. The clinical instructor is always picking on me.
   e. I cannot get to class on time; I am always running behind.
   f. I could not understand what she was talking about, and then when she asked me the question, I looked like such a fool.
   g. I would like to believe I passed the exam, but what's the use?
   h. I don't know what I did to make her angry, but she'd better get over it.
   i. What is the matter with me? I stayed up all night preparing to complete this clinical assignment, and then I got it all wrong.

WEB RESOURCES

The following websites may provide opportunities for additional learning. Give them a try:

Try a quick online learning styles self-assessment at http://ldpride.net/learning-style -test.html

http://ncbi.nlm.nih.gov/pubmed/9282030

http://onlinelibrary.wiley.com/doi/10.1111/j.1744-6198.1994.tb00169.x/abstract

REFERENCES

Cattaneo, L., & Chapman, A. R. (2010). The process of empowerment: a model for use in research and practice. *American Psychologist, 65*(7), 646–659. http://dx.doi.org/10.1037/a0018854.

Chenevert, M. (2010). *Mosby's tour guide to nursing school: a student's road survival kit* (6th ed.). St. Louis, MO: Mosby.

Dossey, B. M., & Keegan, L. (2016). *Holistic nursing: a handbook for practice* (7th ed.). Burlington, MA: Jones & Bartlett.

Knowles, M. S., Holton, E. F., & Swanson, R. A. (2015). *The adult learner: the definitive classic in adult education and human resource development* (8th ed.). New York, NY: Routledge.

Kolb, D. A. (1984). *Experiential learning: experience as the source of learning and development.* Englewood Cliffs, NJ: Prentice-Hall.

Meltzer, M., & Palau, S. M. (1997). *Learning strategies in nursing: reading, studying and test-taking* (2nd ed.). Philadelphia, PA: Saunders.

Merriam, S. B., Caffarella, R. S., & Baumgartner, L. M. (2007). *Learning in adulthood: a comprehensive guide* (3rd ed.). San Francisco, CA: Jossey-Bass.

Nugent, P. M., & Vitale, B. A. (2016). *Test success: test-taking strategies for beginning nursing students* (7th ed.). Philadelphia, PA: FA Davis.

Twiname, B. G., & Boyd, S. M. (2002). *Student nurse handbook: difficult concepts made easy* (2nd ed.). Stamford, CT: Appleton & Lange.

VARK Learn Limited (2016). VARK: A Guide to learning styles retrieved from http://vark-learn.com/.

Watford, L. (1996). *How to study and manage your time effectively when working on the Distance Learning Program, CUNY Distance Learning Program.* New York, NY: City of New York.

CHAPTER

3

Study Habits and Test-Taking Skills

⊖volve WEBSITE

Additional resources are available online at:
http://evolve.elsevier.com/Claywell/transitions

OBJECTIVES

After completing this chapter, the student will be prepared to:
1. Describe positive face-to-face and online class strategies.
2. Describe the components of effective listening.
3. Engage in effective note-taking.
4. Describe how to improve reading skills.
5. Prepare to study effectively using the SQRRR method.
6. Incorporate strategies to improve test-taking.

KEY TERMS

major details
minor details
multiple-choice questions

SQRRR
structured-response questions

| OVERVIEW

Chapter 2 discussed two crucial actions that support self-empowerment: affirmation and the elimination of self-defeating behaviors. Self-empowerment yields fruitful results when paired with a few helpful study habits. Success in college is directly related to your success at developing and maintaining basic study skills.

Even adults need to practice classroom behaviors that promote learning, and they don't necessarily come naturally. This chapter defines skills and tools to help you get the job done.

GENERAL FACE-TO-FACE CLASSROOM BEHAVIOR

You will be better off sitting near the front of the classroom and away from distractions. Resist the urge to talk, unless you are working with a group or engaged in discussion with the class or instructor. If you are tired, bored, or prone to daydreaming, look over previous notes until you can focus on what is going on in the classroom. Copy down each key word and diagram the instructor puts before you. If it is important enough for a professor to write down, take that as a clue and include it in your notes.

EFFECTIVE LISTENING

Listening is not the same as hearing. It is a conscious activity that requires a number of skills.

Before Class

Before going to class, prepare for what you will be hearing, not only by reading the assigned material but by reviewing your notes from the previous class. If there is an outline for the material you are about to hear, briefly scan it just before class begins to prepare you to notice the main points and subpoints as the instructor addresses them.

During Class

Listen and watch for cues that will indicate when the instructor is about to say something he or she does not want the class to miss. Make eye contact and watch for gestures indicating emphasis. Maintain a positive attitude. Even if the teacher makes statements with which you disagree, do not spend the next several minutes thinking of your rebuttal; rather, jot down a word or two and continue to listen. When the time is appropriate, add your comments to the class discussion. Be an active class participant. Students who are active learners retain the information and are able to apply what they have learned. Gaining meaning from new information requires that you interact with it. Ask questions, and actively work with the information while it is new, until it is clear to you. Make it a practice not to leave class with unanswered questions or if you are confused regarding topics or assignments. Maintain your concentration. Think about what is being said. If you are not attentive, your memory will dump the information before you can hook into it. Adults returning to school have many people and responsibilities competing for attention. While you are in class, give the class your undivided attention. Resist the urge to check your phone. Email, social networking, and texting can wait until after class. Put away or turn off anything that might distract you. Allow flexibility. Most teachers provide an outline or agenda in some form for each class meeting. However, if the class is allowed to depart from the plan, do not panic. Stay with the discussion. If you truly begin to lose your train of thought, then ask a question for clarification. This may help both you and the teacher get back on topic. Toward the end of class, but before you leave, make certain all of your questions have been answered.

Immediately After Class

At the end of the session, spend a few minutes reviewing the notes you just took. Add additional clarifying comments. Try to find the answers to any questions that come to mind. If you are unable to find the answers, email your faculty and ask for help.

Instructors do not mind being asked questions and, in fact, appreciate the students who take responsibility for their learning.

EFFECTIVE NOTE-TAKING

Oddly enough, some students ask, "Do we need to take notes on this?" The answer to that is always a resounding "Absolutely yes!" Never miss an opportunity to record what you are learning. Simply hearing a lecture or participating in an experiment or project is not enough for anyone. To fully understand what is being said, you need to be able to review it and reflect on all that has transpired. Most human short-term memories will dump any material that has not been processed within minutes of the event.

Before Class

Read the outline and prepare yourself for what you will hear. You can do this the same way you prepare for listening. Complete your reading assignment before class. Review prior notes and be ready to listen when class begins. Make sure you have plenty of paper and at least two pens or pencils and a highlighter with you in the classroom, out and ready-at-hand on your desk or table. If you are taking notes on a laptop, have a document open, prepared, and saved. Make certain you have your device fully charged or plugged in to avoid interruptions from loss of power.

During Class

Do not try to record a verbatim transcript of the class. Instead, paraphrase what is being said. Write key words and phrases, especially unfamiliar terms, titles, and concepts. Use acronyms and symbols or your own version of abbreviations to increase speed. (Caution: use only abbreviations with which you are familiar; otherwise, you may have a page of gibberish at the conclusion of the lecture.) Write legibly, but do not waste time making it perfect. If you can read it, that is good enough. Use underlining, highlighting, or stars to indicate areas that the presenter signaled as most important. Include examples, pictures, mnemonics, diagrams, and formulas. If your instructor has provided the slideshow electronically, try taking notes on the notes space provided in most slide builder features of slide show software. Finally, take as many notes as possible. Too many notes is not a problem, but too few could leave gaps in your study. FYI 3.1 lists common verbal signals often used by instructors to indicate important information.

After Class

As soon as possible after class, review and expand your notes. You will likely need to add words and phrases and fill in other gaps to give your notes detail.
- Write down any points that you may remember from class that you do not have in your notes. Make connections to content that was covered in prior classes.
- Make note of any conflicting notes or information that does not make sense to you, and ask your instructor about it.
- Compare notes with a classmate.

FYI 3.1 COMMON VERBAL SIGNALS

Most instructors signal, either consciously or subconsciously, what they believe to be most important. Common verbal signals include the following:

- Numbering items ("First, . . . Second, . . .")
- Pointing out the main idea ("Most important . . .")
- Highlighting concepts ("Remember that . . . The basic concept is . . .")
- Giving examples ("For instance, . . .")
- Changing direction ("On the other hand, . . .")
- Repetition
- Referring to text
- Changing tone of voice
- Using qualifying words ("Always," "Never," "Rarely," "Often")

- Read over your notes frequently and especially before the next class.
- Develop your own test questions related to the material for later review.

SUCCESS IN AN ONLINE CLASS

Online learning is a very popular mode of delivering and participating in nursing education. Benefits include the flexibility of anytime, anywhere access as well as a means to attend courses and programs that might not have been available locally. Along with the benefits come challenges for learners and instructors alike, but there are several strategies that you can use to help you enjoy the online experience and capitalize on the benefits.

Online classes, especially those delivered asynchronously, require significant self-discipline and time management skills. Consider creating a written or electronic schedule that both addresses your busy life and carves out specific, reasonable amounts of time throughout the week for reading, searching for references, writing, and completing discussion forums and papers. While the flexibility of an online class is convenient and appealing to busy adults, it can also easily be put off and lead to procrastination. Logging in every day and making progress will help you to stay on track. Getting organized is critical in online classes. Along with the schedule, make a list of assignments, including initial discussion postings and replies and when they are due. Then check them off once complete and submitted. If you have items that require submitting to an anti-plagiarism software such as TurnItIn, back up your personal due date for those assignments at least 3 days so that you can have time to revise (and resubmit) any submissions that come back with a similarity score that is higher than your program accepts. Not only is it important to be organized, but understanding how you might have to adjust your preferred learning style to deal with the heavy text-based structure of online learning is also very important. Content in online classes can be difficult to retain. The more fully you engage in discussions with classmates and the instructor, the better your opportunity for learning as well as the establishment of relationships that can benefit you as you move through the program. Be certain to ask lots of questions and look for ways to apply what you are learning. The best way to apply new information is to think it through in the context of experiences you have already had, taking notes on everything you read (in the text and in the discussion forums) and every recorded lecture you hear. Be certain to jot down things to remind you of past experience that may apply as you go along. Staying in communication with classmates and the instructor not only helps to improve your learning opportunities it also helps you to maintain your own motivation.

Motivation and momentum are critical to your success in the online classroom. The isolation that can happen when all of your studying and interactions are done via the computer, especially when the online learning is conducted asynchronously, is a real threat to your potential accomplishment. Maintain your schedule and engage with others in your class whenever the opportunity arises.

EFFECTIVE READING

One of the most important steps you will take toward a successful college experience is improving your reading skills. Nursing programs have always been, and will always likely be, text oriented and reading intensive. Among the most important keys to effective reading are maintaining your concentration through active reading, identifying main ideas, relating details to a main idea, highlighting appropriately, and improving reading speed.

Maintaining Concentration

Choose an environment for your reading that minimizes distraction. Make it clear to family and friends that for your planned reading session, you are not to be interrupted unless there is an emergency. Turn the phone ringer off and let the answering machine intercept your calls.

Textbooks can be dry and, believe it or not, less than engaging, so you must make a determined effort to stay engaged in what you are reading. It could be that we are more tuned into the audiovisual communication these days and listening to music (even a recorded lecture) or watching a video is preferred to reading, but textbooks, like this one, are still necessary in order to impart large volumes of information as efficiently as possible; therefore, we find the strategies that work and stick with them. One such strategy is to consider that as you read, you are having a conversation with the author. In good conversations, questions are asked on both sides. Stop periodically and ask yourself a question that you would ask the author if you could. Jot the questions down in the margin next to the paragraph for later consideration.

Identifying Main Ideas

Isolating the main ideas of topics is paramount to comprehension. To help you find a main idea, ask yourself questions such as "What is the most important issue or point about this topic?" Most authors signal their main ideas with headings, bold type, or italics. Watch for these cues as you skim the pages before reading in depth. Make a pencil mark in the margin next to the idea, and this will catch your eye and your attention as you read. Look for material that has been placed in boxes. These handy pedagogical features often summarize and highlight key points. Identifying the main points in a mental outline can help organize your reading.

Related to this is isolating the main thing *that an RN must know* in each bit of new information, especially in content that is familiar to you but that you learned and applied in the perspective of an LPN/LVN but now must think of and apply in a new way. When you come upon these points, perhaps mark an RN in the margin of your text or notes to remind you to check your thinking there.

Learning at the Vocational Level vs Higher Education

Nursing school, whether at the vocational or higher education levels, requires tremendous effort and investment of time and effort; however, there is a difference in the depth of learning required in nursing school at the RN level than what you accomplished at the PN/VN level. While many of the topics you will encounter in nursing school will be very familiar and you may be tempted to skim over them, don't do it. Dive in and go deep into the topic, considering all the aspect of what RNs must know to function both autonomously and collaboratively in complex patient-centered care environments. Resist the urge to say, "I already know this," and, instead, look for what you can add to what you already know that takes that knowledge to the next level.

Relating Details to a Main Idea

As you build your mental picture or outline, add the supporting details as bullet points under the related main idea. Reading and trying to remember every single word often frustrate students when they are reading a text. Instead, try to form the idea of the topic in your mind as you read. If you form the idea instead of trying to remember every single word, you can go back and ask yourself what you know about the topic. Say aloud what you learned from your reading. If you find that you stumble over a certain word at first, just skip it and make a note to come back to it. Sometimes if there is a word that is difficult to pronounce, even when reading silently, it might help to give it a mental nickname or abbreviation. This technique might help the flow of your reading. Go back later to deal with the words that tripped you up along the way and perhaps make a note card for each so you can practice. The important thing is to be able to explain the idea of what you are reading and be able to fill in the details at some point.

However, not all details are equally important. Textbooks are often very detailed, much of the time providing so much detail that it becomes difficult to differentiate major from minor details (Meltzer & Palau, 1997). **Major details** are clearly associated with the main ideas and are often considered of primary importance. They should be the focus of note-taking and highlighting. **Minor details** are usually present in support of the major details or only peripherally related to the main idea.

Highlighting Appropriately

Underlining or highlighting your text can be a beneficial tool if you use it appropriately and judiciously. Highlighting is meant to aid in later review. The following are basic guidelines for highlighting written material:

- Read the entire section at least once before you highlight. If you try to underline the first time you read the section, you will often end up underlining entire passages, which will not benefit you when you review.
- Try to create your own sentences by highlighting only certain key words or phrases. Leave out unnecessary words. You may need to write a few of your own words in the margin to make the highlighted words and phrases flow smoothly.

- Try to highlight no more than 20% of the material (e.g., if a section has 50 lines of text, highlight no more than 10).
- Use different ways of highlighting—circles, underlines, asterisks, stars, arrows—to indicate differences in the material. Create a pattern and stick to it.
- Regularly review the material you have highlighted. If you are unable to answer study questions with something you have highlighted, go back and reread the entire passage to look for missed points.

Improving Reading Speed

Evidence relates reading speed to comprehension: the faster you read, the more you understand what you are reading. The same skills may be associated with both increased comprehension and the ability to read material quickly. You can improve reading effectiveness and efficiency by identifying and reducing factors that inhibit reading (FYI 3.2) and by promoting the good habits that enhance reading rate and comprehension (FYI 3.3).

Alter your reading rate according to the type of material. Reading for enjoyment is different from reading for analysis. Although you may read novels extremely quickly, yet with thorough understanding, you will likely find it necessary to decrease your speed for detailed or technical information. Do not become frustrated at needing to

---

FYI 3.2 READING INHIBITORY FACTORS

- Having to read aloud or word by word
- Unfamiliar vocabulary or jargon
- Difficulty making smooth line changes with eyes
- Reading the same material over and over (also called *regression*)
- Lack of engagement with or attention to what is being read
- Lack of experience with reading the amount or type of text you are expected to read
- Trying to remember everything
- Forcing reading acceleration rather than improving reading habits

---

FYI 3.3 IMPROVING READING CONDITIONS AND HABITS

- Visit an optometrist or ophthalmologist. Many times a slow reading rate and poor comprehension are related to visual defects.
- Try not to sound out words during reading. First prepare yourself by going over key terms. Practice saying them aloud until you are comfortable with both their pronunciation and their spelling. Then, as you encounter them in your reading, you will be less likely to stumble and regress (have to reread).
- Stay engaged and focused as you read. Allowing your mind to wander encourages regression and a slower pace, which sets you up for more distractions and regression, and an hour later you've read one paragraph.
- Practice using a broader eye span: look at more than one word at a time. Text is meant to be read as long, streaming sentences and passages. Focusing on one word at a time (or reading word by word) is distracting and inhibits your ability to focus on the idea being presented.

reread to gain complete understanding of nursing and other scientific texts. Frequent review is a necessary part of the discipline for both beginners and experts.

Skimming and Scanning

Among reading tools that are especially effective for reading nursing and scientific texts are skimming and scanning. Nursing texts are generally packed with data and details, and students crawl through the underbrush searching for main points and for what is a "must-know" versus a "nice-to-know." By practicing skimming and scanning before your in-depth reading, your retention of major concepts, ideas, and details will improve (Meltzer & Palau, 1997).

To effectively read a chapter or passage, you must first skim to locate its main ideas or the main concept. This provides the skeleton that you will flesh out with necessary information as you read in-depth later.

Scanning locates unfamiliar or key terms and phrases. It also calls your attention to concepts that are new to you. Scan for definitions, formulas, and pictures that represent or support main ideas.

IMPROVING YOUR STUDY SKILLS

The following is a five-step method for studying that has been used for many years: survey, question, read, recite, and review **(SQRRR).** If applied consistently, the SQRRR formula will help you thoroughly study your material.

Step 1: Survey

To *survey* means to skim the book. Read the headings and subheadings along with the lead sentences that go with each. Read each chapter summary and introduction. Write down any unfamiliar terms as you survey the material.

Step 2: Question

Make *questions* out of the headings and subheadings of each chapter and write them down. Instead of writing "Steps in the Nursing Process," write "What are the steps of the nursing process?" Write a question for each main idea in the chapter. Use any study guides the teacher provides.

Now answer your questions as best you can without returning to the book. Try to reinforce your understanding of any new or unfamiliar terms as you consider the answers to the questions.

Step 3: Read

Read the first section of the book, searching for the answer to the first question you wrote. You may underline a key word here or there. After you have read the entire section, write out what you have found to be the answer to the question. Use your own words. If some terms cause you to stumble, change them, as long as you understand the meaning.

Step 4: Recite

Without looking at the book or your notes, try to say aloud in your own words your explanation or answer. If you are unable to do this just yet, look over the section, your question, and your written answer again until you are able to *recite* the correct response.

Repeat steps 3 and 4 with each section of the chapter. Continue until you complete the assigned reading.

Step 5: Review

Once you have completed the entire lesson this way, *review* daily by reciting aloud the major points of each section. The three stages of review or study are early review, intermediate review, and final review.

Early review is the most efficient and productive form of review. Before you go to class or read new material, do the following:
- Refresh prior material in your mind.
- Say aloud the major concepts of what you already know.
- Engage in early review immediately after class or reading the new material, because review makes the most sense when it is associated with what you already know or have very recently learned. Most forgetting happens immediately after learning. Planning time to engage in early review directly after class is essential.
- Rework your notes. This does not mean to copy—that won't help. Merge the notes you took in class with notes you jotted down during study.
- Organize what you learned by drawing arrows, pictures, or graphs, adding any memory cues that come to mind.
- Associate what you have just learned with what you already know. Speak aloud and link new concepts with prior concepts. In nursing, the curriculum builds, so you should be able to write out how what you've just learned relates to what you already knew.

Intermediate review takes place after early review is completed and focuses on understanding the material. Intermediate review is especially important when you have several weeks before an exam.

Final review takes place in the days immediately before an exam. This is not cramming; final review is not the time to try to catch up on unlearned material. Rather, recite aloud to yourself or a study partner everything you recall regarding the entire semester's material. Space out your review sessions. Three 20-minute sessions are more beneficial than one 60-minute session.

More Study Strategies

The following are some short, straight-to-the-point tactics and strategies for getting the most out of your studying:
- For every hour of class, spend 2 to 3 hours studying, MINIMUM.
- Start your study sessions with the most difficult or boring subjects. We all gravitate toward what we like or what is comfortable and familiar, but you must force yourself to spend quality time working toward understanding the more difficult material. You can't get away with saying, "I just don't get it." You must get it, and the only way to do that is through practice and repetition.
- Do not study for hours on end without breaks or pull all-nighters. Short but frequent study sessions are much more productive. Give yourself and your brain a chance to relax.

- Get up early. Many people are most productive before 9 AM. Your focus will be sharper and your mind clearer. (This assumes, of course, that you went to bed at a decent time.)
- Don't waste your waiting time. Take your notes along in the car and wherever you go. Instead of daydreaming or reading last year's celebrity magazine at the dentist's office, whip out your notes and review. You'll be surprised how important these short, impromptu study times will become.
- Record the class (or ask your professor if there is a podcast of the lectures) and listen to it in the car, while you exercise, or while shopping. Those of you who are kinesthetic learners will find this tactic especially helpful.
- Employ what you've learned to avoid distractions. Claim your right to a conducive study environment, whether at school or at home.
- Study in a group, if possible. Not everyone is a social learner, but we all have different talents for understanding the text and applying experiences. As such, group study is great for processing new information. Studying in groups not only gives the advantage of relating information and concepts in a fun, nonthreatening environment, but it also keeps you from procrastinating because you know your group is counting on you. However, you should avoid the pitfall of being distracted by social conversation while studying in a group setting.

FINDING THE BALANCE

Nursing students often become completely immersed in the rigors and requirements of nursing school. Soon you may feel as though your entire life and those of your family members revolve around your class and clinical schedule. You may also feel that all you ever do is work. Both of these statements are likely true!

Recognize that balance is important to your success. Not only do you need to devote time, energy, and attention to your work and study, but you must also give quality time to your other relationships and interests. To keep your family members and friends, as well as yourself, from burning out, plan time for nurturing. You are at the beginning of a new start in life, or at least in for a dramatic change. You want to be able to enjoy it. Reward yourself and your supporters on a regular basis. Maintain your health through a healthy diet and regular physical activity. Maintain your spirituality. Enjoy the process and experience of growth and becoming.

TEST-TAKING SKILLS

Specific knowledge about types of test questions and how to approach them can be of benefit to the test-taker. The three types of questions you may encounter in didactic testing are structured-response, restricted-response, and essay questions.

Structured-Response Questions

In **structured-response questions,** the correct answers are supplied along with incorrect responses, and the test-taker must select from those provided. Types of structured response questions are multiple choice, multiple response, true-false, and matching.

Multiple Choice/Multiple Response

Multiple-choice/multiple-response questions are common in testing throughout nursing education and are predominant on the NCLEX-RN. A multiple-choice question is made up of the stem and the options, each of which is discussed in detail here. On the new licensing exam, you will find multiple-choice, multiple-response (or select all that apply [SATA]) questions, meaning you are to choose more than one answer that is correct. Chapter 5 of this text covers more detail related to successfully passing the NCLEX-RN.

Question Stem

The stem is the part of the item that asks the question or presents the problem and any conditions that apply. It may be in the form of a complete or incomplete sentence. Polarity, whether it is positive or negative in nature, is also an important characteristic of the stem. A positively formatted question asks about something that is true. Positive stems are used to determine whether the test-taker understands information that is factual and is able to discern related information or actions accordingly. For example, the stem in the following test question is formatted in a positive manner:

You are about to begin a sterile dressing change with your patient. The first three actions you take, in order, are:

a. Wash your hands, gather your equipment, and put on sterile gloves.
b. Gather your equipment, open sterile packages, and wash your hands.
c. Explain the procedure to the patient, wash your hands, and gather your equipment.
d. Explain the procedure to the patient, gather equipment, and wash your hands.

Conversely, a negatively formatted question asks about something that is false. To identify stems with negative polarity, look for words such as "not," "never," "except," "least," or "contraindicated." Negative indicator words will not always stand out, so it is a good practice to underline these and other negative words so as not to miss them (if writing on the test is allowed). The item writer usually employs a negatively formatted question when the test-taker must demonstrate the ability to discern exceptions, errors, and inaccurate or inappropriate information or actions. For example, the stem in the following test question is formatted in a negative manner:

In the elderly, all of the following conditions predispose the patient to urinary tract infections except:

a. Incomplete emptying of bladder.
b. Decreased renal perfusion.
c. Thinning of epidermis.
d. Relaxation of pelvic floor muscles.

The stem may also identify a priority, which you can find by looking for words such as "best" and "first." The options for this type of question stem may all appear to be appropriate, but the top priority is the key. You will be required to determine which is most appropriate or which comes first. The earlier example of a question written in a positive manner is also an example of a question asking you to decide which comes first, second, and third in a series. Because the stem of a multiple-choice question must provide all of the data required to answer the question, you likely will find hints that may lead you to the correct answer.

While reading the stem, be sure to understand who the object of the question is. It is not always going to be the patient or the nurse. One key to success with the multiple-choice question is to read the stem carefully and clearly understand what is being asked.

Question Options

The options are the possible answers in multiple-choice or multiple-response questions. In multiple choice, each test item has one best or correct option. In multiple-response or SATA questions, there will be at least two correct options but only *rarely* will all options be correct. The items also may have multiple incorrect options, known as *distractors* because they are created with the intent to distract the test-taker from the correct answer. This decreases the chance that the test-taker choosing the best option is a coincidence.

Many characteristics about the options might help point out the correct choices. Be wary of options that make wide, sweeping statements. Rarely can we say in nursing that "one size fits all." Instead, look for options with detailed or narrow scopes. Another hint is to look for separate options that contradict each other. Either one is correct and the other is a distractor, or they are both incorrect. If the options all seem reasonable, then reread the stem. You likely will have missed a key word in the stem that points to polarity or priority. Watch for words such as always, all, and complete, which often can signal a wrong answer choice. While considering the options, always remember the basic premise on which nursing stands: the patient is always the top priority. Answers that are patient centered and address the patient needs as a priority are likely good choices. Other strategies include addressing each answer option separately, determining whether it answers the question correctly or not. Even when answering a multiple-response question, consider the options individually rather than by groups.

True-False

In the true-false type of question, the test-taker must determine whether the statement is completely true or completely false. Numerous variations on the true-false format exist; however, regardless of the variation, true-false leaves no room for shades of truth or falsity. The correct or best response should be clearly either one or the other. Read the statement slowly and carefully before choosing.

Matching and Ordered Response Questions

Most often in a matching question, the author arranges the information in the form of two lists or columns. Examine both lists carefully to determine the general relationship between the items in each list. Then, consistently using the same column as your starting point, look for matches you recognize to be absolutely correct. As you make matches, cross them off the list. Once you have made the "guaranteed" matches then work with those of which you are unsure. On the NCLEX-RN, this type of question is also known as an ordered response question type. Ordered response items in computer-based testing involve dragging and dropping options in a correct order, such as in the order of performance, like steps to inserting a urinary catheter. According to Kaptest.com (2016), the appropriate strategy to improve your success with ordered response questions is to form a mental picture of actually doing the procedure and drag and drop the options as you see them occurring in your mind. You can always go back and rearrange if you have misplaced a step.

Restricted-Response Questions

Several forms of restricted-response questions exist. Two familiar types are completion, or fill-in-the-blank, and short-answer questions. You will see fill-in-the-blank questions on the NCLEX-RN exam. The item writer employs these types to test understanding of facts, definitions, formulas, and straightforward concepts. The learner is expected to provide the key words, phrases, or sentences that complete a statement or to provide the answer to the question. The instructor will look for specific information that is considered correct. However, when you are in doubt as to a specific answer, the best rule of thumb is to write more rather than less in the hope that you will supply the desired information. Another strategy to promote your success with fill-in-the-blank items is to carefully read the question as well as any units of measure or other words provided in or adjacent to the answer box so you are fully aware of the type of answer that is expected. The following example is in the form of a fill-in-the-blank question:

Laboratory data that may indicate the presence of an infection include an elevated _____, an elevated _____, and the presence of _____ in the cultures.

Essay Questions

The third major type of question you will likely encounter in nursing school is the essay question, which is most often reserved as a tool for evaluating the student's ability to analyze, synthesize, and solve problems with very complex concepts and related conditions and information. You will not see this type of question in the NCLEX-RN exam, but it is still used in nursing school, so knowing how to best respond to this type of question remains important. To succeed with essay questions, you must be able to articulate in writing what you know. This requires not only that you have a clear grasp of the material but that you have honed your organizational and writing skills such that you are able to communicate your response effectively.

When responding to an essay question, organize your thoughts with an outline that is in the same order as the question. Then write all relevant information you have pertaining to each area of your outline. An essay answer requires more than simply a list of unrelated thoughts, however. Your answer must flow and then end in a clear summary that restates your conclusions. If you recognize that writing is not one of your strengths, you will do yourself a favor by asking your instructor or advisor for assistance. Some colleges have writing labs with faculty members or other tutors who can help you improve your writing ability. The nursing profession requires ability to express ourselves clearly through writing with everything from patient charting and care planning to papers and articles for school courses and publication.

Universal Advice for Optimal Test Performance

Several strategies and behaviors before and during a test may improve your performance. *Preparedness* is the main word to remember. Study, study, study! Read your text and watch any videos prior to coming to class. This way, as you listen to lecture or engage in discussion, you will remember and understand more; in addition, you will already have questions in your mind that you can ask the instructor when it is fresh and you are more likely to assimilate the response. Reread your text and your notes daily and especially right after class. If questions come up, write them down immediately so you remember to ask about them. Use the objectives in the course guide or syllabus as a study guide if the instructor did not provide one. Be certain you can answer each objective in your mind as you go along. Ask your questions! If needed, get help with tutoring. Practice any available tests you can find (check for student resources that may be available with your textbooks) just to get used to taking tests. There are lots of online resources with practice quizzes. Then, once you have prepared academically as much as possible, it is time to prepare in other ways.

Prepare your body, mind, and spirit by following your usual routine in the days before the test. Get plenty of rest and eat a well-balanced diet. All-nighters rarely produce acceptable results. By the time you begin the exam, your brain and your body will be so exhausted that your performance will suffer. The night before, pack everything you will need during the exam so your morning departure is not delayed as you run through the house searching for your calculator or favorite pen.

On the day of the exam, reduce your anxiety by getting to the class on time. Give yourself plenty of time to relax before you begin. Do not get pulled into last-minute study sessions with classmates, but rather meditate or collect your thoughts.

Once the exam begins, read all the instructions and scan the entire test. Note how much time you have to spend on each question. Be aware of timing as you proceed through the test. Answer every question, even if you have to make educated guesses. Leaving a question blank offers no possibility of getting it right. Some instructors offer partial credit, particularly on short-answer or essay questions, so give it your best. Be careful not to overthink the questions or read into the question more than what it is actually asking. Try mentally rewriting the question in your own words and speaking it in familiar terms in your mind. Once you have fully and carefully read the question and you know what it is asking, apply the tips mentioned earlier about how to most successfully answer each question type. Remember that as an RN you will be expected to apply what you have learned, and, most of the time, simply understanding and recalling are not enough; therefore, nursing tests will be at higher levels that require you to apply, analyze, and evaluate nursing care based on what you have learned.

Before turning in your test, check your answers. Reread each question and make sure you have marked/chosen the option or written the answer you intended. Marking wrong answers by mistake can be easy, particularly on tests where you must fill in bubbles or click buttons to indicate your answers. Check them carefully. In written exams, make sure that any erasures are complete and that all writing is legible. Once you have turned in or submitted your test, tell yourself that you have done your best, and let go of the anxiety. Soon you will start studying for the next one.

> 📌 FYI 3.4 **TEST-TAKING STRATEGIES**
>
> - Carefully read all instructions.
> - Glance over entire test to gauge length and become aware of timing.
> - Read every test question carefully—look for key words that tell you priority or timing.
> - Any time priority or timing is mentioned these are important details.
> - Mentally answer the question before looking at answer choices.
> - Read and consider every answer option individually, and beware of key words here, too.
> - Think like an RN as you reason and apply knowledge.
> - Be cognizant of time passing, but do not panic if others finish before you; pace yourself.
> - When you get your results back, learn the correct answers for any incorrect items.

KEY POINTS

After completion of this chapter, you have:
- Learned that to be effective in the classroom and online, you must maintain an active, engaged, and positive perspective.
- Studied effective listening and note-taking skills.
- Improved your study time through practiced and effective reading skills.
- Identified that concentration and the ability to link details to main ideas are critical while studying.
- Learned that reading ability and comprehension are impacted by habits.
- Practiced with the SQRRR method of study.
- Recognized the importance of balance in your work, school, and home lives.
- Learned about different types of test questions and strategies to address each.
- Learned that practicing specific test-taking skills can improve your testing performance.

▋ CRITICAL THINKING QUESTIONS

1. A bird and a cat are sitting on a fence post. The bird is a good distance away from the cat, aware of its perilous perch. The bird looks at the cat and says, "Do you always need to act like a cat?" The cat replies, "What do you mean?"

   The bird further ponders its position and chooses its words carefully: "By nature, you want to eat me. This fact is true. But you were raised in a caring and loving household where you were fed and kept warm. As I sit here on this fence, I believe that if I let you get too close to me, you would take my life because that is who you are."

   The cat looks at the bird and, in a shrewd manner, says, "You're right. I have had a good life, have not had to hunt for my food, and am provided for in a quite luxurious way. But you are also wrong. I have no reason or inclination to want you dead or to eat you. To prove it, come sit next to me. I will not harm a feather on your back."

The bird wisely flies away. As it is leaving, it says, "You are a cat, I am a bird, and I will live to see you tomorrow because I know the difference."

a. Explain the main idea of this story.

b. What assumptions can be made from this story?

c. Explain the point of view of the cat and then the bird. Is there another point of view? Explain.

d. Explain the line of reasoning used by the bird and then by the cat.

2. For the following scenario (in italics), formulate at least eight questions that will help you understand what has happened. Look at your questions and see whether you have made any assumptions.

You walk into your patient's room and find the patient on the floor.

This scenario is incomplete, which you will find to be true for most nursing situations where you will need to make decisions. Each decision you make will require you to gather as many of the facts as you can, and to gather facts, you must be able to ask questions.

3. You wake up the morning of clinical to find that your 3-year-old child has a fever of 102.3°F and is complaining of a "hurt in my throat."

a. What is your top priority?

b. What conflicts are you facing?

c. What steps must you take to meet the requirements of clinical?

4. Having skipped your class, your clinical instructor calls and notifies you that you have no clinical absences left and will need to consider your options.

a. What questions do you need clarified?

b. Write out a script of how you will discuss your options and needs. Identify assertive and nonassertive statements you have written.

c. Write a plan to meet the objectives of clinical in an alternate way.

WEB RESOURCES

http://how-to-study.com/
http://studygs.net/
http://readingquest.org/strat/
http://bigfuture.collegeboard.org/find-colleges/academic-life
www.kaptest.com

REFERENCE

Meltzer, M., & Palau, S. M. (1997). *Learning strategies in nursing: reading, studying and test-taking* (2nd ed.). Philadelphia, PA: Saunders.

UNIT 2

The Profession and Discipline of Registered Nursing

CHAPTER 4

Distinguishing the RN Role from the LPN/LVN Role

⊖volve WEBSITE

Additional resources are available online at:
http://evolve.elsevier.com/Claywell/transitions

OBJECTIVES

After completing this chapter, the student will be prepared to:

1. Discuss the concept of role transition from practical nurse to registered nurse.
2. Describe various role elements that are inherent in the scope of registered nursing practice.
3. Compare and contrast differences in role responsibilities of practical and registered nurses.
4. Describe the process of professional socialization from practical nurse to that of registered nurse.
5. Recognize the differences in the educational preparation of the LPN/LVN and RN.
6. Compare and contrast the differences in the roles of the LPN/LVN and RN.
7. Compare and contrast the scope of practice for the LPN/LVN and the RN.
8. Explain the advantages of obtaining specialty certification in professional nursing practice.

KEY TERMS

advocacy
advocate
American Association of Colleges of Nursing (AACN)
American Nurses Credentialing Center (ANCC)

KEY TERMS—cont'd

associate's degree in
   nursing
baccalaureate degree in
   nursing
care provider
change agent
collaborator
Commission on
   Collegiate Nursing
   Education (CCNE)
counselor
critical thinking
diploma in nursing

doctoral degree
educator
entrepreneur
manager
master's degree in
   nursing
mentor
National Council of
   State Boards of Nurs-
   ing (NCSBN)
Accreditation Commis-
   sion for Education in
   Nursing (ACEN)

professional socialization
researcher
role
role conflict
role model
role transition
scope of practice
standards of professional
   nursing practice
standards of professional
   performance
state nurse practice acts

OVERVIEW

The decision to undertake a course of study that leads to a new role in nursing is not an easy one. It requires a tremendous commitment of time, energy, and financial resources; you may even need to put portions of your personal and professional life on hold while you are in school. Transition and change such as this bring with it uncertainty in many realms, but understanding the differences between the roles will help to lessen the concerns.

Registered nurses wear a wide variety of "hats," and the nature of those hats is probably a little unclear to you at this time. Alternatively, you may not understand what the differences really are between what you do as a practical nurse and what the RNs who practice beside you do. But that will quickly change. You will be exposed to new responsibilities and new ways of thinking that may seem overwhelming at first. However, with practice and experience, you will suddenly find yourself viewing the world of nursing in a completely different way.

This chapter is intended to ease the **role transition** from licensed practical nurse (LPN/LVN) to registered nurse (RN). The road from LPN/LVN to RN is difficult but manageable. A journey of this kind requires an understanding of the major differences between the two roles, especially those related to the thinking processes inherent in each. Before beginning this trip, take time to open your mind to new ways of thinking and behaving. A closed mind will be your greatest obstacle. You have summoned the courage for this great undertaking. If you hang on to that courage as you encounter new territory, you will be successful.

PROFESSIONAL ROLE SOCIALIZATION

Each of us functions in a variety of roles in life—mother, father, teacher, Cub Scout leader, and so on. A **role** carries a set of expectations that define the behavior society deems appropriate or inappropriate for the occupant. With each role comes a set of behaviors that helps us formulate our performance to meet society's expectations. Nurses, both LPN/LVNs and RNs, also have roles. The passage or transition from one nursing role to another involves a change in behavior—a change that must take place over a period of time in order for you, the student, to embrace the new role fully (Schumacher & Meleis, 1994).

In the past, you may have seen pictures of capped nurses in starched white uniforms, or you may have watched television shows in which nurses were portrayed as hospital employees subservient to physicians. These images tend to influence our perceptions of what nursing is all about. Take a few moments to answer the following questions:

How have these early images influenced your expectations of yourself and other nurses?

_____

_____

Did your practical/vocational nursing program support your preformed images about nursing, or did it challenge them? If so, how?

_____

_____

As a practical/vocational nursing student, you acquired certain attributes that you judged to be important to a nurse. You may value characteristics such as a strong work ethic, ability to organize, efficiency, kindness, and dependability as necessary ingredients in the makeup of a good nurse. These are all desirable traits, but as a registered nurse, you'll be adding a broader range of qualities. To be successful as a registered nurse, you must be willing to build on attributes associated with your current understanding of nursing. For example, practical nursing education has provided you with the skills to observe for and report abnormalities in a patient's vital signs. After transition to the registered nursing level, you will have developed problem-solving skills that allow you to act on the information in a manner that will most benefit the patient.

The transition from practical to registered nurse involves shaping, modifying, and adding information in order to achieve a more comprehensive view of patient care. During this process, you will learn new ways of thinking while adapting to and accepting new behaviors within yourself. Take advantage of the learning opportunities provided in your course of study and accept advice from your instructors, for they are your strongest allies at this time in your life. Feedback, positive or negative, is designed to help you move forward toward your goal of becoming a registered nurse.

Because of the importance of making a successful and smooth role transition, a fair amount of research has been done on **professional role socialization**. Zarshenas et al. (2014) found a number of factors that will influence your ability to transition smoothly. These include first a sense of belonging. It is important that you foster that sense of belonging both with classmates as you transition back into nursing school and with new nurse colleagues you may encounter. In addition, the presence of incongruent theory to practice is a source for difficulty. New content learned may not be what you find in your clinical practicums. This may also be extrapolated to mean that theory you previously learned and may currently put into practice as an LPN/LVN may no longer be the current evidence-based practice that is required, and this may cause a rocky transition. Another strong factor is the informal or tacit knowledge you gain from how you perceive others to treat you or what you may believe they think of you. In addition, and perhaps most important for you, is the required shift in your identity from LPN/LVN to RN. You recognize yourself as a "nurse" but it must shift to RN in order for you to fully engage in the role.

This last component is also supported by the study by Melrose et al. (2012) regarding legitimation, or the degree to which you feel legitimate in your new role. It was found by these researchers that LPN/LVNs already have an identity as a nurse but found that it was the clinical experiences during RN school that made all the difference in how well the students took on the new role. Meaning that if the nursing faculty and clinical preceptors treated the student with respect and interacted professionally recognizing the value of previous learning and experience and then took the encounter up to the next level, always discussing what the RN would do and allowing the student to engage as an RN, then the transition to the new role was considered more successfully facilitated. However, not every instructor or clinical preceptor will understand the vast knowledge and experience you bring with you or the struggle to both hold onto and re-shape that learning as they help you to move through RN school.

In cases such as these, you may feel insulted or that your previous learning is being discounted or even ignored. Keep in mind that it is up to you to look for the differences in how you practice as an LPN/LVN and how you are now being taught to practice as an RN. In some environments, there may be very little noticeable difference, but in most cases, the differences are significant. As you travel along the road to transitioning to your new role, you may find that there are slippery slopes and rocky sections that require taking a step back and a deep breath before forging ahead.

Frequently, students encounter feelings of **role conflict,** especially when confronted with incompatible role requirements. Your friends, family, and co-workers have formed an image of you as a nurse on the basis of previous role behaviors. Upon entering a registered nursing program, you may unknowingly begin to change those behaviors as you learn to stretch your mind and assume new characteristics. You may be expected to perform in a new manner in your educational setting, even while those who know you best are still looking for the "old" you.

At this point, it is important to mention a situation that produces a significant amount of role conflict once back in the role of student, and that is for the paramedic to RN transition group. Paramedics, in most states and in the military, function in very autonomous roles under extreme and emergent conditions, having to make decisions based on protocols and algorithms that are already in place, many times without having to consult a physician. Paramedics are licensed and their practice is governed at the state level and varies somewhat from state to state. When a paramedic enters nursing school and takes on the role of student nurse, it is often very difficult to rein in one's previous ways of doing things especially in the clinical area. This may be true for some LPN/LVNs who were practicing in rather autonomous situations. Keep in mind though that once in school and while on student clinical rotations, you are practicing as a student RN under the practice act in your state for that designation and not under the practice act for your previous licensure. This alone can cause confusion and role conflict.

The process of role transition may be stressful when you encounter difficulties in meeting culturally defined role requirements. Uncorrected role strain can lead to chronic frustration and a sense of insecurity. As a student in role transition, consider finding ways to educate your family and friends about the changes that are occurring within you. Share your progress in learning new information and skills with your family. Usually, they will be eager to see the results of your labors, especially if those labors have taken you away from them for periods of time. Add to your circle of friends. Identify other students who are also in role transition and form a support group. You'll be surprised at the strong friendships that are forged from such relationships.

As your journey leads you closer to becoming a registered nurse, you will gradually stop "role playing" as a student, and the new role will become a part of you. That is, it will be internalized. With internalization of the behaviors and attitudes of a registered nurse comes the end of your journey along the path of role transition. But first, you have to begin the journey, and to do that, it will help to take a look at the role of registered nurse in its many aspects.

ROLE ELEMENTS

At this point, the concept of a role may seem a little abstract. You may even be wondering if you are going to be enlightened as to what exactly makes up a registered nurse. (You will.) Right now, however, let's begin with *you*. What do you think? Are registered nurses really so different from practical/vocational nurses? Please take a few minutes to answer the following question:

From your previous experiences, how do you view a registered nurse's duties and responsibilities as differing from those of a practical/vocational nurse?

_____

_____

Actually, the role of registered nurse contains many parts, much like the many sparkling facets of a diamond. Each diamond facet lends its brilliant quality to that of the others to form one shining gem. Without each facet, the diamond would not be as appealing. The many components that make up the role of the registered nurse combine to create the final product, a valuable member (the gem) of the health care team.

Probably the most commonly recognized function of the registered nurse is that of **care provider.** Unit three of this text is dedicated to the provider of care role. Regardless of the setting, nurses are involved in a variety of activities that are aimed at one primary goal: ensuring the best possible health for the patient. Care provider responsibilities in an outpatient clinic may include such functions as health screening, health promotion, and nursing interventions aimed at restoration of health. In the acute care setting, the registered nurse as a care provider must also be concerned with planning care for the entire family, such as on an obstetric unit. Traditionally, the care provider function of nursing—that of actually carrying out interventions that assist patients to meet positive outcomes—has been considered the essence of nursing.

By virtue of their frequent contact with patients and families, registered nurses are exposed to the personal joys and sorrows that occur during times of illness. Faced with navigating a confusing health care system, patients and families rely on nurses for guidance and support at such times. Therefore, the function of the registered nurse as a **counselor** is significant. Registered nurses have an educational foundation of scientific knowledge that assists them in identifying patients' emotional needs. Therapeutic communication skills are a vital aspect of nursing care because many patients have psychosocial needs that are just as important as their physical needs.

In today's rapidly changing world, patients must become more actively involved in their own health care than ever before. This means they need to be as informed as possible about aspects of care once thought to be beyond the comprehension of the general public. The registered nurse, then, is an **educator,** one who is in an excellent position to provide patients with much-needed information about medications, dietary restrictions, treatments, and the like. Whether involved in formal patient education classes, teaching community CPR courses, or answering a new mother's questions about breastfeeding, the registered nurse performs an essential educator function (see Chapter 10 for more on patient teaching).

Nurses make up the largest body of workers in today's health care facilities and are generally looked to for leadership and organizational skills. The **manager** component of registered nursing involves not only supervising other members of the health care team but also planning, managing, and coordinating care for groups of patients, families, and communities. Nurses guide and direct care at several levels, from team leader or charge nurse on a unit to chief nursing officer in an acute care facility. In the community, registered nurses function as case managers and coordinators of groups of patients and staff. To be an effective manager, the nurse should possess sound decision-making and problem-solving skills, which are vital to optimal care planning. Chapter 14 provides a more detailed discussion of nursing leadership and management.

The registered nurse's role as **advocate** requires the nurse to be a protector willing to shield the patient and family from harm. In assuming this duty, the nurse chooses to provide complete, honest information to those in his or her care and to speak up against any harmful or unnecessary forces that might impede progress toward a healthy state. A patient advocate agrees to "take the side" of the health care recipient and "stand up for" the patient's rights to autonomy and self-determination. The oncology nurse who asks for an increase in pain medication for a timid patient is functioning as an advocate, as is the ICU nurse who questions a medical order to perform several procedures in one morning on a fatigued patient.

As a valued member of the health care team, the registered nurse functions as a **collaborator** with physicians, assistive nursing personnel, pharmacists, physical therapists, social workers, and others. Collaboration involves working toward a common goal or end point, which is optimal health or compassionate end-of-life care for the patient and family. Along with other colleagues, registered nurses participate in multidisciplinary meetings to set goals for patients to help achieve earlier discharge from the health care system. Finally, nurses collaborate with patients and families to plan care to ensure cooperation and compliance and with other health care providers to ensure consistent transitional care to reduce the incidence of readmission.

Who is in a better position to sense a needed change in a patient care setting than the registered nurse? As a **change agent,** the nurse must be willing to take risks when others are content with the status quo. Change is often resisted, and a nurse who has the energy, motivation, and interpersonal skills to persuade others to follow suit may not always be popular. However, health care organizations rely on their "frontline workers" to identify problems and make suggestions that could improve patient outcomes, streamline work, and contain costs. The registered nurse who possesses the courage to lead others in change is necessary in order to implement evidence-based care.

Another component of the registered nursing role is that of **role model.** When nurses present themselves to other nursing personnel in a manner that typifies the best attributes of the profession, they are said to be positive role models. Many characteristics have been suggested as desirable traits for registered nurses. For example, a nurse who upholds the American Nurses Association (ANA) Code of Ethics and behaves in a caring, conscientious manner and always places the patient first would be described as a good role model for others. It is particularly important that nursing students and new graduates entering the profession be exposed to favorable role models.

A **mentor** is a trusted advisor. Especially when a nurse is being oriented to a new job, a mentor is important as someone who is available to counsel, teach, and promote professional growth. Generally, a mentor is a more experienced nurse who should be caring, nurturing, and concerned about the new nurse's development. An example of a mentor found in many health care organizations is a preceptor, who is usually responsible for new nursing employee orientation. You may find that you become the mentor or preceptor to new nurses and student nurses quite quickly after assuming your new role. In that role, you will set high expectations of performance and listen carefully and with empathy (Zerwekh & Garneau, 2012). As a steward of the profession, it is our responsibility to encourage and promote nurses. Hopefully, you will find that as you enter your new role, a fine mentor will step up and help you along the way as well.

The **researcher** component of nursing involves investigating possible solutions to nursing and/or patient problems and will be presented in more depth in Chapter 8. Most often, it is registered nurses who have obtained at least a **master's degree in nursing** who engage in nursing research. However, it is the responsibility of all registered nurses to practice evidence-based care and be aware of areas where research is needed to improve care and patient outcomes. For example, staff nurses on a medical unit should be willing to participate in clinical trials of new equipment, with the hope of improving care and reducing skyrocketing health care costs. In addition, staff nurses should be searching the literature to look for the latest evidence upon which to base their practice. Research helps us to find more efficient, effective ways to provide care and helps us to better understand the nature of nursing.

Finally, a fairly new trend seen in nursing is that of the nurse **entrepreneur.** Many nurses have now formed their own businesses in home health, free-standing clinics, schools, and other areas. Nurse entrepreneurs function as consultants, educators, and advisors to organizations and businesses who benefit from their services. This autonomous function of the registered nurse has provided more visibility for nursing to the general public and contributed to a more positive image.

Now, having learned a little about these 11 elements that make up the role of registered nurse, do you begin to see how your role as a practical nurse is about to expand? You may be thinking to yourself, "I do many of these things every day! Sure, maybe I don't get to be the charge nurse or do research, but who cares? I'm still a good nurse."

The issue here is not whether registered or practical nurses are more important or who provides better patient care. As nurses, we are all valuable members of the health care team and as such should focus on those aspects of nursing care that we are best equipped to provide. Registered nurses, by virtue of more lengthy educations, are taught to handle more complex patient care problems, and they have learned the leadership skills necessary for guiding other nursing personnel through day-to-day concerns. In the next section, we'll look more closely at specific differences between the registered nurse and the practical nurse.

DIFFERENCES BETWEEN LPN/LVN AND RN ROLES

In the past, when asked to describe the differences in your duties as an LPN/LVN and those of RNs with whom you have worked, you may have been hard-pressed to come up with many variations in the roles. For example, most LPN/LVNs will answer that the major areas in which RN duties differ from theirs is in supervision, legal responsibilities, and IV therapy. However, there are several areas in which these two types of nurses differ (Box 4.1).

Level of Independence/Autonomy in the Role

In general, in all settings, LPN/LVNs function at the direction of an RN or another authorized care provider, and RNs are authorized to "execute medical orders from select authorized health care providers" (NYSED, 2013 para 5). Additionally, there are a number of situations in which the RN functions independently to provide care, and these include casefinding such as in epidemiology, assessment of abuse, and emergent complications; health teaching such as in health promotion and disease and accident prevention across the life span; health counseling such as in mental health, addictions, and chronic illnesses; restorative care to include bowel and bladder training, ostomy and wound care, assessment, and interventions to rescue those with chronic illness from emergent complications and effects; and supportive care such as palliative and hospice care, management of chronic pain through non-pharmocologic means, and public health care (NYSED, 2013). There may be slight differences from state to state, and therefore it is critical that you are familiar with the scope of practice identified in the nurse practice act in your state.

Educational Level

Traditionally, practical nursing programs focus on teaching the "how to" of patient care, while the emphasis in registered nursing education is on understanding "why" (Hill & Howlett, 2001). Registered nurses are taught to use a variety of thinking skills to understand patient problems and to plan, manage, implement, and evaluate care. Whether a registered nursing program prepares a nurse at the associate, baccalaureate, master's, or **doctoral degree** level, it generally contains the following components that differ from a practical nursing program of study:

- College-level science courses that lay the groundwork for an understanding of psychosocial and physiological aspects of patient care
- College-level liberal arts and general education courses to improve communication skills and encourage a holistic approach to patient care

BOX 4.1 **AREAS OF DIFFERENCES IN LPN/LVN AND RN ROLES**	
• Assessment skills	• IV therapy (in some states)
• Patient teaching skills	• Legal and leadership responsibilities
• Communication skills	• Nursing care planning
• Educational preparation	• Critical thinking skills

- Nursing courses designed to provide an understanding of complex disease processes and patient needs
- Additional clinical hours in which to practice the role of registered nurse under the guidance of an instructor

Registered nurses are educated to function in a variety of settings, such as patients' homes, hospitals, clinics, and long-term care facilities. They have been taught to handle complex patient problems that require a broad scope of knowledge. Even though practical nurses are primarily prepared to practice nursing in a more structured environment under the direction of an RN, they frequently care for patients in the same settings as RNs.

Critical Thinking

Another difference between RNs and LPN/LVNs is in the orientation to the use of critical thinking skills. This book devotes an entire chapter to thinking and judgment. Accredited registered nursing programs are required to provide evidence that **critical thinking** is being taught throughout their curricula. The term *critical thinking* is widely used and broadly interpreted in all aspects of education in the United States. You may be asking yourself, "What exactly is critical thinking?" and "How do I learn to do it?"

Richard Paul (1992), a leading author in the field of critical thinking, defines it as "the art of thinking about your thinking while you are thinking in order to make your thinking better." In other words, critical thinking involves more than simply making routine decisions or judgments. It requires that the nurse be able to evaluate each element of the thinking process to ensure high standards of thinking. In addition, critical thinking involves rationally analyzing information before reaching a conclusion. Complete the short scenario in Box 4.2.

BOX 4.2   PATIENT SCENARIO

Read the following patient scenario, and answer the questions.

Nellie Austin, an 86-year-old patient on a skilled nursing unit, has been repeatedly calling for pain medications since her admission to the unit 1 day earlier. Tom Carey, the nurse on the evening shift, checks her record and finds that she is 5 days post-op from repair of a fractured hip. He notices that she has been receiving oral narcotics for pain management and that her last dose was administered 3 hours previously. The physician's order reads to administer the medication every 4 hours as needed for pain.

Discuss what you would do if you were Ms. Austin's nurse in this situation, giving a rationale for your action(s):

List the steps involved in your thinking process:

Was it difficult for you to analyze the steps involved in your thinking process? Most of us are not taught to analyze and reflect upon how we think. Several choices are possible for this scenario. Tom could have:

- Followed the physician's order and withheld medication for 1 more hour.
- Asked another nurse for advice.
- Called the physician to request additional pain medication.
- Gathered more information in order to choose the best course of action.

Critical thinking calls for gathering all the facts related to the situation and the use of rational judgment to make a decision. Registered nurses must rely on critical thinking skills on a daily basis in order to provide optimal patient care (Alfaro-LeFevre, 1999). "Critical thinking when developed in the practitioner includes adherence to intellectual standards, proficiency in using reasoning, a commitment to develop and maintain intellectual traits of the mind and habits of thought and the competent use of thinking skills and abilities for sound clinical judgments and safe decision-making" (critical-thinking.org, 2015, para 2). Because practical nursing programs are shorter than registered nursing programs, less time is available for discussions of critical thinking and for practice in making sound judgments based on facts or gathered assessment data.

Actually, several kinds of thinking skills should be incorporated into a nursing program of study for the graduate to be best prepared to deal with today's challenging world of health care. Chapter 7 discusses critical thinking; it also describes the need for nurses to possess creative thinking as well as problem-solving and decision-making skills. The registered nurse, as a team leader, is responsible for utilizing clear, analytical thinking abilities to guide others in planning and delivering patient care.

Assessment Skills

Assessment skills, a vitally important area of difference between LPN/LVNs and RNs, also vary with the amount of education and clinical practice time. For legal purposes, registered nurses must complete and sign the nursing assessment portion of a patient's chart. In many instances, however, practical nurses perform a basic nursing assessment, including vital signs; however, in many states, this is considered gathering patient data and measurement (as distinct from assessment, evaluation, and analysis of data) upon which an RN or other authorized care provider can make decisions. Once again you may be wondering how your nursing assessment as an LPN/LVN could be different from that of an RN when you complete the same paperwork on patients. Perhaps this story from a student in an LPN/LVN to RN bridge program will help you understand:

> While I was studying to become an RN, I continued my job as an LPN at the hospital in my hometown. After about 2 months of returning to share what I was learning, I noticed that a good friend, who was also an LPN, began to avoid me. Finally, I stopped her in the hallway one day and asked why she never talked to me at work anymore. She replied, "You act like you know more than me now. I don't see how you can, when you're still doing the same things for patients that you did before you started back to school."

> After considering her comments for a short time, I explained, "Well, you know, I never knew I was acting differently, but I'm glad that I am, because I'm actually learning to be a different nurse than before. For example, when you listen

to a patient's breath sounds, what do you hear?" My friend replied, "I count the respiratory rate and make sure I hear sounds on both sides of the chest." To this I responded, "I do that, too, but now I also know to make sure the breath sounds are equal and to listen for such things as crackles, wheezes, and rubs. Because I'm learning more about disease processes, I can now relate more of what I'm hearing with what I am assessing in my patients."

The registered nurse, with additional theory in pathophysiology and physical assessment, is better equipped than the practical nurse to evaluate a patient's health status. Because of this knowledge base, he or she gathers a wide variety of information during an assessment of the patient and family. Taking into account all aspects of a patient's situation, from cultural and social factors to actual physical and psychological symptoms, the registered nurse utilizes a holistic approach to plan nursing care.

Care Planning

A fifth area of difference between RNs and LPN/LVNs is in nursing care planning. Practical nurses identify common patient problems and participate in assisting patients to achieve expected outcomes in the plan of care. However, registered nurses utilize problem-solving skills to formulate a care plan, establish mutual goals with the patient and family, and oversee the implementation and evaluation of the plan. Nursing diagnosis formulation is widely taught in registered nursing programs, but even if it is introduced in practical nursing curricula, it is generally addressed in less depth. The RN, therefore, is more oriented toward leading other nursing personnel in designing, implementing, and evaluating the nursing plan of care.

The nursing process, reflecting the standards of practice identified by the ANA (2010) that RNs use in patient care, has six steps: assessment, diagnosis, outcomes identification, planning, implementation, and evaluation. The nursing process used by practical/vocational nurses has four steps: assessment, planning, implementation, and evaluation. The major difference between the two is the *analysis* step (diagnosis and outcomes identification). "The work of using critical thinking and clinical judgment to analyze data, make decisions about what that data means, and adapt the plan of care accordingly is uniquely within the domain of the registered nurse. The RN must, however, clearly share results of this analysis as they affect the work of LPNs and other members of the health care team working collaboratively to provide appropriate and timely patient care" (Dickerson, 2009). For more on the nursing process, see Chapter 6.

Legal and Leadership Responsibilities

Legally speaking, there are vast differences in RN and LPN/LVN functions. Even though LPN/LVNs are sometimes found in charge nurse positions in areas that utilize few RNs (such as long-term care facilities), they typically receive little preparation in management theory. Furthermore, state nurse practice acts do not generally recognize leadership or management as a common responsibility of the practical nurse. Team leader, charge nurse, nurse manager, and nurse administrator duties are usually assigned to registered nurses who possess the required education and experience to make the decisions inherent in such positions. The final responsibility for patient care rests with the nurse who functions in a role of authority in any given health care setting. Generally speaking, situations that require a higher level of nursing judgment are assigned to the RN.

In addition, each state has its own nurse practice act (NPA) that governs the practice of nurses (both LPN/LVNs and RNs) in the state. Likely you are already familiar with the NPA in your state of practice as an LPN/LVN. However, you can access these crucial rules and regulations online and, in fact, it is expected that once you achieve licensure, you are accountable for what is in the practice act and will abide by it to the letter. Learn more about nursing and the law in Chapter 12.

Intravenous Therapy

Administration of intravenous (IV) therapy is another area of differing responsibilities among practical and registered nurses. Even though many states have allowed LPN/LVNs to administer IV medications after completing a course in IV therapy, legal considerations continue to suggest that RNs be involved in overseeing the administration of blood and various other IV medications. Some states do require that LPN/LVNs become and remain IV certified, but this does not permit the LPN/LVN to administer all types of IV theory or IV medications. Registered nursing program curricula typically address IV therapy content in greater depth than do practical nursing programs. A greater understanding of drug interactions and complications of intravenous infusions better equips the RN to care for patients on IV therapy.

Communication Skills

Another major area of difference in preparation of LPN/LVNs and RNs is in that of communication skills. Therapeutic communication theory is introduced at the LPN/LVN level in order to prepare students for interacting with patients and families. However, there is limited time to expand upon other aspects of communication that are important to patient care (see Chapter 9). Registered nurses, on the other hand, are exposed to theory on various normal and abnormal communication patterns, as well as mental health disorders. They also have the opportunity to care for patients experiencing behavioral difficulties while in mental health clinical rotations and, therefore, to practice communication skills. The RN completes courses in psychology and sociology in order to form a better understanding of behavioral cues that might influence communication. Therefore, the RN and LPN/LVN have been prepared differently to deal with the communication aspects of the nurse–patient relationship.

Patient Teaching Skills

Patient teaching is an important function of nursing, but LPN/LVNs typically have not received theory regarding teaching-learning principles or been taught to develop educationally oriented mutual goals with patients. Registered nurses are educated to observe for blocks to patient readiness to learning and to prepare an individualized teaching plan for the patient that is realistic and achievable. RNs educate individuals, families, and community groups on wellness topics, provide in-service classes to other health care personnel, and participate in determining evidence-based content for inclusion in teaching sessions. LPN/LVNs are frequently given the responsibility of providing patients with information about diet, medications, and other aspects of self-care but may not have been introduced to principles that enhance learning.

Are you beginning to realize that there are, in fact, many differences in what LPN/LVNs and RNs actually do? You, as an LPN/LVN, may be participating in nursing care planning, delivering and evaluating care, and giving patients discharge instructions for home care. You may have been delegating to assistive personnel as directed by an RN and completing your role as a highly valuable member of the health care team. But now you are journeying toward the full nursing role. Typically, LPN/LVNs who become students in an RN completion program relate that they quickly learn how inadequate their knowledge level was for some of the duties they were asked to perform. As one student stated:

> I've eaten my words many times for saying that I, as an LPN, did the same things as the RN I work with. I'm certified in IV therapy, but it's kind of scary now to see how much I didn't know about the IV medications I've been giving. After my instructor started requiring me to use a medication book to look up the administration rate of IV push medications before giving them, I realized I didn't have all the answers after all!

Each nurse makes important contributions to patient care, regardless of the type of licensure. It is key, however, for you as a practical nurse who is moving into a registered nurse role to be able to see the differences between the two and to be willing to learn new ways of thinking about nursing care. By developing an attitude of eagerness and willingness to assume new responsibilities, you may begin to truly see the benefits of reaching for a higher education. In the next sections, we examine more differences between practical/vocational nursing and registered nursing, including educational preparation and scope of practice.

EDUCATIONAL PREPARATION

Because you are already a licensed practical nurse, you are well aware of the schooling required for you to be eligible to take the NCLEX–Practical Nurse (NCLEX-PN) examination. You likely received your practical nurse education in a hospital, high school, vocational or technical school, or junior or community college. Although the programs have variations, the minimum standard for each program is set by the individual state nursing board, whose goal is to produce graduates with a common base of knowledge and experience that will prepare them to practice as safe and competent beginners.

Only one registered nurse designation exists, and all entry-level registered nurses take the same national examination to achieve RN licensure. In order to gain eligibility to take the NCLEX–Registered Nurse (NCLEX-RN) examination, you may follow any of a variety of educational pathways.

Even though it can be expected that all RNs have a common minimum competency upon exit from a basic program and successful completion of the NCLEX-RN, it is important to understand the differences in the levels of educational preparation. Diploma, associate's degree, and bachelor's degree programs in nursing are designed to provide the education and clinical experience necessary for entry into the profession. Much debate exists about whether diploma and associate's degree nurses are technical nurses and whether professional nursing education isn't actually completed until the bachelor's degree as minimum educational preparation for entry into the profession. Some nursing leaders believe that we should strive for differentiation of practice between the various levels of educational preparation.

In fact, multiple studies over many years found that the higher percentage of bachelor of science in nursing (BSN)-prepared RNs a hospital hired, the lower their mortality rates were in the same time periods. Much of this evidence led to the recommendation by the Institute of Medicine (IOM) that in order to address the highly complex needs of today's patients, 80 percent of the nation's RNs should hold a minimum of a bachelor's degree by 2020 (RWJF, 2014). You may at this time be enrolled in an LPN/LVN to ADN program and that is an EXCELLENT and crucial step, but keep in mind that the BSN is generally preferred as the entry level degree to RN practice, and you may want to immediately make plans to enter an RN to BSN or even RN to MSN program. Your institution may even pay for the tuition and fees as an incentive to keep going!

Some nursing programs allow a layperson to achieve a generic (first-degree) master's degree or a nursing doctorate (ND) before ever taking the NCLEX-RN examination. Advanced practice nurses are educated as clinical nurse specialists (CNS), clinical nurse leaders (CNL), nurse practitioners (NP), or doctors of nursing practice (DNP), or they can have various other master's degrees and doctorates in nursing (Black, 2014). Upon graduation from a nursing program, some states permit new graduates to use the credential designated by the law of your state, such as graduate nurse (GN) or RN applicant (RNA). These are temporary designations that you may use until licensure or, in some cases, until you attempt the examination, whether or not you pass.

Diploma in Nursing

The **diploma in nursing** program is the earliest form of nursing education. Its history is rich and long, with diploma schools prevalent by 1900 (Black, 2014). Such a school is associated with a hospital and, in most cases, the school concentrates on the clinical portion of the program within that hospital. Diploma programs vary in length from 2 to 3 years.

These nursing programs often provide a high ratio of clinical hours to class hours, with the number of nursing credits usually exceeding the general education or liberal arts credits. Diploma schools thus provide a strong clinical-based education, which may translate into shorter orientation times in the work setting. Additionally, diploma graduates often have an acute care background that helps them fill the needs of the hospital associated with the school. Even though diploma graduates may be well prepared to manage the care of their patients, they may not be as well prepared to manage or lead other nurses or peers.

Associate's Degree in Nursing

The first associate's degree program was begun in 1952, and since its inception, the **associate's degree in nursing** program is the most common type of basic nursing education in the United States (Black, 2014). These programs are often seated within community colleges and are usually 2 years in length. The associate's degree nurse is well prepared to give comprehensive bedside patient care in the acute and long-term care settings. The associate's degree nurse is not as well prepared to take on leadership responsibilities or to practice in the school or community health nursing environment. Often the lack of courses in critical care, community health nursing, and leadership, along with a host of general education requirements, separates the associate's degree nurse from the baccalaureate-prepared nurse.

The Associate's Degree in Applied Science (AAS) prepares the nursing student for employment immediately upon graduation. For those planning to transfer to a 4-year program, the Associate of Science (AS) allows students more flexibility in course selection in order to focus on the discipline's requirements.

Baccalaureate Degree in Nursing

The first nursing program on a university campus, and the first program leading to a **baccalaureate** (bachelor's) **degree in nursing,** began in 1919 at the University of Minnesota (University of Minnesota, 2008). Bachelor's degree programs, based in colleges and universities, provide approximately 4 years of study. Typically, a bachelor's degree program requires approximately 120 credit hours, with about half dedicated to nursing courses. The remaining courses are in liberal arts and sciences.

A major difference between baccalaureate and diploma or associate's degree nursing education is the inclusion of leadership courses. The baccalaureate nurse often still requires as much, or perhaps slightly more, time to become comfortable with the technical skills of the patient care area but often acclimates quickly to leadership responsibilities. In order to advance into leadership and other roles with a certain amount of autonomy, a nurse will need to earn a baccalaureate degree. If you prefer to progress to an even more specialized and autonomous role, you will find that a master's degree in nursing is required.

Master's Degree in Nursing

Master's degree in nursing programs are highly specific and prepare students for advanced (very specialized and autonomous) nursing practice in a variety of settings. Registered nurses with master's degrees are found in such fields as higher education, staff development, and administration, as well as such careers as clinical nurse specialist, nurse anesthetist, nurse practitioner, and nurse midwife. The length of a master's program ranges from 1 to 2 or more years beyond the baccalaureate degree for entry into the program, depending on the degree or certifications awarded. Options also exist for the accelerated master's degree by combining 2 years of graduate study with 1 year of an accelerated BSN program.

Doctoral Degrees in Nursing

Doctoral degree programs prepare nurses to become the researchers, teachers, and clinicians who perpetuate and improve the art and science of nursing as a highly specialized profession. Doctoral programs often require at least 2 years of study beyond the master's degree level, a comprehensive examination, and a doctoral dissertation or scholarly project, for a total program length of usually 4 to 7 years. The dissertation is a very rigorous process whereby the student engages in original research, guided by an advisory committee of accomplished faculty members. The research is supported through extensive literature review and presented in the form of a paper and oral defense, often hundreds of pages in length.

The most common doctoral degree was the Doctor of Philosophy (PhD) until 2004, when the American Association of Colleges of Nursing (AACN) announced the intent to move the educational requirements for advanced practice nurse from the master's level to the doctoral level (doctor of nursing practice [DNP]) by 2015. The PhD-prepared nurse generally focuses on research, while the DNP-prepared nurse focuses more on clinical practice (Loomis, Willard, & Cohen, 2007). The AACN considers the DNP to be the entry level into advanced practice registered nursing.

Accreditation

The **Accreditation Commission for Education in Nursing (ACEN)** provides accreditation for both postsecondary and higher degree and certificate programs in nursing. Until 1996, the ACEN was the only official national accrediting organization for master's, bachelor's, and associate's degrees; the nursing diploma; and practical nursing programs (Black, 2014).

The **Commission on Collegiate Nursing Education (CCNE),** organized by the **American Association of Colleges of Nursing (AACN)** in 1996, accredits baccalaureate and higher degree nursing education programs. The accreditation process is intended to demonstrate to the public that a nursing program meets national standards, requirements, and criteria. Accreditation is voluntary. It is important for you to be aware of the accreditation status of a nursing program because some schools will not accept credits obtained from a nonaccredited school of nursing (AACN, 2008).

National accreditation of an educational program is different from state approval of a nursing program. Schools of nursing must have state approval to operate, and the minimum requirements for a nursing educational program are usually found in the state's nurse practice act (Black, 2014).

Specialty Nursing Certification

Specialty certification refers to a high level of knowledge and proficiency by the nurse in specific practice areas. The ANCC offers 46 different certification programs for registered nurses educated at the associate's degree, baccalaureate, or master's levels (Black, 2014).

The **American Nurses Credentialing Center (ANCC),** a subunit of the ANA, is the largest nurse credentialing organization in the United States, and more than 200,000 nurses have been certified since 1990. According to the ANCC, certification validates individual nursing knowledge, builds confidence, increases earning potential, provides career opportunities, and is the best measure of your ability to practice (ANCC, 2010). The ANCC provides opportunities for certification in many nursing specialties. For example, the RN may become certified in medical–surgical, gerontology, pediatric, nursing case management, and psychiatric–mental health. The level of certification depends on the educational preparation of the nurse.

In order to become certified in a nursing specialty, the RN must take a comprehensive examination in that area. In addition, the RN must provide evidence of experience, letters of reference, and other documentation (Black, 2014). More information can be found online at http://www.nursecredentialing.org/Certification.aspx. Additionally, many nursing organizations, such as the Association of Critical Care Nurses, the Emergency Nurses Association, and the American Association of Nurse Anesthetists, offer specialty certification opportunities.

Professional Nursing Organizations

The American Nurses Association represents the nation's 3.6 million registered nurses and advances the profession of nursing by fostering high standards of nursing practice, promoting the rights of nurses in the workplace, projecting a positive and realistic view of nursing, and participating in lobbying efforts on health care issues that affect nurses and the public. Professional nursing organizations serve a vital role in the advancement of the nursing profession (ANA, 2017).

Additionally, many organizations are dedicated to specialty practice such as the Association of Operating Room Nurses, American Psychiatric Nurses Association, American Association of Critical Care Nurses, Association of Rehabilitation Nurses, and numerous others. Belonging to one or many professional organizations provides education, socialization, networking, and collaboration opportunities in nursing.

SCOPE OF PRACTICE

A **scope of practice** is the term used to identify the responsibilities of nurses, depending on their educational preparation and licensure. A nurse's scope of practice is defined by individual **state nurse practice acts,** which are part of the law or code governing that state; however, similarities exist among states. The individual state boards of nursing, which are located within varying government organizations at the state level, commonly exist to protect the consumers of nursing care by regulating the profession. The **National Council of State Boards of Nursing (NCSBN)** is the unifying body for the state boards of nursing.

These lines become blurred, however, in many practice settings, most commonly in long-term care and skilled nursing units. LPN/LVNs are commonly substituted for RNs and perform tasks such as administering IV medications, inserting nasogastric (NG) tubes, pronouncing death, and ventilator care. This is problematic for the RN who is legally responsible and bound by a Code of Ethics, just as the LPN/LVN is accountable for nursing care delegated to unlicensed assistive personnel.

The American Nurses Association's publication *Nursing: Scope and Standards of Practice* (2015) addresses the scope of practice and delineates the practice and professional performance standards and measurement criteria for registered nurses. This publication contains 17 national standards. The six **standards of professional nursing practice** (which make up the nursing process) are assessment, diagnosis, outcomes identification, planning, implementation, and evaluation (ANA). The 11 **standards of professional performance** are ethics, culturally congruent practice, communication, collaboration, leadership, education, evidence-based practice and research, quality of practice, professional practice evaluation, resource utilization, and environmental health. Your performance as a registered nurse will be measured by these standards, and you are encouraged to review them carefully. Standards of practice are also available from the ANA for various nursing specialties and advanced nursing practice. Along with the *Scope and Standards of Practice* (2015), there are two other must-have ANA resources for you to consider adding to your library. They are *Nursing's Social Policy Statement: Understanding the Profession from Social Contract to Social Covenant* (2015) and *Code of Ethics for Nurses with Interpretive Statements* (2015). In fact, not only should you add

---

? EXERCISE 4.1

SCOPE OF PRACTICE AS LPN/LVN	SCOPE OF PRACTICE AS RN

---

them to your permanent library but also read them cover to cover as they represent who we are and what we do, foundationally, as a profession. You will learn in greater depth about both the Social Policy Statement and the Code of Ethics in coming chapters.

Multistate licensure presents another challenge to the practicing RN. Multistate licensure allows nurses in compact states to work in other compact states without obtaining a license in that state. The Nurse Licensure Compact, developed by the National Council of State Boards (NCSBN) and adopted in 1998, facilitates practice across state lines and helps states protect the public's health and safety by ensuring competent nursing care. The nurse licensed in one compact state and practicing in another must adhere to the laws of that compact state, and this requires that the nurse stay abreast of any changes to multistate licensure. More information on multistate licensure can be found by visiting the NCSBN's website or the website of your state board of nursing. Complete Exercise 4.1 to gain further clarity on the difference in scope of practice from LPN/LVN to RN.

Licensed Practical Nursing

According to the American Nurses Association (ANA, 1989), the practice of practical nursing is considered "directed," in that an LPN/LVN functions under the direction of an RN, physician, or other health care provider. Practical nurses are prepared to provide care in settings where patients are experiencing common health problems, and they focus on meeting basic needs. The LPN/LVN is considered the technical nurse (Black, 2014). The LPN/LVN performs basic assessment, or data collection, but does not perform the level of assessment that requires the use of critical thinking and the nursing process.

Registered Nursing

The definition of nursing has evolved over time. Florence Nightingale believed the role of nursing is to put the patient in the best condition possible for healing to take place. In 1955, Virginia Henderson stated:

> *The unique function of the nurse is to assist the individual, sick or well, in the performance of those activities contributing to health or its recovery (or to peaceful death) that he would perform unaided if he had the necessary strength, will, or knowledge and to do this in such a way as to help him gain independence as rapidly as possible.* (p. 7)

In 2015, the ANA defined *nursing* as:

> *The protection, promotion, and optimization of health and abilities; prevention of illness and injury; alleviation of suffering through the diagnosis and treatment of human response; and advocacy in the care of individuals, families, communities, and populations.* (p. 1)

The National League for Nursing has delineated three primary roles of the associate's degree nurse (ADN), which are provider of care, manager of care, and member of the profession. The RN follows the nursing process in all three roles.

Provider of Care

As provider of care, the ADN RN provides competent nursing care to individuals, groups, families, and communities and assists others to achieve or maintain wellness. The RN is critical thinker, teacher, collaborator, and patient advocate and is culturally sensitive to patients and other members of the health care team.

Manager of Care

The ADN RN, as manager of care, prioritizes and manages patient care, is delegator and decision maker, practices legally and ethically, and ensures the provision of treatment interventions by all members of the health care team. Patient **advocacy** and collaboration are also functions of the RN as manager of care. As manager of care, the RN leads others through role modeling and feedback.

Member of the Profession

As a member of the profession, the professional RN assumes individual accountability and responsibility and embraces lifelong learning, is concerned with issues related to quality of care, is responsive to change, collaborates with other health care professionals, and recognizes the holistic nature of persons. The professional RN participates in professional nursing organizations and participates in research and activities that benefit the global community.

Registered nursing practice requires specialized education and experience. The development of improvements in professional practice relies on nursing theory and research. Depending on competency, the RN's authority to perform specific nursing functions is unrestricted.

In the early 1990s, a steering committee of the ANA focused on what nursing should look like in 2010. The committee developed Nursing's Agenda for the Future, which was published in 2002. The committee identified ten domains, or areas of concern, that demanded action: leadership and planning, delivery systems, legislation/regulation/policy, professional/nursing culture, recruitment/retention, economic value, work environment, public relations/communication, education, and diversity. This work was expanded by the ANA working with the Institute of Medicine (IOM) and the Robert Wood Johnson Foundation. In the report of that work, *The Future of Nursing: Leading Change, Advancing Health* (IOM, 2010), four key elements came into focus:

- Nurses should practice to the full extent of their education and training.
- Nurses should achieve higher levels of education and training through an improved education system that promotes seamless academic progression.
- Nurses should be full partners, with physicians and other health care professionals, in redesigning health care in the United States.
- Effective workforce planning and policy making require better data collection and information infrastructure.

As a registered nurse, it is imperative that you are clear on the expectations for members of the profession and find your unique role in helping to sustain it.

Within the RN's roles of provider of care, manager of care, and member of the profession, the RN is also advocate, policy maker, critical thinker, teacher, communicator, leader, and researcher. Nursing is affected by many internal and external factors. For instance, the advancement of technology, the aging population, nursing and nursing faculty shortages, governmental regulations, methods of health care delivery, and globalization will affect the way nursing is practiced in the future. In order to take on the role of critical thinker, it is the RN's responsibility to become a lifelong learner so as to stay fully informed and abreast of changes in health care.

KEY POINTS

This chapter focused on differentiating the role of the LPN/LVN from the role of the RN. There are a number of distinguishing characteristics important to discern as you progress from one role to the other.

- The transition from LPN/LVN to RN is a multifaceted process.
- The RN role is composed of several elements, many of which are already familiar to you.
- The significant differences are encompassed in the expanded scope of practice and include educational preparation, critical thinking skills, assessment skills, care planning, legal responsibilities, communication, and teaching skills.
- The educational preparation and licensure of the roles are similar in process yet different in content and practice. The LPN/LVN has attended school for approximately 1 year, including both nursing classes and clinical, usually culminating in a certificate and in rare cases a degree.
- The RN attends school from 2 to 4 years, composed of nursing classes with extensive clinical practice and liberal arts and sciences.
- The LPN serves the client in a limited role at the direction of an RN or other authorized health care provider.
- The RN serves the client in both autonomous and collaborative roles, participates in the plan of care, possesses advanced assessment skills, utilizes critical thinking, and is aware of his or her legal and professional responsibilities.
- The professional RN will have many roles, including provider of care, manager of care, and member of the profession.

CRITICAL THINKING QUESTIONS

1. Make a list of what you consider to be your LPN/LVN role attributes. How do you think these will change as you move toward becoming an RN?
2. Choose an RN with whom you have worked as an LPN/LVN and compare and contrast each of your responsibilities in patient care. Underline RN role responsibilities that you believe will be the most difficult to learn.
3. Have you experienced any other times in your life when you had a role change? Explain. Describe the emotions you felt during the process.
4. Which people in your life will be your best support systems during this process? Why? Who will be least supportive? Why? How can you best use this information to ease your role transition from LPN/LVN to RN?

5. In your new role as an RN, you will be working with other RNs who may have obtained their licenses through a different educational path than you. One often misunderstands or even belittles a different educational pathway. What measures can you use to understand the strengths of the nurses with whom you work?

6. You are the RN caring for an elderly female who has suffered a hip fracture. The charge nurse RN has been called to the room of another patient in respiratory distress. You discover that the PICC line in your patient has become dislodged. The woman's daughter, who is visiting and is also an RN, insists that you remove the PICC line immediately and insert an IV line. Suddenly a code is called. The LPN/LVN in the room with you tells you that she has experience with both procedures. What would you do and why?

7. Locate your state nurse practice act and read the educational requirements and the scope of practice for the LPN/LVN and the RN. Then, in the left column of Exercise 4.1, write your understanding of your scope of practice as an LPN/LVN. In the right column, relate your understanding of your future scope of practice as an RN.

WEB RESOURCES

http://ncbi.nlm.nih.gov/pubmed/2381479
http://stti.confex.com/stti/bcscience38/techprogram/paper_25393.htm
American Nurses Association, http://nursingworld.org
American Nurses Credentialing Center, http://nursecredentialing.org
The Joint Commission, http://jointcommission.org
National Council of State Boards of Nursing, http://www.ncsbn.org/index.htm
National League for Nursing, http://www.nln.org/index.cfm
Online Journal of Issues in Nursing, http://nursingworld.org/MainMenuCategories/ANAMarketplace/ANAPeriodicals/OJIN.aspx
U.S. Department of Labor, http://bls.gov/ooh/Healthcare/Registered-nurses.htm
Resources for Cross-Cultural Health Care, http://diversityrx.org
Delegation Decision Tree http://pr.mo.gov/boards/nursing/delegationtree.pdf

REFERENCES

Alfaro-LeFevre, R. (1999). *Critical thinking in nursing: a practical approach* (2nd ed.). Philadelphia, PA: Saunders.

American Association of Colleges of Nursing [AACN]. (2008). *Accreditation*. Retrieved from http://www.aacn.nche.edu.

American Nurses Association [ANA]. (1989). *Nursing*. Retrieved from http://NursingWorld.org.

American Nurses Association [ANA]. (2002). *Nursing's agenda for the future*. Retrieved from http://www.NursingWorld.org.

American Nurses Association [ANA]. (2017). *About ANA*. Retrieved from http://www.nursingworld.org/FunctionalMenuCategories/AboutANA.

American Nurses Association [ANA]. (2015). *Nursing: scope and standards of practice* (3rd ed.). Silver Springs, MD: Nursebooks.org.

American Nurses Credentialing Center [ANCC]. (2010). http://ancc.nursecredentialing.org/PromotionalMaterials/products/WHYCERT10.pdf.

American Nurses Credentialing Center [ANCC]. (2017). *ANCC Certification Center*. Retrieved from http://www.nursecredentialing.org/Certification.aspx.

Black, B. (2014). *Professional nursing: concepts and challenges* (7th ed.). St. Louis, MO: Saunders.

Critical Thinking.org (2015). *Critical thinking and nursing.* Retrieved from http://www.critical thinking.org/pages/critical-thinking-and-nursing/834.

Dickerson, P. (2009). *Direction and delegation: maximizing human resources.* Retrieved from http://healthcaretodayonline.com/HCTclassroom/1009coursematerial.pdf.

Hill, S., & Howlett, H. (2001). *Success in practical nursing: personal and vocational issues* (4th ed.). Philadelphia, PA: Saunders.

Institute of Medicine. (2010). *The future of nursing: leading change, advancing health.* Retrieved from http://iom.edu/Reports/2010/The-Future-of-Nursing-Leading-Change -Advancing-Health.aspx/.

Loomis, J. A., Willard, B., & Cohen, J. (2007). Difficult professional choices: deciding between the PhD and the DNP in nursing [Electronic version]. *Online Journal of Issues in Nursing, 12*(1). Retrieved from http://nursingworld.org.

Melrose, D., Miller, J., Gordon, K., & Janzen, K. (2012). Becoming socialized into a new professional role: LPN to BN student nurses' experiences with legitimation. *Nursing Research and Practice.* http://dx.doi.org/10.1155/2012/946063.

Paul, R. (1992). *Critical thinking: what every person needs to survive in a rapidly changing world* (2nd ed.). Santa Rosa, CA: Foundation for Critical Thinking.

RWJF. (2014). *Building the case for more highly educated nurses.* Retrieved from http://www .rwjf.org/en/library/articles-and-news/2014/04/building-the-case-for-more-highly-edu-cated-nurses.html.

Schumacher, K., & Meleis, A. (1994). Transitions: a central concept in nursing. *Image, 26*(2), 119–127.

University of Minnesota, School of Nursing. (n.d.) *About us.* Retrieved from http://www .nursing.umn.edu/about/index.htm.

Zarshenas, L., Sharif, F., Molazen, Z., Khayyer, M., Zare, N., & Ebadi, A. (2014). Professional socialization in nursing: a qualitative content analysis. *Iran Journal Nurse Midwifery Review, 19*(4), 432–438.

Zerwekh, J., & Garneau, A. (2012). *Nursing today: transition and trends* (7th ed.). St. Louis, MO: Elsevier Saunders.

chapter 5

Using Nursing Theory to Guide Professional Practice

⊜volve WEBSITE

Additional resources are available online at:
http://*evolve.elsevier.com/Claywell/transitions*

OBJECTIVES

After completing this chapter, the student will be prepared to:

1. Compare and contrast nursing philosophies, nursing theories, and nursing theoretical models.
2. Discuss the role of nursing theory to the practice of nursing.
3. Evaluate how values and beliefs influence nursing theory.
4. Apply the four universal concepts central to nursing practice.
5. Compare and contrast the nursing philosophies, theories, and models discussed in this chapter.
6. Articulate a personal philosophy of nursing based on personal beliefs and values.
7. Examine level of skill acquisition in past, current, and/or future roles in nursing.

KEY TERMS

adaptation theory	King, Imogene M.	Orlando, Ida Jean
Benner, Patricia	Leininger, Madeleine	**paradigm**
concepts	Levine, Myra E.	Pender, Nola J.
conceptual models	Neuman, Betty	Peplau, Hildegard E.
construct	Newman, Margaret A.	philosophy
deductive reasoning	Nightingale, Florence	role theory
developmental theories	nursing models	Roy, Sister Callista
Henderson, Virginia	nursing philosophies	systems theory
inductive reasoning	nursing theories	theory
Johnson, Dorothy E.	Orem, Dorothea E.	Watson, Jean

OVERVIEW

Many students enter their first theory class with the predetermined idea that nursing theory is only for faculty members and researchers and that everyday nurses do not need to know about it. However, nursing theory is the foundation on which practice as a registered nurse is based. It is also the source from which new knowledge is generated, expanding and defining best practices and thereby improving outcomes for patients. Every nurse must engage in evidence-based practice—that is, practice guided by diverse theories that help the nurse interpret the evidence and direct his or her decision making. Theoretical works provide a systematic approach to professional practice that is focused on the patient (Alligood & Tomey, 2010).

Numerous philosophies, models, and theories have built the foundation and expanded the knowledge unique to the profession. Most have in common four universal concepts central to nursing practice: person, health, environment, and nursing. These themes are described, defined, ordered, and interrelated in distinctive, meaningful, and powerful ways as nursing theorists endeavor to continue the development of nursing's unique body of knowledge.

BACKGROUND

In the 1850s, **Florence Nightingale** envisioned nurses as educated women during a time in history when women were neither educated nor employed in public service. She adamantly believed that nursing knowledge was distinct from medical knowledge. It was not until the 1950s that serious discussions began about the need for the development of nursing theories (Alligood & Tomey, 2014). Four general types of theoretical works discussed in this chapter are philosophies, conceptual models and grand theories, theories, and middle-range theories.

A **philosophy** is a cohesive explanation in an attempt to identify overarching assumptions and beliefs about humans, our world, and the nursing discipline. In other words, a philosophy is a school of thought or study that seeks to clarify an approach in nursing, a worldview and generally more broadly understood, though to date, there is no singular, universally accepted nursing philosophy; indeed, there are many (McEwen & Wills, 2014). *Philosophies* are expressions of personal thoughts, beliefs, and values. Nursing philosophies express beliefs about nursing and nursing-related values (Black, 2014).

A philosophy may also be defined as a broad, global explanation of a phenomenon of interest that contributes to nursing knowledge by giving direction to the profession and providing a basis for theoretical understanding (Alligood & Tomey, 2014). For example, professional nursing values include caring, integrity, a nonjudgmental attitude, listening, accountability, empathy, knowledge, teamwork, and patient advocacy. Nursing philosophies serve as guides for professional practice and influence professional behaviors (Black, 2014). Nursing philosophies include the works of Nightingale, Henderson, Watson, and Benner.

Theory, on the other hand, is developed within specific contexts, seeking to explain a phenomenon, using concepts and definitions making it possible to systematically collect data, determine goals and predict outcomes, and identify standards, processes and parameters for nursing intervention and evaluation of care. They address particular situations, people, and things in objective and often scientific ways that may be verified empirically, often tested quantitatively (McEwen & Wills, 2014). The theories you will see in this text were chosen from dozens that support nursing practice. The theorists include Peplau, Orlando, Pender, Leininger, and Newman.

Theories are an integrated set of concepts and statements that can be used to explain, describe, predict, or control a phenomenon. Theories may be developed using inductive or deductive reasoning, and both are valid forms of logic. **Deductive reasoning** proceeds from the general to the specific. Here the reasoning progresses such that you would use true broad premises or principles to logically progress to a more detailed conclusion. It requires that the initial generalizations be correct. An example of deductive reasoning would be:

1. All members of Class A are purple.
2. Mary is a member of Class A.
3. Therefore, Mary is purple.

With induction, reasoning proceeds from the specific to the general. That is, an observation is made, patterns are recognized, which leads to a tentative hypothesis, and then finally a general conclusion about a broad theory or generalization. An example of **inductive reasoning** would be:

1. Twenty males between the ages of 19 and 35 had symptoms of posttraumatic stress disorder (PTSD) after returning from war.
2. Therefore, all males between the ages of 19 and 35 returning from war will have symptoms of PTSD.

Middle-range nursing theories focus on answering specific nursing practice questions. They can describe phenomena, explain relationships, and predict the effects of one phenomenon on another. To be useful in practice, theories should be clear, simple, generalizable, important, and accessible (Alligood & Tomey, 2014). Nursing research is the vehicle by which nursing theories are tested.

Concepts are the building blocks of nursing theory, which are initiated based on a personal philosophy or belief about nursing and may be abstract or concrete. They allow the theorist to describe and classify a phenomenon of interest. A concept can be thought of as an idea and must be clearly defined to reduce misunderstanding (Alligood & Tomey, 2014). The term **construct** is often used interchangeably with *concept*, but a construct is generally thought of as being more abstract.

Conceptual Models are representations (composed of concepts) depicting phenomena occurring in reality presenting from specific viewpoints and perspectives that strive to help users to understand or grasp the phenomenon or system in a concrete manner whether directly or only indirectly observable (McEwen & Wills, 2014). Models can be one-dimensional or multi-dimensional and often involve input, output, directionality, and boundaries. The models you will see in this chapter were created by Johnson, King, Levine, Neuman, Orem, and Rogers.

THEORIES IN SUPPORT OF NURSING

Nursing theory, as you have seen, is built upon several important adapted scientific theories.

Developmental, or Physiological, Theories

Developmental theories teach nurses that all systems in the human body are interdependent. Many such theories help us understand the hows and whys of health and illness. For example, Maslow's Theory of the Hierarchy of Needs states that humans have certain basic needs, such as basic physiological needs (air, food, shelter, water, sexual expression, safety, and love and belonging) that must be met before we can focus on more advanced, abstract needs, such as self-esteem or self-actualization (Black, 2014). As nurses, we prioritize our care based on the basics needed to sustain life before we move on to other considerations. Multiple levels of needs may occur simultaneously, but a good rule to remember is that if the patient is unable to breathe, restoring that basic need takes priority over concerns about self-esteem.

Another developmental theory is Erikson's Theory of Psychosocial Development, which says that the six stages of psychosocial development are influenced by biological, social, and environmental factors. The stages range from infancy, which Erikson labeled the stage of *trust versus mistrust,* through the lifes pan to elder adulthood, labeled *ego integrity versus despair* (Erikson, 1980). According to this theory, humans, based on several influencing factors, experience either the positive or the negative aspect of each developmental stage, and we as nurses must adapt our care to the specific age and developmental stage in order to promote the person's positive development and overall health.

Systems Theory

Systems theory, principally developed by Ludwig von Bertalanffy in the 1920s, defines the interdependence of environments in and around us. What this means for nursing is that we must understand that all parts of a system are connected, that a change in one part will have an effect on another. For instance, a person with low blood pressure will have multiorgan involvement. Similarly, if one person in a family is ill, then all members of that family will react to that illness. Systems theory can also be applied to organizations, groups, and professions.

Systems theory has identified the following fundamental concepts and characteristics of systems:
- All living organisms are systems.
- Interrelated parts act together toward the purpose of the whole.
- Because the parts are connected, a change in one component will necessarily ripple to other components, much like the effect of a pebble dropped into a pond.
- Systems have boundaries.
- Systems are both affected by and have an effect on the environment, both internally and externally.
- Systems self-correct based on reactions (CurrentNursing.com, 2012).

Role Theory

Role theory helps you, as a nurse, function therapeutically in interactions and helps you understand behaviors in your patients, their families, and yourself. A role defines the expected behaviors of people in the particular role.

Roles change over a lifetime, and at any one time a person may occupy several roles. This theory can be applied to you at this very moment. As you move from the role of practical nurse into that of registered nurse, you will experience role transition and possibly role confusion as you expand your nursing practice.

Adaptation Theory

Adaptation theory helps the nurse understand the ability of living things to adjust (or adapt) in response to continuous internal and external stimuli (Alligood & Tomey, 2010). In studying adaptation theory, you can begin to understand how and why humans cope (or do not cope) with physical, developmental, emotional, intellectual, social, and spiritual stressors.

NURSING PHILOSOPHIES

Discussing only a few **nursing philosophies, nursing theories,** and **nursing models** is difficult because they are in many cases interrelated, but for a beginning understanding, at least several major theorists and their works need to be briefly introduced.

Florence Nightingale: Philosophy of Nursing

Florence Nightingale, called "the Lady with the Lamp" for her ministrations to British soldiers during the Crimean War, determined in the 1850s that nursing knowledge differed from medical knowledge and that nursing duties should not include errands and chores, as was prevalent at the time, but rather focus on the personal care of the patient (Alligood & Tomey, 2014).

Nightingale described the nurse's function as one that puts the patient in the best condition for nature (God) to act upon him or her. Her theory of nursing focused on the environment and described in detail the concepts of light, cleanliness, ventilation, warmth, diet, and noise (Nightingale, 1860). These concepts have provided the foundation for nursing practice and current nursing theories (Alligood & Tomey, 2010).

Nightingale's theory focused on three major relationships: environment to patient, nurse to environment, and nurse to patient (Alligood & Tomey, 2014). Nightingale believed that nurses manipulate the environment every day to enhance patient recovery (Nightingale, 1860). She also believed that good education was necessary for good practice and that nursing was a respected occupation that required advanced education (Alligood & Tomey, 2014).

> ≫ **APPLICATION TO PRACTICE 5.1**
>
> The nurse caring for the patient in the ICU will ensure that noise is minimal in order to facilitate healing and recovery.
>
> The home health nurse will ensure a safe and clean environment for the patient recovering from surgery.

Virginia Henderson: Definition of Nursing

Virginia Henderson is well known for the definition of *nursing,* which states that nursing's primary responsibility is "to assist the individual, sick or well, in the perfor-mance of those activities contributing to health or its recovery (or to a peaceful death) that he would perform unaided if he had the necessary strength, will, or knowledge and to do this in such a way as to help him gain independence as rapidly as possible" (Henderson, 1966, p. 7).

Henderson is further credited with integrating the view of holism into nursing. She believed that humans have needs that are not only biological but also psychologi-cal, sociocultural, and spiritual. In her 1966 work *The Nature of Nursing: A Definition and Its Implications for Practice, Research, and Education,* Henderson described 14 needs and inherent rights of the individual, which have served as an early yet endur-ing guide for nursing practice. These 14 fundamental needs are breathing, eating and drinking, eliminating, moving, sleeping and resting, selecting clothing and dressing, regulating body temperature, maintaining adequate hygiene, remaining free from harm and avoiding harming others, communicating, learning and seeking general fulfillment, worshiping, working, and playing (Henderson, 1966). These 14 needs can be broadly categorized into a holistic view of persons in terms of physical, psycho-logical, emotional, sociological, spiritual, or developmental needs (Black, 2014).

> ### ⟫ APPLICATION TO PRACTICE 5.2
>
> The nurse working in the long-term care setting will work independently and with the interdisciplinary team to ensure that an individual's 14 fundamental needs are met.
>   The nurse working in a rehabilitation facility will act independently and holistically to perform tasks that the patient is unable to do for himself or herself.

Jean Watson: Philosophy of Science and Caring

Jean Watson's Theory of Caring first originated in 1979 (Watson, 1997). It emerged from her own values and beliefs and was guided by her commitment to the caring-healing role of nursing and its mission to help sustain humanity and wholeness as the foundation of health and nursing's purpose for existence. She was influenced by the works of nursing theorists, nurse scholars, psychologists, and philosophers.

Watson states that her original work was organized around ten "carative" factors that attempted to honor the human dimensions of nursing's work and the subjective experiences of the people nurses serve (Watson, 1997). These ten carative factors are values, faith and hope, compassion for self and others, trusting, rapport, encouraging and accepting emotional expression, analytical decision making, collaborative teach-ing and learning, supportive environment, and meeting needs (Alligood & Tomey, 2014). Watson's work has evolved, but it "continues to make explicit that humans can-not be treated as objects, that humans cannot be separated from self, other, nature, and the larger universe" (Watson, 1997, p. 50). Watson believes that if an individual works from a caring-healing paradigm, then it must be lived out in daily life through a commitment to self-care.

Her theory continues to evolve and is widely accepted by the nursing community. In 1986, the University of Colorado's School of Nursing founded the Center for Human Caring, the first of its kind (Watson, 1997). You can obtain more information on the Center from http://hschealth.uchsc.edu/son/faculty/caring.htm.

> ## ▶ APPLICATION TO PRACTICE 5.3
>
> The nurse working in the psychiatric mental health setting will focus on creating a nonjudgmental, trusting relationship while meeting psychological, social, and physiological needs.
>
> The nurse working on the medical floor will assess the patient's spiritual beliefs and strengths and perceptions in order to determine the patient's ability to cope with illness.

Patricia Benner: From Novice to Expert

Patricia Benner's philosophy focuses on clinical nursing practice and her belief that nursing knowledge accrues over time (Benner, 2001). Her theory is heavily influenced by the work of Hubert and Stuart Dreyfus, who developed the Dreyfus Model of Skill Acquisition.

Her model describes five levels of skill acquisition: novice, advanced beginner, competent, proficient, and expert. The novice nurse, or level 1, applies to the student nurse or a skilled nurse being placed in an unfamiliar area. The advanced beginner (level 2) is considered the new graduate nurse who demonstrates marginally acceptable performance and relies on more experienced nurses. The nurse functioning at the competent level, level 3, can multitask, plan, and set goals and has the ability to think abstractly and analytically. The proficient nurse (level 4) is able to see the whole (rather than the parts) of a situation, recognizes subtle changes, and focuses on long-term goals. The expert nurse, the final level, has the ability to recognize patterns and responses that are automatic and integrated. The nurse reaches this level only after extensive experience (Benner, 2001). Complete Exercise 5.1, at the end of this chapter, to assess your level of skill acquisition in both your current role and your new role as an RN.

> ## ? EXERCISE 5.1
>
> Using the Novice to Expert Philosophy assess your level of skill acquisition as an LPN/LVN and explain how you've come to believe you have attained that level. Then looking forward to your future role as an RN describe the level at which you believe you will enter your new role and how long you believe it will take you before you attain the next levels. What milestones do you expect to achieve and by when? What evidence will support your attainment of each level?

> ## ▶ APPLICATION TO PRACTICE 5.4
>
> The manager of a medical–surgical unit assigns an expert nurse to precept a new graduate.
>
> The hospital facility establishes a clinical nurse ladder for advancement using Benner's levels, which describe the specific behaviors required for proficiency at each level.

The essential concepts of Benner's model include "competence, skill acquisition, experience, clinical knowledge and practical knowledge" (McEwen & Wills, 2014, p. 232). It is through testing and refinement of formal and tacit knowledge in practice situations that expertise develops. Further, Benner identifies the following seven domains of nursing practice:

- Helping role
- Teaching or coaching function
- Diagnostic client monitoring function
- Effective management of rapidly changing situations
- Administering and monitoring therapeutic interventions and regimens
- Monitoring and ensuring quality of health care practices
- Organizational and work-role competencies (Benner, 2001 as cited in McEwen & Wills, 2014, p. 232)

NURSING THEORIES

Hildegard E. Peplau: Theory of Interpersonal Relations

Hildegard Peplau, known as the mother of psychiatric nursing, published her Theory of Interpersonal Relations in 1952 in her landmark book *Interpersonal Relations in Nursing.* Peplau's theory was grounded in practice and based on the belief that the goal of nursing should be directed toward reducing dependence and encouraging autonomy (Peplau, 1952). Her psychodynamic approach explored the meanings and functions of behaviors and experiences and that the concepts of nurse, patient, health, and environment are interconnected and should be viewed within the context of the environment. Peplau believed that the interpersonal relationship occurs in interlocking and overlapping phases known as *preorientation, orientation, working,* and *termination* (Forchuk, 1993). Understanding this relationship will provide the most holistic patient care, and both the nurse and patient will grow.

Peplau believed that the only way nursing was going to make strides toward becoming an independent profession was for nurses to engage in scientific research. She also believed that good education was necessary for good practice and that nursing was a respected occupation that required advanced education (Alligood & Tomey, 2010).

> ### ▶▶ APPLICATION TO PRACTICE 5.5
>
> The nurse working in the psychiatric mental health setting will utilize Peplau's theory to establish a therapeutic relationship, establish trust, and promote independence.
> The nurse working with the homeless patient will assess the behaviors and experiences that have meaning to the patient through therapeutic communication skills.

Ida Jean Orlando: Nursing Process Theory

Ida Jean Orlando's theory of effective nursing practice was first proposed in 1961 and later revised in 1990 as a nursing process theory. Orlando believed that the goal of the nurse is to meet the immediate needs of the patient and relieve distress or discomfort

(Black, 2014). A major assumption by Orlando was that nursing practice should be autonomous. Orlando believed that nurses must also explore the patient's thoughts, feelings, and perceptions and that assessment includes verbal and nonverbal behaviors. She believed that using the nursing process in the provision of nursing care provides an overall framework for nursing and is effective in achieving a good outcome (Alligood & Tomey, 2014).

>> **APPLICATION TO PRACTICE 5.6**

The nurse caring for the patient in the operating room must be able to accurately and rapidly assess the patient.

The nurse working on a medical floor will approach the patient in pain by observing verbal and nonverbal cues in order to determine the patient's needs.

Nola J. Pender: Health Promotion Model

Nola J. Pender developed the Health Promotion Model based on the belief that the patient assumes an active role in managing his or her own health. Her model focuses on wellness and clarifies the nurse's role in health promotion. Her model was first presented in 1982 in her book *Health Promotion in Nursing Practice,* later reviewed in 2002 (Alligood & Tomey, 2014).

Pender's Health Promotion Model for nursing practice focuses on ten determinants of health promoting behavior: prior related behavior, personal factors, perceived benefits to an action, perceived barriers to an action, perceived self-efficacy, activity-related effect, interpersonal influences, situational influences, commitment to a plan of action, and intermediate competing demands and preferences. Changes in health care have increasingly emphasized preventing disease and promoting health, and wellness promotion has become a major focus of nursing education (Alligood & Tomey, 2014).

>> **APPLICATION TO PRACTICE 5.7**

The nurse working in the wellness clinic will provide teaching to the patient who is obese.

The nurse caring for the patient with newly diagnosed type II diabetes will provide instruction on the importance of diet and exercise in managing diabetes.

Madeleine Leininger: Culture Care Theory of Diversity and Universality

Madeleine Leininger first began to study transcultural nursing in the mid 1950s when she was working as a clinical nurse specialist in psychiatric nursing. Leininger's Culture Care Theory of Diversity and Universality was derived from her studies of anthropology and nursing (Leininger, 1996). Leininger stated that the central goal of the theory is "to provide culturally congruent nursing care in order to improve or offer a different kind of nursing care service to people of diverse or similar cultures" (p. 72).

Leininger has distinguished the term *transcultural nursing* as a major area of nursing that focuses on the comparative study of diverse populations with respect to their own individual values and expressions, with very notable patterns of health-illness that are predictable (Alligood & Tomey, 2014). Leininger believed that the art of nursing must take into account a creative discovery about the cultural community as individuals, families, and groups and their expressive ability of caring, values, expressions, beliefs, actions, and practices that are based on their cultural lifestyles. In doing so, Leininger believes that nurses can deliver the appropriate level of care based on these aspects of individual cultures with a noted increase in nursing satisfaction performance, healing, and well-being (Alligood & Tomey, 2014).

Transcultural nursing not only involves being aware of different cultures, but it involves planning nursing care based on that knowledge (Black, 2014). Leininger (1996, p. 75) stated, "Nurses need to realize that humans are complex beings who want their holistic views of life, care, culture, and health to remain together and do not want to be viewed as fragmented organs or body parts." Given the changing demographics of our country, the registered nurse will find that the provision of health care services will no doubt entail delivery to a patient population who is diverse and may not speak English at all. It is crucial that the registered nurse be aware and knowledgeable in the concepts of cultural competence and integrate those concepts along with other chosen nursing theories appropriate to practice.

> ### ▶▶ APPLICATION TO PRACTICE 5.8
>
> The nurse working with the Hispanic population will be familiar with the particular cultural values and beliefs of this population.
>   The nurse caring for the Chinese patient will ensure that the patient is given a choice of culturally appropriate foods.

Margaret A. Newman: Theory of Health as Expanding Consciousness

Margaret Newman's theory, Health as Expanding Consciousness, focused on patterns, life processes, and wholeness (Black, 2014). Newman saw the life process as a progression toward higher levels of consciousness and health and believed that health and the evolving pattern of consciousness are the same. She described the environment as being the larger whole, of which the individual is unaware. The interactions that occur between the environment and the person are key processes, and both health and illness can be seen as the manifestation of the pattern of the person-environment (Alligood & Tomey, 2014).

Newman (1999) stated that nurses need to learn to listen to the rhythm of another person's interactive pattern, which may be irregular, difficult to sense, or chaotic at times, but that nurses need to "hang in there" with clients (patients) until a new rhythm emerges. Newman emphasized the importance of silence and listening in order to discern these patterns:

> *The nature of nursing is found in the nurse's relationship with the client, a relationship characterized by a rhythmic coming together and moving apart as clients encounter disruption of their organized, predictable state and moving through disorganization and unpredictability to a higher, organized state. (p. 228)*

Newman (1999) stated that if we want to get in touch with this pattern, we need to listen to the silence and to listen with our hearts.

>> **APPLICATION TO PRACTICE 5.9**

The nurse forms meaningful relationships and facilitates the patient's identification of inner strengths while caring for the patient with cancer.
   The nurse teaches the patient strategies for focusing on self-awareness and positive outcomes.

NURSING MODELS

Dorothy E. Johnson: Behavioral Systems Model

Dorothy E. Johnson's model, the Behavioral Systems Model, focuses on human behavior. She believes that a person (or system) is composed of seven interrelated behavioral components (subsystems) that function together to form a whole. These seven subsystems of the behavioral system are attachment, dependency, ingestive, eliminative, sexual, aggressive, and achievement behaviors; an eighth component, restorative behavior, was added later. Johnson's work was influenced by Nightingale, systems theory, and behavioral scientists (Alligood & Tomey, 2014). In Johnson's theory, the goal of nursing is to assess the internal and external environments and to assist the patient in selecting mutual goals and developing interventions (Black, 2014).

>> **APPLICATION TO PRACTICE 5.10**

The nursing researcher compares the coping abilities and perceptions of children raised in their own homes and those raised in foster homes.
   The nurse assists the patient in identifying maladaptive behaviors that are contributing to illness and disease.

Imogene M. King: Theory of Goal Attainment

Imogene M. King's Interacting Systems Framework and Theory of Goal Attainment, first published in 1981, included the characteristics of general systems theory, which are goals, structure, functions, resources, and decision making (King, 1994). It was based on her belief that humans are composed of three interacting systems (personal, interpersonal, and social) and that they can lead to goal attainment, representing outcomes (King, 1996). According to King (1996), human beings are the focus of nursing care, and the goal of the framework is health for individuals, families, communities, and the world. King states that the theory "provides a process for human interactions that lead to transactions and to goal attainment for individuals, families, and communities. The structure is human beings transacting with their environment" (p. 62). The goal of her theory is health for individuals, groups, and society (King, 1994).

King's theory has been used extensively in nursing research and practice. Some examples of the application of King's model to practice are the use of her theory to deliver quality nursing care in the changing health care environment, implementing managed care in a hospital setting, using the theory in ambulatory care in patients with cancer, restructuring case management, developing documentation systems, or designing a method of evaluating patient teaching.

> ## ⟫ APPLICATION TO PRACTICE 5.11
>
> The nurse plans goals and outcomes collaboratively with the patient after a careful assessment of personal, interpersonal, and social environments.
>
> The nurse providing group teaching will observe the personal, interpersonal, and social interactions among the participants.

MYRA E. LEVINE: CONSERVATION MODEL

The Conservation Model, theorized by **Myra E. Levine,** is based on three concepts: wholeness, adaptation, and conservation. Conservation is guided by four principles: conservation of energy, conservation of structural integrity, conservation of personal integrity, and conservation of social integrity. The ability of an individual to adapt to his or her environment depends on the individual's ability to manage the fight or flight response, the inflammatory response, response to stress, and perceptual awareness (Alligood & Tomey, 2014).

Levine believed that the health or well-being of the patient (wholeness) is sustained through adaptation, a process of change where conservation is the outcome (Alligood & Tomey, 2014).

> ## ⟫ APPLICATION TO PRACTICE 5.12
>
> The nurse caring for the patient with AIDS will plan interventions aimed at conserving the patient's energy and facilitating rest.
>
> The nurse caring for the patient with a leg amputation realizes that the patient must go through changes in order to adapt to the disability.

Betty Neuman: Healthcare Systems Model

Betty Neuman's Healthcare Systems Model, based on general systems theory, theorizes that a person is a complex system that responds to stressors originating in both the internal and external environments (Alligood & Tomey, 2014). The Healthcare Systems Model guides nursing practice at three levels of prevention: primary, secondary, and tertiary (Neuman, 1996). Neuman believed that nursing should treat the whole person where systems (individuals, group, family, or community) are seen as being in constant change or motion and where interventions are aimed at maintaining stability (Alligood & Tomey, 2014).

Neuman's model has been widely accepted as an organizing framework for nursing care and has been used extensively in research. Research studies, for instance, have focused on the needs of family members of a critically ill patient, the spiritual needs of adults following surgery due to cancer or cardiac disease, coping strategies used by adult cancer survivors, and the effects of a back exercise regimen in municipal workers who had experienced back injuries. Neuman's model is used in practice for the development of nursing documentation, tools, and nursing care plans and has been used in many settings such as critical care or intensive care units, emergency departments, psychiatric and mental health units, medical–surgical units, rehabilitation units, an orthopedic practice, a hospice, a children's daycare center, and in-home care (Neuman, 1996). Neuman states, "The purpose of nursing practice is to assist clients to retain, attain, or maintain optimal system stability" (p. 69).

> ### ▶▶ APPLICATION TO PRACTICE 5.13
>
> The community health nurse will assess individuals at all three levels to treat illness and promote health.
> The nurse caring for the patient with a stroke will take care to ensure family visitation.

Dorothea E. Orem: Theory of Self-Care Deficit

Dorothea E. Orem's Theory of Self-Care Deficit is a general theory composed of three theories: theory of nursing systems, theory of self-care deficit, and theory of self-care. Orem's work was first published in 1959 and revised most recently in 2001 in the fifth edition of her book, *Nursing: Concepts of Practice.* In this model of practice, the outcome of all nursing actions should be to promote the capacity for self-care in all individuals; activities of self-care are defined as purposeful, ordered, and learned; and the degree to which a person is able to participate in this is called *self-care agency.* In contrast, *self-care deficit* is the degree to which the patient is unable to perform self-care (Alligood & Tomey, 2014).

Orem believed that self-care must be learned and performed deliberately and continuously (Alligood & Tomey, 2014). Appropriate care for the patient is developed through three operations to determine a self-care deficit: diagnostic, prescriptive, and regulatory. Diagnostic operations would include establishing the nurse–patient relationship; prescriptive operations occur when self-care needs and deficits are determined by the nurse and reviewed with the patient; and regulatory operations refer to planning care (Black, 2014).

> ### ▶▶ APPLICATION TO PRACTICE 5.14
>
> The home health nurse ensures that the plan of care includes interventions aimed at promoting independence.
> The nurse caring for the patient following a heart attack will adjust the plan of care until the patient no longer needs assistance.

Sister Callista Roy: Roy Adaptation Model

The Roy Adaptation Model, developed by **Sister Callista Roy,** is based on adaptation and adaptive behaviors that are produced by altering the environment. Roy believed that the goal of nursing is to promote adaptive responses through a six-step nursing process (Black, 2014). These steps are assessing behaviors, assessing stimuli, formulating a nursing diagnosis, setting goals to promote adaptation, implementing interventions, and evaluating whether the goals have been met. Roy developed her theory based on the social and behavioral sciences and systems theory (Alligood & Tomey, 2014).

After the nurse has assessed adaptation and adaptive behaviors, he or she can then develop nursing diagnoses to guide goal setting and interventions aimed at promoting adaptation. Roy viewed the person as a biopsychosocial adaptive system with physiological, self-concept, role function, and interdependent modes (Black, 2014).

> ## ⟫ APPLICATION TO PRACTICE 5.15
>
> The nurse caring for the new mother and newborn will plan interventions to facilitate bonding, promote adaptation to the situation and environment, and decrease harmful stimuli.
> The nurse caring for the individual following a national disaster uses the six-step nursing process to plan interventions to decrease environmental stimuli and promote adaptation.

OTHER THEORISTS

Many other theorists have contributed to the body of nursing knowledge that we claim today, each deserving of celebration. Although more theorists are not mentioned in this text, you should seek out and understand the development of nursing theory and its influence on nursing practice of the present and future. You are encouraged to visit the various nursing theory websites listed at the end of this chapter.

Individual philosophies influence nurses daily by their individual written or unwritten informal philosophies. It is helpful to begin a personal philosophy of nursing, which can be reviewed and revised over time. Writing and periodically reviewing your personal philosophy of nursing reveal personal and professional growth over time. Collective philosophies are those found in schools of nursing and hospital settings and are the collective beliefs that guide the practice of nurses in that setting (Black, 2014). Box 5.1 compares individual and collective philosophy statements.

In Exercise 5.2, consider how the nursing theories in this chapter can be applied to your daily practice. Provide examples and explain how they apply to your former role as an LPN/LVN and your future role as an RN.

BOX 5.1 COMPARING INDIVIDUAL AND COLLECTIVE PHILOSOPHIES

INDIVIDUAL PHILOSOPHY	COLLECTIVE PHILOSOPHY
I believe that the nurse–patient relationship is central to all nursing practice.	We agree with the philosophy of Watson and will use it to guide our practice.
I believe in the value of education and am committed to lifelong learning.	We believe that meeting the needs of our patients is our primary nursing goal.
I believe that nursing is both an art and a science.	We believe that each patient deserves quality care through the delivery of evidence-based practice.

❓ **EXERCISE 5.2**		
THEORIES	**FORMER LPN ROLE APPLICATION**	**FUTURE RN ROLE APPLICATION**

KEY POINTS

After completion of this chapter, you have learned:

- A commitment to theory-based practice provides a systematic, knowledgeable approach to patient care and contributes to the professional growth of the nurse and the nursing profession as a whole.
- Nursing theory provides a systematic, knowledgeable approach to patient care and serves as a tool for critical thinking and decision making in nursing practice.
- To be useful to your practice, nursing theories should be clear, simple, generalizable, important, and accessible. It will be up to you to choose the nursing theory most in line with your beliefs and appropriate to your practice.
- One of the most significant benefits of applying nursing theory to practice is its usefulness in developing the plan of care. The focus of your care and the interventions that you plan will be different for the dying patient, the patient demonstrating health-seeking behaviors, the surgical patient, and so on.
- Nursing theory provides the rationales for why you do what you do and serves to guide nursing practice.
- Developing a personal philosophy of nursing will require examination of your personal beliefs and professional practice and will reveal your growth as a nurse.

CRITICAL THINKING QUESTIONS

1. Which nursing theory would you choose to implement in an acute care mental health facility and why?
2. The nurse manager of the medical–surgical floor has asked you to evaluate three nursing theories or models that could be implemented to improve patient care. Choose three nursing theories (or models), and compare and contrast the theories you choose. State which theory or model you would implement and why.
3. Dorothea Orem's general theory of nursing describes nursing as a complex form of deliberate actions whose goals are to provide a helping human health service. How would you apply her theory to your current practice setting?
4. Identify the concepts of person, environment, health, and nursing as subject matter common to all theories of nursing and explain how they interact with one another.
5. Holistic patient care is a common theme among various nursing theories, nursing philosophies, and nursing models. Choose a nursing theory, philosophy, or model and apply it to a school-age girl with sickle cell anemia.

6. Madeleine Leininger's Culture Care Theory of Diversity and Universality is applicable to practice in association with any nursing theory or model. How would you apply concepts of this theory when delivering care using Nola Pender's Health Promotion Model? What about Betty Neuman's Health care Systems Model?

7. Jared provides care based on his assessment of the following patients. Which nursing theory might drive the care for each of the patients described below? Demonstrate how the theory would apply.
   A. 431: A 68-year-old female with surgical repair of a hip fracture. Jared notes that the patient lives independently in her home and that her two sons live nearby in the same community. She will be discharged tomorrow, and Jared prepares to address her needs.
   B. 432: A 32-year-old female posthysterectomy. The patient is upset and tired, having been up all night because of her roommate (a dementia patient who screamed throughout the night). Jared arranges to have the dementia patient moved into a single-bed room.
   C. 433: A 66-year-old male with chronic congestive heart failure. Jared identifies the need for prevention of further disease-related problems and promoting optimal health. He initiates teaching the patient about diet, exercise, fluid restriction, medications, and signs/symptoms of disease progression.
   D. 434: A 70-year-old male rehabilitating from a stroke and experiencing right-sided weakness. Jared rearranges the room to promote accessibility to certain items such as the phone, call light, and water cup. He also arranged the patient's get-well cards on a bulletin board so that the patient could see the well wishes.
   E. 435: A 40-year-old female with surgical repair for bladder cancer. Jared's assessment identifies needs in the following systems: elimination, ingestion (pain), and sexuality. He focuses his care on each subsystem in order to restore balance.

WEB RESOURCES

Hahn School of Nursing and Health Science: Nursing theory page http://sandiego.edu/academics/nursing/theory

Margaret Newman, http://healthasexpandingconsciousness.org/index.html

The Virginia Henderson International Nursing Library, http://nursinglibrary.org/vhl/

REFERENCES

Alligood, M. R., & Tomey, A. M. (2014). *Nursing theorists and their work* (8th ed.). St. Louis, MO: Elsevier Mosby.

Benner, P. (2001). *From novice to expert: excellence and power in clinical nursing practice.* Upper Saddle River, NJ: Prentice-Hall.

Black, B. P. (2014). *Professional nursing: concepts & challenges* (7th ed.). St. Louis, MO: Saunders.

CurrentNursing.com. *Nursing theories.* (2012). Retrieved from http://currentnursing.com/nur
sing_theory/systems_theory_in_nursing.html.

Erikson, E. (1980). *Identity and the life cycle.* New York, NY: Norton.

Forchuk, C. (1993). *Hildegard E. Peplau: interpersonal nursing theory.* Newbury Park, CA:
Sage Publications.

Henderson, V. (1966). *The nature of nursing: a definition and its implications for practice,
research, and education.* New York, NY: MacMillan.

King, I. M. (1994). Quality of life and goal attainment. *Nursing Science Quarterly, 7*(1). Retrieved from Academic Search Premier full text database.

King, I. M. (1996). The theory of goal attainment in research and practice. *Nursing Science
Quarterly, 9*(2). Available from Academic Search Premier.

Leininger, M. (1996). Culture care theory, research, and practice. *Nursing Science Quarterly,
9*(2). Available from Academic Research Premier.

McEwen, M., & Wills, E. M. (2014). *Theoretical basis for nursing* (4th ed.). Philadelphia, PA:
Wolters Kluwer.

Neuman, B. (1996). The Neuman systems model in research and practice. *Nursing Science
Quarterly, 9*(2). Available from Academic Research Premier.

Newman, M. A. (1999). The rhythm of relating in a paradigm of wholeness. *Image: Journal of
Nursing Scholarship, 31*(3). Available from Academic Search Premier.

Nightingale, F. (1860). *Notes on nursing: what it is and what it is not.* New York, NY: Appleton.

Peplau, H. (1952). *Interpersonal relations in nursing.* New York, NY: Putnam.

Watson, J. (1997). The theory of human caring: retrospective and prospective. *Nursing Science
Quarterly, 10*(1). Available from Academic Search Premier.

Providing Patient-Centered Care Through the Nursing Process

ⓔvolve WEBSITE

Additional resources are available online at:
http://evolve.elsevier.com/Claywell/transitions

OBJECTIVES

After completing this chapter, the student will be prepared to:

1. Compare and contrast the steps of the nursing process.
2. Formulate an actual, potential, and wellness nursing diagnosis.
3. Discuss the five realms that may affect a patient's health status that should be addressed in order to complete a thorough nursing assessment.
4. Formulate and prioritize nursing diagnoses in the practice setting.
5. Apply the nursing process to the practice setting.
6. Formulate and apply reasonable and measurable outcomes to patient care in the practice setting.
7. Compare and contrast the responsibilities of the RN with the role of the LPN/LVN in assessment and developing the plan of care.
8. Compare and contrast nursing assessment of the individual, family, and community.
9. Explain collaborative problems with respect to formulating the nursing diagnosis in the practice setting.
10. Formulate a plan of care.
11. Explain use of concept mapping in developing plans of care.

KEY TERMS

actual problem	interview	observation
assessment	NANDA-I	outcome identification
concept map	NIC	physical assessment
critical pathway	NOC	planning
evaluation	nursing diagnosis	potential problem
identifying criteria	nursing process	subjective data
implementation	objective data	validating

OVERVIEW

The nursing process is a critical concept necessary for the provision of optimal patient-centered nursing care. The application of nursing process theory in daily practice is what sets nursing apart from other health care disciplines. In this chapter, you first learn about patient-centered care and why the nursing process is central to the concept. You'll also learn about the evolution of the nursing process as an applied theory. The chapter then introduces you to the six steps involved in the nursing process: assessment, diagnosis, outcomes identification, planning, implementation, and evaluation (FYI 6.1).

FYI 6.1   LPN AND RN ROLES IN THE NURSING PROCESS

PHASE OF NURSING PROCESS	LPN ROLE	RN ROLE
Assessment	Gather basic objective and subjective data to be analyzed by the RN.	Complete and analyze a comprehensive assessment of the patient within the physiological, psychological, social, cultural, and spiritual realms.
Diagnosis	Understand the diagnoses the RN has assigned and what that means for the patient's plan of care. LPNs do not create/assign nursing diagnoses.	Fully analyze assessment cues into relevant groups of identifying criteria and formulate individualized nursing diagnoses.
Outcome Identification	Able to identify day-to-day goals for recurring care for stable patients.	Identify all expected outcomes for patients in the full range of acuities and care settings.
Planning	Clearly understand the priorities and interventions identified in the plan of care that are the LPN/LVN's responsibilities. Able to plan recurring care for stable patients.	Prioritize nursing diagnoses and individual interventions, as well as alternatives, to be carried out by the health care team.
Implementation	Carry out specified interventions as directed by the RN.	Direct and carry out nursing interventions, participate in the implementation of collaborative interventions, and follow up on those interventions appropriately delegated to other members of the health care team.
Evaluation	Provide the RN with basic assessment data that reflect measures indicated in the plan of care.	Comprehensively evaluate the patient's progress toward achievement of outcomes and adjust the plan of care accordingly.

HISTORICAL PERSPECTIVE

Some say it was Lydia Hall, in 1955, who first introduced a process for nursing practice that included observation, administration of care, and validation. In 1958, Ida Jean Orlando created a process model for nurses to use to plan the care of medical patients and referred to the concept as the **nursing process** by 1961. Several other Orlando contemporaries were beginning to integrate this three-step (assessment, planning, and evaluation) model into practice. In 1967, Yura and Walsh developed a four-step nursing process that became the foundation for the problem-solving process familiar to modern-day nurses, including assessment, planning, implementation, and evaluation (Craven, Hirnle, & Henshaw, 2017). The American Nurses Association (ANA, 1973) added a fifth item to the nursing process concept, when concurrently with the first meeting of the group that would later be known as the North American Nursing Diagnosis Association (NANDA), now known as NANDA International, Inc. (**NANDA-I**, where the NA no longer stands for North American), diagnosis was distinguished as a separate functional step. Nursing diagnosis quickly became a central theme of study for nursing theorists, and in 1980, actual and potential nursing diagnoses were considered essential to practice. In fact, the mission of NANDA-I is "to facilitate the development, refinement, dissemination and use of standardized nursing diagnostic terminology" (NANDA-I, 2016, para. 5).

The study of the nursing process continues to advance and refine nursing practice. In 1991, the ANA added yet another chapter to the book of nursing innovation by introducing outcome identification as a new step in the nursing process. The six steps of the nursing process as it is now known include assessment, diagnosis, outcome identification, planning, implementation, and evaluation. You may think of the nursing process as a problem-solving method that combines the art and science of nursing.

Take this time to assess what you believe your roles to be in the nursing process by completing the statement in Exercise 6.1.

NURSING PROCESS

Excellent critical thinking skills lead to good clinical judgment and are crucial in providing nursing care for patients with complex health conditions. Critical thinking is more than problem solving in that it is a complex, purposeful, and disciplined process that is driven by the needs of the patient and family. Black (2014, p. 156.) states, "The

---

? EXERCISE 6.1

My role as the RN in the nursing process involves _____, and this is different from my current LPN/LVN role in that _____.

Repeat this sentence for each stage of the nursing process.

nursing process is a method of critical thinking focused on solving patient problems in professional practice."

The **nursing process** is composed of the five phases known as assessment, diagnosis, outcomes identification/planning, implementation, and evaluation, also known as ADPIE (ANA, 2016). It is through this process that nurses deliver carefully planned, high-quality, patient-centered care that is holistically and continually evaluated and refined.

Assessment

The first step of the nursing process, **assessment,** involves the collection of both objective and subjective data about an individual, family, or community. Registered nurses gather information specific to the patient's physiological and psychological status, as well as sociocultural, economic, and lifestyle factors, along with the adequacy of support systems in the community and home environment (Hinkle & Cheever, 2014; ANA, 2016).

For the patient, you need to examine five realms to thoroughly complete the assessment: physiological, psychological, social, cultural, and spiritual. You must survey each realm for factors that may affect the patient's health status. If you concentrate on only one or two areas, you will likely miss important data, make inappropriate nursing diagnoses, and carry out inappropriate or incomplete nursing actions.

The RN gathers data from many areas, along with information about the patient's current and past health concerns. A thorough health history is completed upon the patient's admission into the health care setting or at the nurse's first interaction with the patient (or significant other). The history is obtained either through the primary source (the patient), through a secondary source (those who know the patient, such as family or friends), or through the patient's past medical record. The history often contains valuable insights into what is currently happening or what may happen concerning the patient's health.

Assessment is accomplished through a number of mechanisms. The nurse observes the patient and the surrounding situation, interviews both primary and secondary sources, examines the patient from head to toe in a systematic manner, and interprets laboratory data. The RN's assessment will contain both objective and subjective data. **Objective data** contain information that is observed and leaves little room for interpretation; they are facts that can be measured and verified. Examples of objective data are vital signs, size and location of a wound, color of drainage, or any assessment that does not require personal perspective or opinion to document.

Subjective data contain information experienced and described only by the patient and cannot be verified as to its characteristics or easily quantified. Examples of subjective data include such feelings and experiences as the patient's pain, fear, nausea, and uneasiness. In instances of subjective data collection, the best practice is always to write exactly what the patient says, using quotation marks, rather than to paraphrase, which is when the RN documents in his or her own words what the patient has said. Be careful not to use your own opinion words, just the facts.

The nurse must understand that every time he or she interacts with the patient in any way assessment is taking place. While the nursing process as a whole may seem elaborate or confusing to the beginner, part of what the new RN comes to understand is that the nursing process is so integral to minute-to-minute practice that it often occurs without conscious awareness. The process behind nursing practice requires a whole new way of thinking, which soon becomes second nature. This manner of thought is not uncommon to adult students who make critical decisions in everyday life. What is likely to be different is that the nurse needs to have the ability to keep multiple patients' many problems and requisite assessments, interventions, and evaluations in mind concurrently, all the while planning for what comes next for every patient. Although assessment may become second nature, the nurse must still think carefully and deeply about it. Because assessment is carried out every time the patient is seen, it becomes as natural as breathing, and no less important. However, the level of rigorous and meticulous care in managing the assessment makes the difference.

Data Collection Methods

Data collection is accomplished by several different methods, including interview, observation, and physical assessment.

The **interview** is a dialogue or question-and-answer session with the patient or people accompanying the patient. Through the interview, you obtain the complete nursing history, which includes demographics; the chief complaint, normal health-seeking behaviors, current state of health, and medications; and developmental, social, environmental, and family history. You may wish to interview the patient and the significant other separately to verify data and to gain perspective on a particular situation, or the patient may desire to be interviewed alone. In each case, provide as much privacy as possible, remembering that voices easily penetrate the curtain drawn around the bed. During the interview, seat yourself at the same level as the interviewee. Keep in mind that the patient may be tired or in pain and not able to talk for long periods of time.

Observation is the collection of data through seeing, listening, smelling, touching, and generally sensing the patient and the immediate environment as well as the larger context of the situation.

Physical assessment is the collection of objective data through inspection, auscultation, palpation, and percussion. The nursing health assessment differs from the medical physical assessment by determining functional abilities and deficits in order to focus the plan of care and help identify the outcome priorities.

The nurse must individualize and prioritize the nursing assessment according to each patient's situation. The assessment will have different perspectives and focuses with pediatric patients compared with adults and from one setting to another.

In 1987, Marjorie Gordon proposed a guide for establishing a comprehensive nursing database for data collection. Gordon used the word *pattern* to refer to a sequence of recurring behaviors. She proposed 11 categories of functional health patterns that make a systematic and standardized approach possible. The 11 categories identified by Gordon are health perception and health management, nutrition and metabolism, elimination, activity and exercise, cognition and perception, sleep and rest, self-perception and self-concept, roles and relationships, sexuality and reproduction, coping and stress tolerance, and values and beliefs (Gordon, 2016). Each will be discussed briefly.

- *Pattern of health perception and health management* describes a patient's perceived pattern of health and how health is managed. In order to assess this category, for instance, the nurse asks the patient to describe his or her health and what the person does to improve or maintain health.

- *Nutritional-metabolic pattern* describes the patient's pattern of food and fluid intake relative to metabolic need. Assessing this category should focus on questions related to the patient's customs, current health status, height and weight, and diseases or illnesses that may affect nutritional-metabolic function.
- *Pattern of elimination* describes patterns of excretory functions.
- *Pattern of activity and exercise* describes patterns of exercise, activity, leisure, and recreation.
- *Cognitive-perceptual pattern* looks at sensory deficits, the ability of the patient to express himself or herself, level of education, pain perception, decision making, and cognitive functions.
- *Sleep-rest pattern* involves the patient's perception of the quality and quantity of sleep.
- *Self-perception and self-concept pattern* involves body image, self-esteem and feelings, and nonverbal data.
- *Role-relationship pattern* assesses the patient's perception of current major roles and responsibilities, satisfaction with family, work, and social relationships.
- Assessing *sexuality-reproductive pattern* seeks to understand patterns of satisfaction and dissatisfaction with these areas.
- *Coping/stress tolerance pattern* describes coping, handling stress, support systems, and perceived ability to handle situations.
- *Value-belief pattern* includes assessment of religious affiliation, spirituality, values, and beliefs related to health.

Virginia Henderson, a nurse theorist, identified 14 needs of the individual: breathing, eating and drinking, eliminating, moving, sleeping and resting, selecting clothing and dressing, regulating body temperature, maintaining adequate hygiene, remaining free from harm and avoiding harming others, communicating, learning and seeking general fulfillment, having spirituality, working, and playing. Further, Henderson believed that people, both ill and well, had nursing care needs in order to maintain balance achieved by attending to the 14 basic needs (McEwen & Wills, 2014). This holistic approach assesses the biological, psychological, sociocultural, and spiritual needs of the individual. Both of these methods will assist you in identifying dysfunctional patterns.

Organization of Data Collection

Nursing assessments must be organized in a clear, systematic manner that permits logical progression of the data. Organization of the data promotes accurate and comprehensive determination of the plan of care and subsequent prioritization of nursing interventions. Furthermore, clearly documented nursing assessments are valuable tools for communicating and collaborating with other members of the health care team in the provision of total patient care.

Validating Assessment Data

Validating, or verifying, assessment data is necessary to ensure accuracy. Be alert to instances where what the patient is stating is markedly different from what you are observing or when specific measurable data lack initial objectivity. Methods of data validation range from repeating what you believe you understand of the patient's story for clarification to asking another nurse to check a suspicious vital sign or interpret a 6-second telemetry strip.

> ## CASE STUDY
>
> A patient with type 2 diabetes mellitus is admitted to the hospital because of necrosis of his left great toe, secondary to poor circulation. The patient is noted to have decreased dorsalis pedal and posterior-tibial pulses in the left foot. The foot and ankle have a mottled appearance, and the skin is dry and shiny. The characteristic lack of hair of the lower extremities is suggestive of long-standing peripheral vascular disease. The patient states that he is experiencing severe pain in the left foot and leg, which he rates at 7 on a 1 to 10 pain scale. He is scheduled for surgery to remove the great toe and surrounding involved tissue. The overall outcome priority is to provide an environment that will optimize the surgical intervention, while establishing a level of comfort and safety that promotes a return to a level of function higher than the current level of wellness.

Diagnosis

The clustering of cues, or data points, gathered in the assessment phase helps define the care priorities and the associated "problems," or nursing diagnoses. "The nursing diagnosis is the nurse's clinical judgment about the client's response to actual or potential health conditions or needs" (ANA, 2016, para 3). Every **nursing diagnosis** must be substantiated by **identifying criteria,** also known as *defining characteristics.* For a nursing diagnosis to be accepted, often numerous signs and symptoms together make up the actual diagnosis. These identifying criteria must be present in the patient to assign that diagnosis. Caution and attention to detail are crucial here because many diagnoses are similar but have different interventions and different outcomes. Also, patients will almost always have multiple diagnoses.

Nursing diagnoses may be actual, potential, or wellness oriented. An **actual problem** or diagnosis is substantiated by the patient's current signs and symptoms. This problem is identified as requiring specialized nursing interventions or collaborative interventions from the rest of the health care team. Actual problems have three parts to the nursing diagnosis: the problem, the "related to" statement, and the "as evidenced by" statement. The NANDA-I identifies these steps using the acronym PES:

P = Problem
E = Etiology
S = Signs and symptoms

Collaborative problems are medical problems or complications that require collaborative interventions with the physician and the health care team. With collaborative problems, nurses monitor the patient to detect changes in patient status or for the onset of complications (Hinkle & Cheever, 2014). An example of a collaborative problem is *Decreased tissue perfusion, left lower extremity.* Note that the problem statement is not written in terms of a nursing diagnosis, but is reflective of the fact that a collaborative effort by members of the health care team will be needed to treat and monitor the condition.

A **potential problem** or diagnosis is understood by the nurse as likely to develop, although not currently evidenced specifically in the signs and symptoms. Potential problems require the nurse to be vigilant in planning care so that actual problems are avoided. Note that potential problems are written with two parts because a problem does not exist and therefore will not have an "as evidenced by" statement.

Wellness diagnoses are statements about strengths and can be written in one or two parts. For instance, an example of a wellness diagnosis might be *Increasing ability to avoid stressful situations* or *Increasing ability to avoid stressful situations related to initiation of stress-reducing activities.* Using a wellness diagnosis will help the nurse focus on the patient's strengths in order to sustain wellness and improve health (Stolte, 2005). The NANDA-I has also created wellness diagnoses (e.g., *Readiness for enhanced sleep*).

Nursing diagnoses are written in a format that places the problem as related to an etiology, or cause, of the problem. At this point, some schools add the "as evidenced by" statement. The identifying criteria or defining characteristics follow as evidence that this problem or diagnosis is substantiated by assessed signs and symptoms. Also, remember that you must never state a medical diagnosis in the related portion of your diagnosis. Ackley and Ladwig (2014 p. 5) suggest five steps to formulate a nursing diagnosis:

1. Highlight or underline the relevant symptoms.
2. Make a short list of the symptoms.
3. Cluster similar symptoms.
4. Analyze/interpret the symptoms.
5. Select a nursing diagnosis label that fits with the appropriate related factors and defining characteristics.

The nursing diagnosis includes the problem, etiology, and signs and symptoms. The problem is the NANDA-I diagnostic label (e.g., *Spiritual distress*). The etiology (or cause) is what causes or contributes to the development of a problem (e.g., *Spiritual distress related to death of husband*). The signs and symptoms, or defining characteristics, refer to the problem. The complete nursing diagnosis for spiritual distress may be written *Spiritual distress related to death of husband as evidenced by tearfulness and subjective comment "Why did God let this happen?"*

One mistake a beginning nurse can make is identifying patient problems without supporting data. Also, the beginning nurse might identify potential problems but give supporting data for actual problems. In either case, the nurse must take care to use data correctly to individualize the plan of care.

Prioritizing

After the nursing diagnoses have been developed, prioritization occurs. When prioritizing nursing diagnoses, the most critical problems receive the highest priority. Using Maslow's Hierarchy of Needs, importance is first given to physical needs (Hinkle & Cheever, 2014). Safety is always a priority. When assigning priorities, the nurse must consider the urgency of the problem(s).

No evidence exists that this is an actual injury that has already occurred, yet the problem statement will alert nurses to be extra vigilant in patient care. For instance, providing the patient with assistive devices and orienting him or her to the environment will decrease the risk for injury.

The assessment process requires identifying and ordering cues to determine the level of care needed to identify patient problems and outcome priorities. Many institutions continue to use the NANDA-I list of standard nursing diagnoses in the development of the plan of care (a list of the latest NANDA-I nursing diagnoses is provided at the Evolve website for this book).

You may need to clarify findings when collaborating with other health care workers on a patient's plan of care. For example, you as a nurse would diagnose a patient with hypoxemia as having *Ineffective tissue perfusion*. However, you would need to communicate to a respiratory therapist the patient's need for a respiratory treatment. This communication will include specific signs and symptoms with which the patient is presenting, rather than the nursing diagnosis. A common health care language may soon be developed to identify problems and implement collaborative plans of care more clearly.

The plan of care includes independent, dependent, and collaborative interventions, which are coordinated by RNs. Evaluation of the plan of care is also the responsibility of RNs, using data collected from many sources, including licensed practical nurses and unlicensed assistive personnel. RNs direct the data collection process and implementation of the interventions through delegation of duties to the resources available to them. Determining the plan's effectiveness includes the evaluation of the team effort in carrying out the plan. Decisions regarding changes in the plan will be the RN's responsibility.

Outcome Identification/Planning

After prioritizing nursing diagnoses or collaborative problems, as the first stage of outcome identification, identify measurable and achievable immediate, intermediate, and long-term goals with the patient and family (Hinkle & Cheever, 2014; ANA, 2016). Examples of these goals for a patient with the nursing diagnosis of *Altered nutrition, more than body requirements* are:

Immediate: Patient will tolerate an 1800 calorie/day American Heart Association (AHA) diet.

Intermediate: Patient will plan three meals/day for 1 week using the 1800 calorie/day AHA diet.

Long-term: Patient will remain on the 1800 calorie/day AHA diet after discharge.

Outcomes are specific and make the goal measurable (Black, 2014). Whether using NANDA-I or another reference when identifying problem areas and building the plan of care, the nurse identifies the criteria for evaluating the intervention outcomes. Every diagnosis is associated with specific, individualized, and expected outcomes. These expectations must be measurable and clearly communicated, along with signs of attainment or nonattainment, as well as dates and times for evaluation. Precise articulation of the expected outcome criteria will ensure that each nurse or team member assessing the patient will be looking for the same clues, which may signal a need for a change in the plan of care or reevaluation of the outcome priority. The expected outcome is written in positive, patient-centered terms and must be realistic and measurable.

Measurability means that the outcome can be consistently evaluated. An example of a measurable goal would be *The patient will be able to ambulate 50 feet by (a certain date)*. As another example, an outcome may be related to the goal of decreasing a patient's infection. Two measurable outcome criteria would be *Will remain normothermic as evidenced by PO temperature between 97°F and 99°F and WBCs will remain within 5000 to 10,000 mm³*. Any nurse caring for the patient on the day designated for evaluation of the outcome will know by what measures the patient has attained or failed to attain the outcome and will adjust the plan of care accordingly. A measurable outcome for the diabetic patient in the case study might be:

Patient's pain will decrease to ≤2 on a 0 to 10 pain scale by (a certain date).

The Center for Nursing Classification and Clinical Effectiveness at the College of Nursing at the University of Iowa (2008) developed the Nursing Outcomes Classification **(NOC)** and also published it in 1992 (Moorhead, Johnson, Maas & Swanson, 2013). There are 490 NOC outcomes grouped into 32 classes and 7 domains in the fifth edition of NOC. The seven domains include functional health, physiological health, psychosocial health, health knowledge and behavior, perceived health, family health, and community health. Using NOC defines outcomes that focus on the patient, identifies risk adjustment factors, and provides measures for comprehensive outcomes that respond to nursing intervention. NOC can be used by nurses in all settings as well as other disciplines. NOC is used in other countries and has been translated into at least eight languages.

Using the NOC system, an outcome for the diabetic patient with pain would be stated:

"Patient will use a pain rating scale to identify level of pain intensity by (time frame)."

Planning

Planning involves establishing goals and outcomes and determining appropriate interventions. The plan of care, developed during the planning phase of the nursing process, includes the process of identifying the interventions needed for the patient to regain a level of independence at or higher than he or she had before admission into the health care setting. Inherent to the planning process is prioritization of the nursing diagnoses as well as the collaborative patient care issues. This process is often simultaneous with the actual development of the diagnoses and outcomes. RNs will likely be compelled into action by prioritizing the urgent issues. Nursing diagnoses then are listed in order of priority (life and limb).

Establishment of the outcome priority is a planning mechanism. This concept may help the beginning RN understand that optimal nursing care involves constant assessment and reevaluation of the plan of care and substantiation of the outcome priority at any given moment. Planning involves the setting of both measurable and achievable short-term and long-term goals or outcomes (Hinkle & Cheever, 2014; ANA, 2016). This substep often occurs when identifying outcome criteria. Short-term goals are outcomes that are likely, or required, to be achieved in the acute setting before discharge to a subacute setting is permitted. Long-term goals are outcomes that, although they are being addressed, are not likely to be achieved until some later time in a nonacute setting.

A serious element of planning patient care is determining whether the RN can legally order the nursing care that the patient requires. Here the RN is accountable to ensure that appropriate medical and ancillary interventions are prescribed and carried out in a collaborative manner. Knowing what you can and cannot do autonomously as an RN is imperative to safe practice.

Planning ultimately involves mapping out specific, individualized nursing actions that aim to achieve the desired outcomes associated with the nursing diagnoses. To appropriately plan interventions, the RN must consider all aspects of the patient, including age, culture, gender, and past experiences with health care. Planning includes ensuring that ethical and established standards of practice are maintained. Interventions should extend beyond the patient to include the environment and family unit. Including such context as the larger patient situation is essential to complete planning (Hinkle & Cheever, 2014).

In some institutions a **critical pathway** for one of the most common and predictable diagnoses may be initiated. This is a plan of care that assists RNs in defining, within time frames, the expected level of care needed, some specific nursing and medical interventions, and the evaluation intervals. Critical pathways for many diagnoses are developed from patient norms within a particular health care concern and are often specific to the facility, unit, and even physician. They are effective tools for nurses to use as guides, but you must be alert for patient problems that fall out of the pathway and need individualized attention. Care mapping, another method of planning patient care, is used for patients with highly complex conditions because the use of outcomes is more realistic than specific time frames (Hinkle & Cheever, 2014).

For the diabetic patient in the case study, the nurse has gathered the following objective data: (1) patient's complaint of severe pain in the left foot; (2) 1+ pedal and dorsalis pedis pulses; (3) foot temperature cool to touch; (4) great toe dry, black appearance, with no nail noted, and second toe with a 2-cm-diameter black area; and (5) decreased sensation of the foot. Additional information gathered from the history reveals a decrease in eyesight as a result of bilateral cataracts and a decrease in hearing.

From these data, the following actual problems can be identified. Note that many problems are indeed collaborative problems because the etiologies (or sources of the problems toward which interventions are addressed) are often outside the realm of nursing. Such is the case here. The patient has severe pain in the left foot, which is an actual problem and can be written as such:

Collaborative problem: *Pain LLE, actual, related to the complications of the disease process, as evidenced by the patient's subjective report of a pain level of 7 on a scale of 0 to 10.*

A potential problem in the above scenario is the patient's failing eyesight and hearing, which may compromise the patient's ability to respond to an unfamiliar environment, causing injury. In this case, the nurses can reduce the impact of the etiologies by addressing the failing hearing and eyesight in the manner in which they communicate with the patient and addressing the impaired mobility by manipulating the care environment. Therefore, the patient is at risk for injury, and the problem statement is written:

High risk for injury, related to failing eyesight, decreased hearing, unfamiliar surroundings, and impaired mobility.

Interventions for the diabetic patient related to pain would include:

- Administer pain medication as ordered.
- Assess patient's level of pain q1 hour using a pain scale of 0 to 10.
- Provide support, reassurance, and understanding in order to facilitate the patient's expression of feelings.
- Decrease environmental stimuli to promote rest.
- Teach patient nonpharmacological methods to decrease or manage pain.

The Center for Nursing Classification and Clinical Effectiveness at the College of Nursing at the University of Iowa developed the Nursing Interventions

Classification **(NIC).** NIC was first published in 1992 (Bulechek, Butcher, & Dochterman, 2013). The 2013 edition of the NIC contains 554 nursing interventions that are grouped into 30 classes and 7 domains: basic, physiological, behavioral, safety, family, health systems, and community. Each intervention is coded and linked with NANDA-I nursing diagnoses. NIC is recognized by the American Nurses Association, the National Library of Medicine, the National League for Nursing, the Joint Commission, and the Cumulative Index of Nursing and Allied Health Literature (CINAHL) and can be used in all settings and all specialties. In addition, NIC has been translated into at least 12 languages and is used in at least 12 countries (Bulechek, Butcher, & Dochterman, 2013).

An example of a nursing intervention using the NIC system is *Performing prompt and comprehensive assessment and management of pain, including location, characteristics, onset and duration, frequency, quality, intensity, and precipitating factors.*

Using the nursing process to assess the diabetic patient in the case study, we have developed a nursing diagnosis, set a measurable outcome related to that diagnosis, and planned interventions intended to meet the goal or outcomes. The next step is implementation of the plan of care.

Implementation

Implementation, the carrying out of the plan of care, requires a multidisciplinary approach. Licensed practical nurses collect data, implement actions specific to the patient care needs, perform basic teaching, record data as well as interventions, and report to RNs the progress the patient is making. RNs are responsible for delegating and coordinating the care given, implementing advanced interventions, evaluating and updating the plan of care and the associated outcome priorities, and engaging in and documenting patient and family education. Documentation is an important part of this phase.

The RN serves as gatekeeper and all-around organizer of all care and interventions that the interdisciplinary health care team provides, and therefore continuity of care (through discharge and transition to home or the next level of care) is assured (ANA, 2016). As interventions are administered and completed, evaluation becomes an ever-present and crucial part of the role. Accountability for both independent and interdependent functions remains a part of the role of the RN.

Evaluation

Evaluation is the process of examining the effectiveness of the plan of care and adjusting it to ultimately meet the needs of the patient (ANA, 2016). Outcome achievement is determined as part of the evaluation. Assessment and evaluation occur simultaneously and continually; therefore, it is clear that the steps of the nursing process are cyclic and not linear. Unique, inventive changes in the plan of care are necessary when RNs carefully examine the patient's response to nursing interventions—that is, what the patient did or did not demonstrate. LPN/LVNs assist in the evaluation process by reporting progress and assessment data promptly and accurately. The RN interprets the data and adjusts the plan of care to best meet the patient's needs. An appropriate plan of care may require no changes if the patient's condition is progressing as expected.

Now that you have studied the chapter, complete the sentences in Exercise 6.2.

? | EXERCISE 6.2

Developing a Care Plan from a Concept Map

An 80-year-old patient is brought to the emergency department after fainting at home. His serum digoxin level is 2.3 ng/mL. He is transferred to a medical telemetry nursing unit. The next day, the nurse asks the patient to tell her about his routine for taking his daily digoxin tablets. He states that he was told to check his pulse every morning before taking a pill. He does this in his kitchen because the clock on the wall has big numbers and he can see the second hand go around. The nurse asks him how long he measures his pulse. He replies, "I keep counting the beats until I get to 60. Sometimes it takes a long time. Then I take my heart pill." Later he tells the nurse that he hates "having so many pills to take" and admits having trouble remembering to take his pills. He states that he sometimes can't remember which pills to take with breakfast and which to take at night.

Student Name:

Date of Care:

Patient Diagnosis:

NURSING DIAGNOSIS (IN ORDER OF PRIORITY)	GOALS	NURSING INTERVENTIONS	RATIONALE WITH CITED REFERENCES	EVALUATION

From Ignatavicius: *Evolve Resources for Medical-Surgical Nursing*, 8th Edition

CONCEPT MAPPING

Care plans are the essential means by which nurses plan, prioritize, organize, standardize, and customize and communicate safe, evidence-based, patient-centered holistic care. Learning to create them and use them is a necessary practice in nursing school. A concept map creates a visual representation of the client's pathophysiology, medical treatments, and nursing needs. It allows you to see the relationships between clusters of data and concepts associated with the case and to efficiently analyze what you see. This way, you can see how best to identify the patient problems and thus establish nursing diagnoses based on your assessment data. Further, it helps you to see how to prioritize the outcomes and determine your interventions and how they relate to the rest of the treatment plan and assessment data (Schuster, 2015). Concept maps, also known as mind maps and cognitive maps, originated in the field of education as a way to help students find meaning with complex concepts and systems.

Developing a Concept Map

Fig. 6.1 illustrates a simple example of a concept map in diagram form with a very basic level of information included that you might see in the early development of a concept map related to an elderly male patient with a diagnosis of COPD. If you search online for "concept maps nursing" and look at the "images," you will see hundreds of colorful and elaborate examples of how a concept map can look. In each case, however, there are similar steps to developing a concept map. Because of your

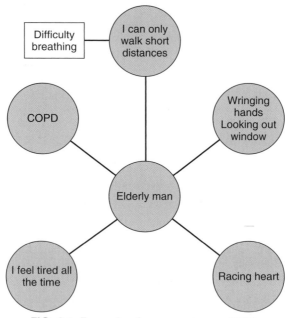

FIG. 6.1 Example of a concept map, 2008.

previous experience with patients, you can draw upon a real example as you think through the process. Let's go through the steps now and, as we do, think of a specific patient, perhaps one with COPD as in Fig. 6.1, and consider what other data points you might be able to add to the basic example provided.

First, what do you know about the patient as far as why he or she came to need medical and nursing care? Fill in the middle circle (or box; the shape does not matter) with the medical diagnosis. Then underneath, in the same circle, list what areas of assessment are key for this particular diagnosis. Be certain to consult your textbooks and keep a reference list (perhaps on the back of the paper) as you will likely need to supply any resources you used to help you develop your concept map.

Next, analyze and categorize your data (Schuster, 2015). Based on what you find as you look up the medical diagnosis in your textbooks, you will find the nursing diagnoses that are most often relevant to the pathophysiology the patient exhibits. Write each of these nursing diagnoses in a separate circle around the diagram, reserving one circle for information and data that you are not sure how to categorize and will come back to later. Then begin to sort and place the data that seem to pertain to each diagnosis within the appropriate circle. These data include what you gathered from the medical record including assessment data, lab results, medications, and other treatments. Sometimes symptoms and other data will apply to more than one circle; write them in both (Schuster, 2015).

Third, it is time to confirm the diagnoses and then prioritize. You may need to consult a nursing diagnosis textbook for help. Number the circles in order of priority. Even though you have identified your top priority, remember that all of the problems are important and the priorities will change as you go through your shift and thus the concept map will also change as to continually assess, treat, and evaluate your patient. To

Nursing Diagnosis 1	
Nursing Intervention	Patient Response Evaluation Data
Monitor I & O hourly	Urine Output 45-60 cc per hour, NPO, NS at 100 cc/hour
Assess bowel sounds q 4 hours	Bowel sounds active in all quadrants

FIG. 6.2 Nursing Intervention Table.

help you think critically through the complexity of the patient problems, you may [?] find that it is helpful to draw lines between related concepts and issues to demonstrate relationships among the problems, assessment data, and treatments (Schuster, 2015).

In step 4, you will create a table that lists nursing interventions for each nursing diagnosis. (The table may look something like Fig. 6.2.) Be certain that you have consulted your reference texts and noted the citation of each reference in your running list. Here you list all treatments that evidence says pertain to and are appropriate for this specific patient, keeping in mind the whole person and how this specific patient may differ from those in the textbook.

Step 5, which would be done during your clinical day, involves writing in the patient's responses to your interventions as well as the evaluation data you may collect as directed by your list of interventions. In addition, this is where you write your patient's progress toward the intended outcomes of care and get an idea of whether or not the plan needs to be adjusted (Schuster, 2015).

As you become familiar with creating concept maps, you may find that other templates or forms and processes better suit the way you think and the way you like to analyze or make connections among data. The more you play with it, the more you will learn. Now that you have learned about both care plans and concept maps, it is time for you to practice creating a care plan based on a concept map. In the following exercise, create a concept map based on the hypothetical case study provided, or if your instructor allows, write one of your own based on past experience.

KEY POINTS

After completion of this chapter, you have learned:
- The nursing process has evolved over many years to a six-step model of assessment, diagnosis, outcomes identification, planning, implementation, and evaluation.
- The complex task of creating an individualized plan of care is crucial to the role of the RN.
- The RN retains full accountability for ensuring that the plan of care is carried out in a sensitive and effective manner.
- Meticulous attention is paid to assessment and evaluation to ensure that, from minute to minute, all patient needs are anticipated, identified, and being met.
- The nursing process, as a method of critical thinking, is crucial to excellence in patient care.

- A concept map creates a visual representation of the patient's pathophysiology, medical treatments, and nursing needs. It allows you to see the relationships between clusters of data and concepts associated with the case and to efficiently analyze what you see.

CRITICAL THINKING QUESTIONS

1. For the following scenarios, what are the identified nursing diagnoses or problem statements?
   a. An 8-year-old child newly diagnosed with insulin-dependent diabetes will be going home.
   b. A 72-year-old with COPD, recovering from pneumonia, is currently on 2 L of oxygen per nasal cannula, with a pulse oximeter reading between 90% and 94%. The patient becomes dyspneic and tachycardic while getting up to use the bathroom and returns to baseline after 10 minutes of rest.
   c. A 24-year-old female in her third trimester of pregnancy with pan-edema and blood pressure of 150/88 mm Hg and 160/99 mm Hg on two occasions 4 hours apart. She complains of not being able to get her rings off and of a headache.
   d. A newborn within 24 hours of birth will be going home.
2. For the following situations, what assessment questions would you need to ask?
   a. You complete a 0700 blood sugar reading on your patient and get a level of 265.
   b. You get a blood pressure reading of 190/110 mm Hg on an individual who is attending a wellness fair.
   c. The health care aide reports that a patient who was admitted to your unit to rule out GI bleed just had a 100-mL emesis.
   d. You walk into a room to do an assessment on your patient and find him sitting on the floor next to the bed.
   e. After waking your patient, you assess your patient's lungs and note fine crackles bilaterally in the bases.
   f. You are assessing a 6-year-old patient who has just had a full liquid dinner, and you note that the patient is blue around the lips.
3. You are scheduled to discharge a patient home. The patient has an ongoing problem identified as "Impaired mobility related to decreased tissue perfusion, left lower extremity secondary to peripheral vascular changes as evidenced by diminished pedal pulses, complaint of cold feet, pain, numbness, and tingling of the toes." Design a discharge plan of care, including the necessary teaching.

WEB RESOURCES

North American Nursing Diagnosis Association, http://nanda.org

Knowledge-Based Terminologies Defining Nursing, http://www.nanda-i-nic-noc.html

University of Iowa School of Nursing, Center for Nursing Classification and Clinical Effectiveness, http://www.nursing.uiowa.edu/center-for-nursing-classification-and-clinical-effectiveness

SmartDraw, http://www.smartdraw.com/specials/flowchart.asp

Concept Draw, http://www.conceptdraw.com/en/products/mindmap/main.php
SMART Ideas, http://www.smarttech.com/products/smartideas/index.asp
Inspiration, http://www.inspiration.com/productinfo/Inspiration/index.cfm
Knowledge Manager, http://www.knowledgemanager.us/KM-KnowledgeManager-eng.htm

REFERENCES

Ackley, B. J., & Ladwig, G. B. (2014). *Nursing diagnosis handbook: an evidence-based guide to planning care* (10th ed.). St. Louis, MO: Mosby.

American Nurses Association. (2016). *The nursing process*. Retrieved from http://www.nursingworld.org/EspeciallyForYou/What-is-Nursing/Tools-You-Need/Thenursingprocess.html.

American Nurses Association. (1973). *Standards of practice*. Washington, DC: Author.

Black, B. P. (2014). *Professional nursing: concepts & challenges* (7th ed.). St. Louis, MO: Saunders.

Bulechek, G., Butcher, H., Dochterman, J., & Wagner, C. (2013). *Nursing interventions classification (NIC)* (6th ed.). St. Louis, MO: Elsevier.

Craven, R. F., Hirnle, C. J., & Henshaw, C. M. (2017). *Fundamentals of nursing: human health and function* (8th ed.). Philadelphia, PA: Wolters Kluwer.

Hinkle, J. L., & Cheever, K. H. (2014). *Brunner and Suddarth's textbook of medical-surgical nursing* (10th ed.). Philadelphia, PA: Lippincott.

Gordon, M. (2016). *Manual of nursing diagnosis* (30th ed.). Burlington, MA: Jones & Bartlett Learning.

McEwen, M., & Wills, E. M. (2014). *Theoretical basis for nursing* (4th ed.). Philadelphia, PA: Wolters Kluwer.

Moorhead, S., Johnson, M., Maas, M., & Swanson, E. (Eds). (2013). *Nursing outcomes classification (NOC)* (5th ed.). St. Louis, MO: Elsevier.

North American Nursing Diagnosis Association–International. (2016). *NANDA-I Defining the knowledge of nursing: About us*. Retrieved from http://www.nanda.org/about-nanda-international.html

Schuster, P. M. (2015). *Concept mapping: a critical-thinking approach to care planning* (4th ed.). Philadelphia, PA: F.A. Davis.

Stolte, K. M. (2005). *Wellness: nursing diagnoses for health promotion*. Philadelphia, PA: Lippincott-Raven Publishers.

University of Iowa. (2008). *NIC and NOC*. Retrieved from http://nursing.uiowa.edu.

Yura, H., & Walsh, M. B. (1967). The nursing process: assessing, planning, implementing, and evaluating. In *Proceedings of the Continuing Education Series Conducted at the Catholic University of America*.

Critical and Diagnostic Thinking for Better Clinical Judgment

⊖volve WEBSITE

Additional resources are available online at:
http://evolve.elsevier.com/Claywell/transitions

OBJECTIVES

After completing this chapter, the student will be prepared to:
1. Define critical thinking.
2. Explain the importance of critical thinking in nursing.
3. Identify the types of reasoning based on critical thinking.
4. Describe the role of cultivated thinking in critical thinking.
5. Compare inductive and deductive reasoning.
6. Explain the eight elements of reasoning in critical thinking.
7. Identify attributes of critical thinkers.

KEY TERMS

assumption	cultivated thinking	point of view
available information	curiosity	purpose
clinical judgment	deductive reasoning	question at issue
concepts	implications	rational thought
consequences	inductive reasoning	reasoned thought
creativity	inference	reflection
critical thinking	intuitive thought	

❘ OVERVIEW

"Knowing a great deal is not the same as being smart; intelligence is not informa-
tion alone but also judgment, the manner in which information is collected and
used."

(Carl Sagan)

As you transition to the role of RN, it becomes increasingly important to make sound clinical decisions based on your knowledge, experience, and skill. Thinking critically is a skill that you learn and hone throughout your nursing program and subsequent career. **Critical thinking** is purposeful and rational and sets out to accomplish a specified goal (Paul, 1995). The only way to become a critical thinker is to learn the process and practice it.

This chapter explores many aspects of critical thinking, such as its practical application to nursing. The elements of critical thought as well as attributes of the critical thinker are presented. Situations requiring the RN to think critically and anticipate the associated outcomes are presented.

DEFINITION OF CRITICAL THINKING

Critical thinking has been described in many ways, such as a way of knowing, a habit of mind, a rational thought process, and a scientific process (Boychuk Duchscher, 1999). It is considered a skill that is necessary in the nursing process. Gordon (2000) found several definitions for critical thinking. For the purposes of this text, the following definition is offered:

> *Critical thinking is a purposeful, goal-directed process of inquiry that utilizes available facts, principles, theories, and abstractions to analyze, make inferences, solve problems, or arrive at decisions.*

This definition is operational, meaning that it has a base in practice and that implications exist for nurses within their scope of practice. To simplify, consider the following model of critical thinking, called Pearson's RED. In this simple but powerful model, R is for recognize symptoms, E is for evaluate arguments, and D is for draw conclusions (Pearson Education, 2012).

PURPOSE OF CRITICAL THINKING

All individuals think. Each time we engage in a decision-making process, we have an intended outcome in mind. However, we make decisions every day that do not lead to the expected or intended outcomes. How often have we decided to purchase a product based on what we have heard in commercials, only to be disappointed in the product after using it? Our decision might have become biased by the emotion of buying the product or by the carefully crafted bravado of the advertising firm. If we had researched the product by other means before giving in to our impulses and purchasing it, we might have discovered general consumer dissatisfaction in the item, and our choice might have been different.

We assume that every nurse wants the health care consumer—the patient—to receive the best care possible. The nurse makes multiple decisions on a daily basis that will affect the patient's outcomes. The nurse must make these decisions using a critical thinking process. Complete Exercise 7.1, answering the questions related to critical thinking.

Need for Critical Thinking

Hansten and Washburn (1999) indicate that the nurse must be able to think critically as a way to decrease errors and sentinel events and assist in cultivating an

---

? EXERCISE 7.1

List words you would use to define critical thinking:
List the characteristics of a nurse you believe is an expert:
Describe in detail a situation that demonstrates this nurse's expertise:
When telling the story, how many of the words you listed as defining critical thinking did you use?
What additional words have come to mind now that you have told the story?

---

improved patient care system. The nurse needs to give careful, complex consideration to what must be done and how best to do it (Greenwood, 2000). This conscious effort is facilitated through a critical thought process. Boychuk Duchscher (1999) reports that as nursing is guided by theoretical concepts, the process of inquiry into these concepts is applied through critical thought. Furthermore, the process of evaluating nursing care occurs through critical thought. The nurse should challenge his or her own previously established thoughts and labels. This process becomes especially important for you as you transition from LPN/LVN to RN. Your previous experiences may hinder your ability to learn anew or to reconsider prior beliefs. An insightful, reflective thought process distinguishes the nurse as a careful thinker.

TYPES OF REASONING EMBEDDED IN CRITICAL THINKING

Reasoned Thought

Reasoned thought is discriminating and prudent and does not allow emotion, feelings, or prejudices to skew decisions. Individuals who practice reasoned thought recognize when negative factors may be interfering with their ability to think clearly. The practice of reasoned thought is an intricate part of the critical thinking process.

Clinical Judgment

Clinical judgment is perceptive understanding of a situation based on knowledge, empirical data (i.e., data that can be observed or experienced), theory, and scientific inquiry. Clinical judgment requires a series of decisions based on changing observations and collected data. Chase (1995) states, "Clinical judgment is the complex cognitive process by which a clinician interprets patient behaviors and builds a communicable description of the status of the patient." Through clinical judgment, the nurse makes decisions on whether to proceed with or revise a course of action. The inquiry (investigational or exploratory) subprocess necessary for sound clinical judgment is critical thinking.

The nursing process emerges as the framework for the RN to design care based on the inquiry process. The standard of care dictates that the nurse assess, analyze, plan, implement, and evaluate a plan of care for each patient. Careful thought is continually given to the process to expose faults. Critical thinking sets the standard for careful thought, and careful thought must be the practice standard for the nurse.

Nursing care is becoming research based and guided by theory and practice standards. As nursing requires a more scientific approach, the RN must become more knowledgeable with regard to following standards of care. The RN's role, which involves collaboration with physicians and other health care providers, is more autonomous in nature than that of the LPN/LVN. The complexity of the current health care environment requires more carefully prepared nurses—nurses who can think clearly, carefully, and purposefully. The nurse who can think critically is better prepared for the increasing demands of his or her responsibilities.

Experience, knowledge, and skills are required in order to think critically (Paul, 1995). Critical thought is a disciplined, rational, and self-directed activity that uses standards and criteria (Paul, 1995; Paul, Elder, & Bartell, 1997). Critical thought assists the nurse in making more effective clinical decisions. The nurse who engages in critical thought will meet more of the patient's needs and affect positive patient outcomes.

RELATED THINKING SKILLS

Many related thinking skills, such as cultivated thinking and deductive and inductive reasoning, support the critical thinking process.

Diagnostic Thinking

Diagnostic thinking is flexible and embraces complexity. Its base is in the scientific process, but it uses both analytical and intuitive cognitive processes. Clearly, differences exist between novice and expert nurses with regard to the ability to use diagnostic thinking. However, the ability to grasp and analyze the complexity of any given situation, using all the data at hand to make both inferences and deductions, is required of a diagnostic thinker.

Cultivated Thinking

People who engage in critical thought can be said to practice **cultivated thinking,** which is organized, enlightened, and educated. By organizing the thought process, the individual is able to make sense of information. Relevant data are sorted and prioritized in a coherent manner. The nurse uses the nursing process to gather assessments and cluster relevant data to identify actual and potential patient problems.

The cultivated thinker does not assume that he or she has gathered all the pertinent information yet. The cultivated thinker is not arrogant and recognizes traits that interfere with the ability to gain knowledge. This type of thinker seeks the latest and best information available to make the most appropriate decisions. The RN who continues to update the data and stay well informed will best meet patients' needs.

Deductive Reasoning

The nurse must logically analyze situations every day, and how this is done demonstrates the ability to solve problems. Collection of data, part of the assessment phase of the nursing process, is followed by analysis to formulate a plan of care. The process of going from broad information to specific details, or general to specific, is **deductive reasoning.** Taking general assessment data, drawing conclusions, identifying problems or needs, and formulating a plan of care are the steps in the deductive reasoning process. The nursing process is an example of deductive reasoning because it involves taking data and deducing a plan of care.

Specific data lead to specific nursing diagnoses. The North American Nursing Diagnosis Association–International (NANDA-I) provides the standard nursing diagnoses for nurses to follow. Standard nursing diagnoses require specific assessment data to support their use. The nurse who uses deductive reasoning sets out to prove the result through supporting data. The data will likely measure and describe a physical or psychological problem that interferes with the patient's ability to satisfactorily perform activities of daily living. The problem usually also implies a need for assistance with the activity.

For example, a patient has a problem that prevents him from shaving himself, tying his shoes, or fixing his meals. He is not physically able to compensate for the problem, so he is in need of assistance. Data support the nursing diagnosis *Impaired physical mobility* by deduction.

Inductive Reasoning

The nurse uses **inductive reasoning** when a patient presents with symptoms or problems the nurse has seen before. From the assessment data gathered, the nurse makes inferences (i.e., conclusions or assumptions), asks further questions, and makes decisions. The nurse, using inductive reasoning, goes from specifics to generalities and infers the likely outcomes based on supporting data.

For example, an RN has been working with a patient on the nursing unit for a 12-hour shift. The nurse recognizes that each time the patient is turned to the left, her blood pressure drops 15 mm Hg. The same RN has seen this phenomenon in several other patients and makes the inference that patients with right-sided heart failure (the medical diagnosis) will experience a blood pressure drop if turned to their left side. If this patient and others with the same diagnosis do indeed become hypotensive, then the nurse becomes more confident of the reasoning. However, from the data gathered, the RN cannot yet come to a certain conclusion or formulate a nursing diagnosis. The nurse may go on to use these data, however, to support a nursing diagnosis, perhaps *Fluid volume deficit, relative, related to decreased right ventricular function.*

The strength of the inference is based on the extent of the RN's knowledge and experience. The RN with limited experience and with developing knowledge may rely on only the proven, is less comfortable with uncertainty, and looks to others for validation of decisions. While gaining experience and expertise, though, the nurse becomes better able to use cues from the patient and the environment to make stronger and more accurate inferences.

ELEMENTS OF REASONING AND CRITICAL THOUGHT

Richard Paul (1995) lists eight elements as the basis of critical thought: purpose, question at issue, point of view, available information, concepts, assumptions, implications or consequences, and inferences or answers to the original purpose.

Purpose

The **purpose** recognizes that all thought has an agenda or asks the question "What are you trying to accomplish within the context of your thought process?" An assumption exists that not all aspects of a thought are fully understood until the entire process is complete. The purpose of the inquiry thus is to answer the original question.

Question at Issue

The **question at issue** defines the purpose clearly and accurately. The question is relevant to the purpose and will allow the rest of the process to follow logically.

Point of View

All thinking stems from a **point of view.** An enlightened thinker is able to interpret data and clarify meaning from several points of view—that is, to explain or illustrate how the data can be understood from multiple positions. The RN will be able to recognize that a routine treatment may seem strange and frightening from the patient's point of view. In gathering the data to support this assumption, the nurse will ask questions to better understand how the patient is responding to the demands of the treatment. If the nurse does not understand that all thought is based on particular points of view or does not try to look at the problem from varied perspectives, then nonoptimal outcomes may result. An unenlightened nurse may make erroneous assumptions that label the patient as problematic and noncompliant.

Available Information

The thought process must be based on **available information,** data that are at hand, and will give a greater understanding of the problem. Gathering historical and assessment data from the patient, as well as seeking all available secondary-source information, will assist the critical thinker to support the plan of care and understand the potential outcomes. Information also comes from the theoretical knowledge base of the nurse.

Concepts

As the thought process develops, **concepts** will form that begin to explain the problem at hand. A concept is an idea, theory, or mental image of something that does not yet have a tangible representation. Concepts are the structural components of the thinking process, helping us understand complex ideas, events, actions, and entities, defining and shaping our thought processes. As critical thinkers, we must be aware of how our concepts are influencing our thought processes.

Assumptions

Conceptual mental images help the thinker draw assumptions about the events, objects, or actions that are taking place. An **assumption** is an educated guess, hypothesis, or stated or unstated belief that is accepted or held as a truth without proof. Often the thought process will be based on assumptions that are taken for granted or presumed to be true but not tested or proven. In critical thinking, assumptions are challenged through inquiry as to their genuineness or their basis in reality. The RN must test assumptions before they are proven. All assumptions must be checked against the available data. If an assumption cannot be verified, then it may need to be discarded.

Implications and Consequences

Implications or **consequences** are defined through outcomes. Implications or consequences can be expected or unexpected, but each must be considered. For example, an expected consequence of bathing a patient is clean, intact skin that has a greater ability to fight infection or breakdown. Another consequence of bathing may be fatigue or chilling, which could place undue stress on the patient. The implications and consequences of thoughts, actions, and interventions must be checked and understood before completing the intervention. Every action or intervention has implications or consequences. The individual engaging in critical thought must ask the question "What are the implications of this train of thought?" or "If I continue on this path, what will be the consequences?"

Inferences

At the completion of the systematic process of critical thought, inferences are drawn. An **inference** is the conclusion that results from, or is a summary of, the process. The nurse may be confident in the decisions made if the process is completed diligently (Paul et al., 1997).

FYI 7.1 illustrates a case study and questions related to the eight elements of reasoning and critical thought.

STRUCTURE OF CRITICAL THOUGHT

Now that the elements of critical thought have been defined, consider the structure of the thought process. Critical thought is fluid and circular. The nursing process, at first glance, may appear linear in nature. Evaluation of the plan is expected throughout the process, yet one cannot logically design nursing interventions before problems are identified. The critical thinking process assumes that questions are formed for each step of the nursing process, asked, and answered. For example, if in the process of gathering information the nurse makes certain assumptions, then the critical thinker must process these assumptions by determining their relevance to the issue at hand and whether they are based on available data, research, or theory. Complete Exercise 7.2, answering the questions related to the structure of the thought process.

ATTRIBUTES OF THE CRITICAL THINKER

The nurse who engages in critical thought does so on a foundation of knowledge and other specific attributes that support the process, including curiosity, diligence in the pursuit of evidence and information, rational thought, reflection, and creativity.

⚡ FYI 7.1 USING THE EIGHT ELEMENTS OF THOUGHT

A 68-year-old male patient with type 2 diabetes mellitus is being admitted for evaluation of a nonhealing wound to the left foot. To plan the patient's care using the elements of thought, the nurse would ask the following questions:

- *Purpose:* What must be accomplished with this admission? What would the priority goal be? What would be the intent of any intervention?
- *Question at issue:* What problems are present? Are any problems high priority? What is already known about the problems?
- *Information:* What empirical data (evidence) are present to support the questions at issue? What previous experiences or knowledge can be drawn upon to assist in this situation?
- *Point of view:* What are the problems as identified by the patient or the patient's family? What was going on that gave rise to the problem? What is the top-priority problem from the physician's point of view? Are the identified problems compatible or in conflict with one another? How is the top-priority problem addressed once relevant points of view have been considered?
- *Concept:* What is the main intention of the plan that is developing? Does scientific foundation or theory support the concept?
- *Assumptions:* Are any assumptions not supported by the information at hand? Are developing assumptions being ignored? What has been done or is being done to validate the assumptions being formulated?
- *Implications and consequences:* If the plan is continued, what will happen? If the interventions are implemented, what are the potential consequences? How will the interventions that are delegated or are completed by the nurse affect the patient's outcome or well-being?
- *Inferences:* What are the actual conclusions to the plan? Were these conclusions expected? Do the same questions have other answers to consider?

❓ EXERCISE 7.2

Besides ensuring the Five Rights of medication administration, what questions must you ask before giving any medication?

You enter the room of your patient to encourage him to cough and deep-breathe. What are you trying to accomplish by this intervention?

Before delegating a bed bath to a certified nurse assistant, what questions must you ask? What must you know about the patient and the nurse assistant?

You decide that your patient may be developing pneumonia. What information might you be using to come to that conclusion?

Curiosity

Curiosity drives the nurse to seek knowledge in regard to the situation at hand. Curiosity is the desire to understand what something is or how it works, to be compelled to explore beyond what is immediately obvious. Curiosity may also imply skepticism, or the need to challenge beliefs in search of other possible conclusions or truths.

This relentless pursuit of truth is an attribute of the curious mind. Retaining an open mind, looking freshly at the world (and our patients), and practicing discovery every day demonstrate curiosity at its fullest.

Curiosity stimulates the RN to apply all available facts, principles, and theories, as well as specific knowledge of the situation to formulate the plan of care. Not having prejudged the situation shows the nurse to be an abstract thinker, able to derive unique solutions to best address the problems of the patient.

Diligent Pursuit of Evidence and Information

A critical thinker diligently seeks relevant evidence and information as part of the process of decision making. Collaborating with experts and consulting other references while developing the plan of care are important. The critical thinker continually assesses and responds to the patient's changing condition and makes autonomous decisions as to immediate action, within the appropriate scope of practice.

Rational Thought

Another attribute of the critical thinker is **rational thought,** which is fueled by knowledge gained through study and experience. Employing rational thought helps the nurse predict likely outcomes of planned actions or interventions, thus making sound clinical decisions based on all available information.

Reflection

To become comfortable with the process of thinking critically, the critical thinker should practice **reflection,** looking back and reconsidering ideas, thoughts, beliefs, and actions. The nurse evaluates not only the plan of care and the patient's response to nursing and medical interventions but also his or her own thought process. Reflection helps the nurse improve practice through careful self-critique of prior scenarios. In reflecting, the nurse asks whether he or she has been prejudicial or rational, considerate of other points of view or single-minded, focused on the inquiry or distracted, and flexible or rigid in the thought process.

Creativity

An important attribute of the critical thinker is **creativity,** the ability to be innovative, resourceful, and inventive. Paul (1995) presents the argument that creative thinkers use critical thinking, and critical thinkers must use creative thinking principles. Creative thinking is linked to inductive reasoning in that creative thinkers recognize patterns that are present but understand that outcomes are often uncertain until tested. Each new idea generated by the creative thinker increases the number of potential outcomes to consider. If ideas are limited to those that are already accepted, then the possibilities are limited as well. Unique solutions to ambiguous problems can be found when the nurse begins by thinking creatively.

Intuitive Thought

Intuitive thought, often linked to critical thinking, involves one's sixth sense, instincts, or insight. Intuition implies perceptiveness, the ability to see or sense subtle

---

? EXERCISE 7.3

Describe a typical day as an LPN/LVN within the unit where you work.

Identify techniques you have learned to organize your day, prioritize the tasks you must accomplish, and make sure you have administered medication to your patients safely.

In the previous item, describe where you now see elements of critical thinking or where the inclusion of an element of critical thinking would make a positive difference in your practice.

---

patterns or characteristics. The intuitive nurse synthesizes data gathered from all senses and interprets the data based on experience. Some nurses refer to this as their "gut feeling." This ability to organize minimal or vague data in order to come to conclusions is observed in the nurse who is considered an expert.

Complete Exercise 7.3, answering the questions related to the attributes of the critical thinker.

FOSTERING CRITICAL THOUGHT

Much as critical thinkers are described as having multiple attributes, the process of critical thinking is similarly multidimensional and nonlinear. With this in mind, Paul (1995) believes that the process of critical thought is rooted in discipline, which is exemplified by being true to the standards of thought and testing one's thought process for clarity, accuracy, specificity, relevance, logic, consistency, depth, and significance (FYI 7.2).

Hansten and Washburn (1999) believe it is the individual RN's responsibility to develop critical thinking skills. The process of acquiring these skills includes being open-minded, valuing intuition, having the ability to self-examine and challenge one's own thought process, and having the courage to take a stand even if it is unpopular or involves a change. Furthermore, to foster critical thinking in employees, organizations must adopt a culture that accepts and encourages it.

Atay and Karabacak (2012) studied the use of concept maps to help students develop critical thinking skills, thus improving their ability to link theory into practice. They found that the group that created several concept maps over the span of a semester, instead of using the traditional columned format of the care plan, scored significantly higher on a critical thinking abilities inventory after the test. A concept map allows the student to visually group information into meaningful patterns and models, thus clarifying how practice is guided by theoretical knowledge.

FYI 7.2 THE NURSE AS A CRITICAL THINKER

- Practical nursing education helps the nurse recognize important, pertinent data collected and the need to convey this information to the appropriate individual.
- The nurse who thinks critically has several attributes: curiosity, rationality, reflection, independence, creativity, fair-mindedness, and focused and flexible thinking.
- The nurse who uses critical thinking attributes to their fullest will facilitate optimal patient outcomes.

KEY POINTS

After completion of this chapter, you have learned:

- Critical thinking is a skill the RN must understand and incorporate into practice.
- The purpose of critical thinking is to ensure that the decision-making process will lead to the best possible patient outcomes.
- The RED model of critical thinking includes R for recognize symptoms, E for evaluate arguments, and D for draw conclusions.
- Critical thinking opportunities are embedded throughout the nursing process, and taking advantage of them will improve nursing care.
- To realize success in both personal and professional life, the nurse must consistently practice the process of critical thinking.

CRITICAL THINKING QUESTIONS

1. From a clinical experience as a student or as an LPN/LVN, describe a situation that you feel could have been solved in a better way if sound reasoning had been used instead of emotions or feelings. How might the situation have been different, in relationship to outcomes, if rational thought had been used?

2. In response to a call light, you enter a room to find a 68-year-old patient on the floor next to the bed. The patient is in his first day post-operative for surgical resection of the colon, he had slept all night without complaint, and the report states that he had not been agitated or confused but doing well.
   a. What assumptions, if any, can you make about this situation?
   b. What are the questions that you need to ask?

3. A 65-year-old female was admitted to your division today with exacerbation of CHF. The patient was dyspneic and complained of heaviness in the chest and swelling in her feet and ankles. Cardiac enzymes are negative. Chest X-ray was negative for pneumonia. The patient states that she needs to go outside to smoke. Past medical history includes an acute MI two years ago with stent placement. Using the eight steps of critical thought, consider what information you need to plan this patient's care and what may be the priority of care based on what you already know.

4. Critical thinking involves the process of reflection. Think of a patient scenario from your past clinical experience. Write out the details of that situation, of course omitting any patient identifiers, and through the process of reflection, determine how the situation might have been handled differently for an improved outcome.

5. Now think of a situation where conflict occurred on the nursing division. Through the process of reflection, how might things have been handled differently for an improved outcome?

6. You are in the middle of a dressing change for a patient with a sacral pressure ulcer positive for MRSA when you realize that you do not have everything you need to complete the dressing change; the client is already in position, which tends to be uncomfortable, and the old dressing has already been removed. Using the process of critical thought, what are several options open to you to address the situation most effectively? What questions do you need to ask to examine your situation?

WEB RESOURCES

http://criticalthinking.org
http://austhink.org/critical
http://thinkwatson.com/think-red/red-critical-thinking-model

REFERENCES

Atay, S., & Karabacak, U. (2012). Care plans using concept maps and their effects on the criti-cal thinking dispositions of nursing students. *International Journal of Nursing Practice, 18,* 233–239.

Boychuk Duchscher, J. E. (1999). Catching the wave: understanding the concept of critical thinking. *Journal of Advanced Nursing, 29*(3), 577–583.

Chase, S. K. (1995). The social context of critical care clinical judgment. *Heart & Lung, 24*(2), 154–162.

Gordon, J. M. (2000). Congruency in defining critical thinking by nurse educators and non-nurse scholars. *Journal of Nursing Education, 39*(8), 340–351.

Greenwood, J. (2000). Critical thinking and nursing scripts: the case for the development of both. *Journal of Advanced Nursing, 31*(2), 428–436.

Hansten, R. I., & Washburn, M. J. (1999). Individual and organizational accountability for development of critical thinking. *Journal of Nursing Administration, 29*(11), 39–45.

Paul, R. (1995). *Critical thinking: how to prepare students for a rapidly changing world.* Santa Rosa, CA: Foundation for Critical Thinking.

Paul, R., Elder, L., & Bartell, T. (1997). *California teacher preparation for instruction in critical thinking: research findings and policy recommendations.* Sacramento, CA: Commission of Teacher Credentialing.

Pearson Education. (2012). RED model for critical thinking. Retrieved from http://thinkwatson.com/think-red/red-critical-thinking-model.

CHAPTER

8

Practicing Evidence-Based Decision Making

⊖volve WEBSITE

Additional resources are available online at:
http://evolve.elsevier.com/Claywell/transitions

OBJECTIVES

After completing this chapter, the student will be prepared to:
1. Define evidence-based practice.
2. Identify gaps and barriers to implementing evidence-based nursing practice.
3. Identify high-quality electronic resources for locating evidence-based nursing practice.
4. Develop a sound clinical question utilizing the PICO format.
5. Discuss the hierarchy (levels) of evidence.
6. Articulate the role of the RN in research and research utilization.
7. Describe the research process.

KEY TERMS

active variable
attribute variable
best practices
clinical question
concept
critical appraisal
dependent variable
empirical data
evaluation

evidence summary
Evidence-Based Medicine
    Reviews (EBMR)
evidence-based
    practice
experimental design
hypothesis
independent variable
operational definition

performance
    improvement
PICO
population
qualitative study
quality assurance
quantitative study
quasi-experimental
    design

120

KEY TERMS—cont'd

reliability	sample size	variable
research design	systematic review	
sample selection	validity	

OVERVIEW

A growing expectation exists that nursing should become a research-based profession. Utilization of research is a role expectation and standard of care for an RN in the planning and implementation of care for patients. State nursing boards and The Joint Commission (TJC) are more insistent that policies and procedures have a foundation in scientific research. It is essential that nurses become skilled in reading, understanding, and critically evaluating published research studies. The objective of integrating evidence-based practice (EBP) with nursing care is to empower the nurse to become a competent consumer of research. As an RN, you should be able to search the nursing literature and to determine whether research findings are available to assist in patient care. Therefore, an RN must be able to understand basic research as it applies to the practice as well as practice standards.

This chapter addresses fundamentals of research and research utilization. Components of and steps in the research process are explained. The chapter also gives examples of how research is applied to nursing practice, provides the reader with a better understanding of EBP, and directs the nurse and new graduate where to find evidence-based resources, as well as how to accurately evaluate the strength of the evidence.

Economic factors, the variability of care, and the rising cost of health care have been the driving forces in the call for EBP. Consumers and governmental agencies are insisting on transparency, accountability for effectiveness, and efficiency in health care. One of the many responses to the call for quality of care has been that of the American Nurses Credentialing Center's (ANCC) Magnet Recognition Program. The ANCC awards those hospitals who meet the criteria for providing quality patient care and recruiting and retaining nurses. While it has been proposed by the Institute of Medicine (IOM) report that all health care organizations adopt an EBP paradigm, this proposal will most likely encounter some opposition due to the nature of organizational change itself. To achieve magnet status, the facility must apply the credentialing standards of care that were developed by the ANCC in the daily practice of patient care (ANCC, 2017).

The significance of achieving magnet status indicates a hospital that succeeded in creating an atmosphere that nurtures EBP in nursing practice. The nurses are free to exercise professional autonomy. The particular hospital becomes known for its effective and efficient nursing care. There are 39452 magnet facilities around the world (ANCC, 2017). The task remains for each nurse to individually add to the body of nursing knowledge and practice by adopting a personal attitude of EBP. The first step is to become knowledgeable and skilled in the EBP process.

WHAT IS EVIDENCE-BASED PRACTICE?

Evidence-based practice is the integration of the best available evidence, combined with clinical expertise, which enables health practitioners of all varieties to address health care questions with an evaluative and qualitative approach. The American Nurses Association (ANA) has developed standards that guide nursing practice and establish a general framework for integrating the science (evidence-based) of nursing into daily practice. The National Guideline Clearinghouse offers a huge collection of peer-reviewed, current scientific (evidence-based) clinical guidelines. It is critical for the RN to become familiar with standards that support clinical decisions in nursing practice to ensure the delivery of safe and professional care (Cassey, 2007).

The New York State Association 2006 Research Report concurs with the ANA in its statement that nurses must consider the correlation that exists between evidence-based practice and standards of care. Standards of care are continually changing; therefore, the nurse must be involved in evidence-based practice to effectively meet the standards.

DEFINING EVIDENCE-BASED PRACTICE

The overall aim of evidence-based practice is to standardize practice by maximizing good practice, reducing costs, and improving quality of care. *Evidence-based practice* refers to the integration of the best available research and clinical expertise in the context of patient characteristics, culture, patient preferences, and values. EBP is a problem-solving approach to nursing practice that involves the conscientious use of current best evidence in making decisions about patient care. One of the various definitions offered for evidence-based practice is the integration of individual clinical expertise with the best available external clinical evidence from systematic research. It is important for the RN to understand the underlying process of EBP and possess the skill to apply that knowledge to nursing practice. Evidence-based nursing practice (EBNP) is the process by which nurses make clinical decisions using the best available research evidence, their clinical expertise, and patient preferences (Sackett et al., 2000).

Several electronic databases are available with a wide variety of current evidence-based research that is relevant to nursing. The literature reveals that most nurses have a lack of knowledge regarding the research process, a deficit in accessing and utilizing resources, and little experience in planning patient interventions or outcomes. Organizational culture is a major barrier to incorporating evidence-based practice into health care decisions. A lack of administrative support often leaves nurses feeling disempowered to initiate change even when current evidence-based research is available. Patients are often without basic health care coverage, which has resulted in patients requiring more complex health management. Nurses often feel there is little to no time to do "research EBP," allowing the practitioner to address health care questions from an evaluative and qualitative approach. The nurse does not have to conduct research studies; however, all nurses are expected be competent in assessing current and past research in order to differentiate between high-quality and low-quality literature.

The gap between research findings and integration into daily practice is approximately 17 years. Gilbert, Salanti, Harden, and See (2005) provide the following example:

> *Prior to the 1990s, it was recommended that infants sleep on their stomachs despite evidence in the 1970s that this contributed to sudden infant death syndrome (SIDS). (p. 874)*

The role of the RN in health care institutions is ideal for creating an environment that embraces the **evaluation** and implementation of EBP policies and procedures. It is important that the nurse present research findings and research evidence that will lead to improved patient outcomes.

DEFINING ATTRIBUTES OF EVIDENCE-BASED PRACTICE

There are three key features unique to evidence-based practice. First, EBP is problem solving in its approach that takes into account the clinical experience of the nurse. *Clinical experience* refers to the nurse's ability to use clinical skills and past experience to identify the patient's health state and diagnosis and both the risks and benefits of the prospective interventions.

Second, EBP combines researched evidence with knowledge and theory. The use of patient-centered researched evidence allows for accuracy and precision of diagnostic tests and prognosis markers, in addition to the effectiveness and safety of therapeutic treatment.

Third, evidence-based practice allows for patient values to be expressed and incorporated in treatment regimens. Patients bring their individual preferences, concerns, and expectations to the clinical setting.

PUTTING EVIDENCE-BASED PRACTICE TO WORK

EBP allows the RN to assess current and past research, clinical guidelines, and other information resources in order to identify relevant literature while differentiating between high-quality and low-quality findings. The practice of EBP includes five fundamental steps, which were first described in 1992.

The five-step process forms the basis for the integration of clinical evidence and nursing practice. EBP utilizes a five-step process to provide a structured method that enables the nurse to understand the underlying principles of EBP, implement evidence-based policies, and have a critical attitude to the patient care provided. Without these skills and attitudes, nurses who are unable to meet this minimum requirement will find it difficult to provide patients with **best practices** (Guyatt et al., 2000). Table 8.1 summarizes the five-step evidence-based practice process.

Getting Started

The first step in the evidence-based practice process is to become proficient in effectively searching appropriate resources. The RN must decide what details are important to the problem or concern. A well-built **clinical question** includes the following components, the patient's disorder or disease, the intervention or finding

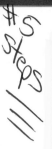

TABLE 8.1   EVIDENCE-BASED PRACTICE PROCESS

Step 1: Construct a relevant, answerable question from an identified clinical concern.
Step 2: Search the literature for the best external evidence that addresses the clinical concern.
Step 3: Critically appraise the evidence for validity and applicability.
Step 4: Apply the evidence to your clinical concern.
Step 5: Evaluate your performance.

under review, a comparison intervention (if applicable—not always present), and the outcome.

Step 1: Construct a Relevant, Answerable Question from an Identified Clinical Concern Case

An answerable question is one that is focused on a specific patient-centered concern by the RN. Once a specific concern has been identified, the nurse pulls the important details that are relevant to the clinical question. Example: In children with acute otitis media, should watchful waiting be considered instead of treatment with antibiotics? In this example, the problem is a child with otitis media; the intervention is antibiotic therapy; the comparative intervention is watchful waiting/observation; and the outcome is the resolution of acute otitis media. The type of question formulated determines which resources should be accessed (University of Alaska, Anchorage, Consortium Library, n.d.).

Background questions. Background questions seek general knowledge about a disease or disease process, and foreground questions ask for specific knowledge to inform clinical decisions or actions. The two characteristics of background questions are (1) who, what, when, where, and (2) focus on a disorder, test, or treatment. Background questions are not asked to determine a specific clinical condition or a specific patient. Example: What causes sleep apnea? How often should postmenopausal women have a Pap smear?

Foreground questions. Foreground questions have four key components: patient- or problem-centered focus on knowledge about managing patients with a disease, intervention, comparative intervention (an optional step, only used if relevant), and clinical outcome. Example: In young children with streptococcal pharyngitis, is amoxicillin as effective as penicillin in short-term antibiotic therapy?

Developing the clinical question is the most important step in the evidence-based practice process. The RN must develop a clinical question that encompasses the key components to ensure that the question addresses an answerable concern that can be converted into relevant application. It must be practical, and the answer must have the potential to produce meaningful applications to treatment.

PICO. PICO is an acronym used to describe a format of the four elements required to formulate a good clinical question (*P*, patient or problem; *I*, intervention; *C*, comparison; *O*, outcomes). Employing the PICO approach allows for a systematic method of identifying important concepts when formulating the clinical question. Every component of the PICO model may not be utilized in every case. However, regardless of the type of resource used, the PICO model is effective in strategically guiding the

TABLE 8.2 **PICO**	
P	**PATIENT, POPULATION, OR PROBLEM**
	How would you describe a group of patients similar to yours? What are the important characteristics of the patient, such as the primary problem, disease, comorbidity, sex, age, or ethnicity?
I	**INTERVENTION, ISSUE OF INTEREST**
	What is the main intervention or therapy under consideration? Include exposure to disease, a diagnostic test, patient perception, and any risk factors.
C	**COMPARISON OF INTERVENTION (IF APPLICABLE)**
	Is there an alternative to compare with the intervention? Include no disease, placebo, or diagnostic test.
O	**OUTCOME TO BE MEASURED OR ACHIEVED**
	What is the clinical outcome, including a time frame?

PICO Example
P-Population-In patients 65 and older with a new diagnosis of *Type 2 Diabetes*, how well does
I-Intervention-patient education material regarding nutrition placed online and freely available 24/7/365, compared to
C-Comparison-paper based instruction handed to client at first post-diagnosis visit, improve the
O-Outcome-feeling of self-efficacy in addressing nutritional changes.

Adapted from the Ebling Library, University of Wisconsin-Madison (2004; retrieved from http://ebling.library.wisc.edu).

development of the clinical question. The "Evidence-Based Nursing: Evidence-Based Practice in the Health Sciences" presented by the Information Services Department of the Library of the Health Sciences-Chicago, University of Illinois-Chicago, is a free resource to enhance the nurse's skill in developing relevant answerable clinical questions. The tutorial can be accessed at http://ebp.lib.uic.edu/nursing/. Table 8.2 provides a clinical scenario using the PICO format.

Clinical question categories. The clinical question will fall into various categories that are classified according to use. Remember the earlier principle: the type of question will influence the type of search strategies and resources to be used.

Diagnosis: This category emphasizes how to select a diagnostic test or interpret the results of a particular test. Example: In patients with suspected dementia, what is the accuracy of the Cornell Scale for Depression in Dementia compared with the Geriatric Depression Scale?

Therapy: An inquiry into the most effective treatment for a particular condition. Example: In estrogen hormone replacement therapy for postmenopausal women, does traditional medical treatment or alternative therapy with Chinese herbal therapy improve patient symptoms better?

Harm or Etiology: Questions what the harmful effects of a particular treatment are or how the harmful effects can be avoided.

Prognosis: The focus is on the disease process, screening, and risk reduction. Example: What is the normal grief process in healthy women who suffer a miscarriage, and are there any factors associated with longer than normal grieving?

Prevention: Interested in how to modify patients' risk factors to reduce the risk of disease. Example: Does the influenza vaccine reduce the risk of pneumonia in patients diagnosed with a compromised immune system?

Qualitative: Emphasis is on understanding a clinical phenomenon (i.e., an occurrence, circumstance, or fact that is perceptible by the senses) as the patient experiences and values it.

Step 2: Search the Literature for the Best External Evidence

The clinical question has been identified, and the question has been categorized. It is now time to track down the evidence. This is often a challenging process for the RN due to time constraints and lack of resources and research skills. It is usually best to begin with a broad literature search in familiar electronic databases. Librarians are often a valuable resource when researching the literature. Several indexes, journals, and databases are available from which to begin the literature search. The following are electronic resources that place strong emphasis on evidence-based practice studies and tools. The best of these is the **Evidence-Based Medicine Reviews (EBMR)** from Ovid Technologies (http://ovid.com). EBMR is a group of several electronic databases that include MEDLINE, HealthStar, The Cochrane Library, National Guideline Clearinghouse, and the Agency for Healthcare Research and Quality (AHRQ).

MEDLINE. MEDLINE is the largest biomedical research literature database (over 10 million references) for general information. MEDLINE compiles information from Index Medicus, Index to Dental Literature, and International Nursing Index. Because of its large size, it is challenging to find a specific topic.

HealthStar. HealthStar indexes published literature on health sciences, technology, administration, and research. Its focus is on both clinical and nonclinical aspects of health care delivery. HealthStar indexes material from journals, book chapters, and government documents.

The Cochrane Library. The Cochrane Library is an electronic library designed to help make informed health care decisions. The program showcases the Cochrane Collaboration and others interested in EBP. It contains four growing databases:

- The Database of Abstracts of Reviews of Effectiveness
- The Cochrane Controlled Trials Register
- The Cochrane Review of Methodology Database
- The Cochrane Database of Systematic Reviews, which is one of the most popular databases in the Cochrane Library. It evaluates individual clinical trials and condenses systematic reviews from over 100 medical journals. The database provides an efficient method of interpreting the results of many studies. The Cochrane Library can be accessed at http://cochrane.org.

National Guideline Clearinghouse. The National Guideline Clearinghouse provides evidence-based clinical guidelines. The Clearinghouse also offers recommendations from the American Medical Association, the American Nurses Association, and the Agency for Healthcare Research and Quality, at http://guideline.gov.

Agency for Healthcare Research and Quality. The AHRQ has contributed to evidence-based practice by the establishment of 12 Evidence-Based Practice Centers (EPCs). Evidence-Based Practice Centers develop evidence guidelines and technology assessments on various clinical topics (http://ahcpr.gov).

Evaluating the strength of a study. Both the experienced RN and the new graduate lack a thorough understanding of the research process. Information literacy is a fundamental skill that the nurse must develop. *Information literacy* is defined as "the ability to recognize when information is needed and have the ability to locate, evaluate, and effectively use the information" (Information Literacy Competency Standards for Higher Education, American Library Association, 2017). As professionals and lifelong learners, nurses must become information literate. The Association of College and Research Libraries (ACRL) has a well-constructed website that provides helpful resources on information literacy. The ACRL can be accessed at http://ala.org/acrl/.

The Oncology Nursing Society (ONS) (2008) employs Sackett's (2000) method in rating the strength of the evidence. Sackett's method includes assigning hierarchy (i.e., levels) of evidence to studies based on the methodological quality of their design, validity, and applicability to patient care. Levels of evidence refer to ranking the strength of the evidence and are measured on scales of 1 to 3, 1 to 4, or 1 to 5.

Level 1 Evidence: Represents the most valid reports addressing patient-oriented outcomes. A level 1 ranking also indicates that specific quality criteria were met based on the study type.

- Randomized trials with at least 80% follow-up
- Inception cohort studies for prognostic information
- Systematic reviews of level 1 evidence reports

Level 2 Evidence: Addresses patient-oriented outcomes, using some method of scientific investigation. Level 2 evidence implies an association rather than reliable evidence. Example: hormone replacement therapy was associated with reduced cardiovascular events in large cohort studies (level 2 evidence) but was then shown not to be preventive (and to possibly increase the cardiovascular risk) in randomized trials (level 1 evidence).

- Randomized trials with less than 80% follow-up
- Nonrandomized comparison studies
- Diagnostic studies without adequate reference standards

Level 3 Evidence: Represents reports that are not based on scientific analysis of patient-oriented outcomes.

- Case series
- Case reports
- Expert opinion
- Conclusions extrapolated indirectly from scientific studies

The **systematic review** or meta-analysis of randomized controlled trials (RCTs) and evidence-based practice guidelines is considered to be the strongest level of evidence on which to guide practice. The weakest level of evidence is the opinion from authorities and/or reports of expert committees.

Critical appraisal requires knowledge of the research design and statistics. The evidence is assessed according to the strength of the evidence (Salmond, 2007). Critically appraising the evidence means to examine its validity, beginning with the overview. The overview will probably contain limited support for the conclusions. The nurse should look at the reference list to draw a conclusion regarding the validity of the study. Determining the criteria for inclusion is valuable in examining if the investigators reviewed the appropriate research.

The nurse must also review the study to ascertain if the investigators missed any relevant studies. There should be some type of notation by the researcher stating if any of the information was obtained from unpublished studies. If so, was the study's validity investigated?

Specific critical appraisal tools exist to aid the nurse in appraising research studies for each category of research study. The nurse remembers that there are three basic questions that are universal for any type of research study. Critique appraisal tools differ slightly in design and layout, but each tool asks these same questions of the research study: Is it worth looking at the results of this study? Can I trust the results (reliability)? What are the results? Are the results relevant for the patient? Duke University sponsors a free access website to an interactive online tutorial that allows the practitioner to work through an evidence-based practice scenario at http://hsl.unc.edu/Services/Tutorials/EBM.

The role of the RN is a critical link in bringing research-based changes into clinical practice (Pipe et al., 2005). The article "Implementing Evidence-Based Nursing Practice" (2005) reports the following:

> Nursing has a strong tradition of focusing on Carper's four fundamental patterns of knowing to provide excellent patient care. These four ways of knowing are (1) empirical knowing, (2) ethics, (3) personal knowing, and (4) aesthetic knowing. Empirical knowing is ideal for use in the EBP process in that it focuses on "methods" of critically appraising and applying available data and research to understand and inform clinical decision making. (p. 366)

The following critical appraisal tool has been developed by the Center for Evidence-Based Medicine and can be accessed at http://cebm.net/index. Each type of critical appraisal tool can be downloaded free of charge. This example represents the questions to ask in a systematic critical appraisal.

1. *Was the review question clearly stated?* This information can be found in the title, abstract, or final paragraph of the introduction.
2. *Is it likely that relevant studies were missed?* Did the search strategy include both Medical Subject Headings (MeSH) terms and text words? The methods section should describe the search strategy. The results section will outline the number of studies retrieved, excluded, and why.
3. *Were the criteria used to select articles for inclusion appropriate?* The eligibility criteria used should be specific regarding the patients, interventions, exposures, and outcomes of interest. This information can be found in the methods section.
4. *Were the included studies sufficiently valid for the type of question asked?* The article should describe how the quality of each article was assessed. The methods section

should describe the assessment quality and the criteria used. The results section should provide information on the quality of the individual study.

5. *Were the results similar from study to study?* The results of the study should be similar or homogeneous. The results section should state whether the results are heterogeneous and discuss possible reasons.

6. *What are the results?* Systematic reviews should provide a summary of the data **(evidence summary)** from the results of a number of studies.

LIMITATIONS OF EVIDENCE-BASED PRACTICE

The literature supports the apparent lag time from research to application. Many countries have conducted primarily quantitative studies to explore the reasons for this finding. The following list describes the most common barriers cited in a presentation by Janet Bingle (2007).

The Evidence

- Accessibility by the end user (nurse); inadequate access to clinical researched evidence and guidelines
- Large volume of research to sift through
- The research language
- Complex data retrieval systems

The Individual

- Resistant to change

The Health Care System

- Systemic barriers such as policies, procedures, and financial accountability
- Physician idiosyncrasy versus disciplined inquiry
- Cost/benefit issues
- Bureaucratic structures

Nursing

- Split between education and service (lack of time)
- Lack of consensus about nursing responsibilities
- Lack of communication among nurses and researchers
- Lack of skills in locating, reading, and appraising nursing research data
- Lack of organizational support

Nurses should be active on patient care, quality improvement, and policy and procedures committees. Participation on these committees allows the nurse to function as advocate, change agent, and disseminator of information to peers, patient, family, and hospital administrators.

The RN should also understand that sound nursing judgment has its basis in scientifically tested rationale. For the RN to utilize research in his or her practice, he or she should have a basic understanding of the investigational process and how it applies to practice. Estabrooks (1999), in conducting a literature search, reports numerous studies that called for nursing to be research-based. The author concludes that RNs had difficulty applying research to practice, which is using the scientific process to gain knowledge that has direct application to the practice of nursing or health care. This is not to say that all nurses must conceive of and conduct new research, but certainly all nurses need the ability and the empowerment to appropriately institute change based on research findings. The RN must base specific interventions and all aspects of the nursing process on scientific research.

APPARENT GAPS IN RESEARCH UTILIZATION

Carroll and colleagues (1997) and Mackay (1998) report on the apparent gap in research and research utilization by nurses. Carroll and colleagues suggest that nurses have a lack of knowledge of the availability of research applicable to nursing practice. They also suggest that nurses lack educational preparedness to understand research, which is an apparent barrier to research utilization.

Mackay has suggested several other barriers to research utilization by nurses, including lack of support from administration and lack of the authority to institute changes based on research. In some instances, there is no forum in which research-based practice change proposals can surface and there exists no clear method of launching a trial. In an age where most staff nurses are pressed to the limits of time and energy already, incorporating research into practice often falls to the convenience of tradition. This apparent dichotomy with regard to research utilization frustrates the RN faced with decisions about patient care.

Research, Both Simple and Necessary

The simplest research the RN will take part in is **quality assurance** (QA) **or performance improvement** (PI) studies, which use data to determine whether patient outcome criteria are being met, charting is complete, or procedures are being done per protocol. The result of these studies is to assist the staff in achieving consistently excellent quality care. Problems in these studies provoke questions that may be answered through the scientific approach.

COMPONENTS AND PROCESS IN A RESEARCH STUDY

Research as a discipline has its own methodology and terminology that may seem confusing at first. An RN who has learned to read research critically and understand how it may be applied to the clinical setting will be able to exercise better clinical judgment in planning and implementing the nursing process. Components of a research study, at a basic level, include concepts, variables, and a literature search. From these flows an elementary research process.

Concepts

Basic research is the process of refining a **concept,** which is an abstract idea taken from an observed behavior or characteristic so as to make it usable or applicable. Consider the behavior of a patient exhibiting pain. The concept is *pain,* which is defined uniquely by the individual and manifested by the behavior. The pain is an abstraction because another individual cannot experience it in the same way. The concept of pain can be studied as a means to better understand similarities and differences in multiple patients' manifestations of pain. The research attempts to define pain in terms of common behaviors, refining the concept so it can be applied to a population of people rather than just an individual.

Variables

Types of Variables

A **variable** is a concept, idea, or attribute that is captured and defined within a research study. Variables are so named because they vary from subject to subject, as with height and weight, propensity to exercise, and personal preferences. Variables are the unique characteristics between one human being and another. Another example of a variable is people's environment, which varies from point to point, from minute to minute, and from day to day. When conducting research, the researcher attempts to control the variables, statistically account for them, or explain them in relation to what is being studied.

Two types of variables are found in research studies: active and attribute variables. The researcher is attempting to manipulate an **active variable** in an attempt to determine whether this will have the desired effect on the outcome. The researcher has no control over an **attribute variable.** For example, determining the type of dressing most likely to improve patient outcomes would require the RN researcher to study the differences between at least two types of dressings. The dressings would be randomly used on different patients, with one group receiving one type and another receiving the second type. The dressings would be the active variable because the researcher is manipulating them. The attribute variables would be the condition of the patients, their sex, and other preexisting characteristics over which the researcher does not have control.

In addition, the researcher makes a distinction between a variable that influences a presumed effect, called the **independent variable,** and a variable that is influenced, called the **dependent variable** (Exercise 8.1). The purpose of the research study is to determine the apparent relationship between the independent variable and the dependent variable. For example, imagine a study looking at length of stay of patients with a certain disorder. The interest is in understanding why patients have varying lengths of stay (dependent variable) and the apparent

---

? EXERCISE 8.1

Upon completion of this activity, student will be able to conduct a critical appraisal using the evidence-based practice process. Follow the directions below to begin this activity.

1. Read the article "A Systematic Review of the Effectiveness of Antimicrobial Rinse-Free Hand Sanitizers for Prevention of Illness-Related Absenteeism in Elementary School Children." A complete electronic version of this article can be freely accessed online at http://biomedcentral.com/1471-2458/4/50.
2. Use the Systematic Review in Chart 8.1 to evaluate the article.

Courtesy of Centre for Evidence-Based Medicine, Old Road Campus, Headington, Oxford, U.K. Website accessible at http://biomed.lib.umn.edu/learn/ebp/index.html.

CHART 8.1 SYSTEMATIC REVIEW: ARE THE RESULTS OF THE REVIEW VALID?

WHAT QUESTION (PICO) DID THE SYSTEMATIC REVIEW ADDRESS?

WHAT IS BEST?	WHERE DO I FIND THE INFORMATION?
The main question being addressed should be clearly stated. The exposure, such as a therapy or diagnostic test, and the outcome(s) of interest will often be expressed in terms of a simple relationship.	The *Title, Abstract,* or *final paragraph of the Introduction* should clearly state the question. If you still cannot ascertain what the focused question is after reading these sections, search for another paper!

This paper: Yes □ No □ Unclear □

Comment:

IS IT UNLIKELY THAT IMPORTANT, RELEVANT STUDIES WERE MISSED?

WHAT IS BEST?	WHERE DO I FIND THE INFORMATION?
The starting point for comprehensive search for all relevant studies is the major bibliographic databases (e.g., MEDLINE, Cochrane, EMBASE) but should also include a search of reference lists from relevant studies and contact with experts, particularly to inquire about unpublished studies. The search should not be limited to the English language only. The search strategy should include both MESH terms and text words.	The *Methods* section should describe the search strategy, including the terms used, in some detail. The *Results* section will outline the number of titles and abstracts reviewed, the number of full-text studies retrieved, and the number of studies excluded, together with the reasons for exclusion. This information may be presented in a figure or flowchart.

This paper: Yes □ No □ Unclear □

Comment:

WERE THE CRITERIA USED TO SELECT ARTICLES FOR INCLUSION APPROPRIATE?

WHAT IS BEST?	WHERE DO I FIND THE INFORMATION?
The inclusion or exclusion of studies in a systematic review should be clearly defined a priori. The eligibility criteria used should specify the patients, interventions, or exposures and outcomes of interest. In many cases, the type of study design will also be a key component of the eligibility criteria.	The *Methods* section should describe in detail the inclusion and exclusion criteria. Normally, this will include the study design.

This paper: Yes □ No □ Unclear □

Comment:

CHART 8.1   SYSTEMATIC REVIEW: ARE THE RESULTS OF THE REVIEW VALID?—cont'd

WERE THE INCLUDED STUDIES SUFFICIENTLY VALID FOR THE TYPE OF QUESTION ASKED?

WHAT IS BEST?	WHERE DO I FIND THE INFORMATION?
The article should describe how the quality of each study was assessed using predetermined quality criteria appropriate to the type of clinical question (e.g., randomization, blinding and completeness of follow-up).	The *Methods* section should describe the assessment of quality and the criteria used. The *Results* section should provide information on the quality of the individual studies.

This paper: Yes ☐ No ☐ Unclear ☐

Comment:

WERE THE RESULTS SIMILAR FROM STUDY TO STUDY?

WHAT IS BEST?	WHERE DO I FIND THE INFORMATION?
Ideally, the results of the different studies should be similar or homogeneous. If heterogeneity exists, the authors may estimate whether the differences are significant (chi-square test). Possible reasons for the heterogeneity should be explored.	The *Results* section should state whether the results are heterogeneous and discuss possible reasons. The forest plot should show the results of the chi-square test for heterogeneity and, if present, then discuss reasons for heterogeneity.

This paper: Yes ☐ No ☐ Unclear ☐

Comment:

What were the results?

How are the results presented?

Courtesy of Centre for Evidence-Based Medicine, Old Road Campus, Headington, Oxford, U.K. Website accessible at www.biomed.lib.umn.edu/learn/ebp/index.html.

---

causative factor (independent variable) for the differences. If the researcher notes a specific problem that seems to cause the increased length of stay, this problem will be designated as an independent variable to see whether an actual relationship exists. The researcher may also spin off further research to see whether the length of stay might be the reason for patients to have specific problems. Here the dependent variable would be the problem the patients are having, and the independent variable would be the length of stay.

Defining Variables

In an attempt to control the research as much as possible, the researcher defines the variables. The "tighter" the definitions are, the more precise the research can be. An **operational definition** of a variable specifies the operations associated with collecting the data on that variable, or how the researcher will measure the variable. These operational definitions are expected to be firm so the researcher can formulate a tight research project. The researcher who is going to measure weight as one of the dependent or independent variables must determine whether the weight will be in grams or pounds as well as the type and manufacturer of the scale. The researcher may also need to define when weighing will be conducted, such as a specific time each day or before or after a particular procedure. Thus, the variable—weighing time—becomes a unique entity to the particular study and is controlled as much as possible through the operational definition so as to account for discrepancies that might occur.

When the operational definition is too tight, it might interfere with generalizing the research results in practice. For example, a researcher describes a specific instrument that was used to affect an outcome that is available only for this study. The study supports the usefulness of the instrument to assist the patient to wellness, but because the instrument is not widely available, the findings have little value except to the original researcher.

Literature Search

As part of the conceptualization of the study, the researcher does a literature search to determine whether prior research has been done on the defined problem. The literature search can also identify past research that can be transferred to the current situation. The literature search can assist in defining the variables, formulating a hypothesis, establishing tools that may be needed to collect data, and clarifying the problem. It may define the theory or identify additional variables that may need to be considered or controlled. The literature search will also suggest areas that are not as well supported by research. Once the research is completed, the literature search serves to support the findings.

RESEARCH PROCESS

FYI 8.1 lists the steps in the research process. This section provides a detailed discussion of each step.

Making Predictions

The researcher begins the process of research by making an assumption as to the relationship between the dependent variable and the independent variable. Such assumptions are turned into a **hypothesis,** which is a written prediction made by the researcher with regard to the variables. It directs the research by setting limits to the study because the researcher will try to prove or disprove the prediction. Generally, the hypothesis results from a question the researcher has with regard to a specific concept. These questions often come from practice situations where **empirical data,** or objective evidence, would suggest a relationship between the variables. The research is designed to gain as much control as possible to determine whether a relationship exists. The following is an example of a hypothesis:

Menopausal women who include 40 mg of isolated soy protein in their daily diets report fewer hot flashes and more uninterrupted sleep than those whose diet contains no isolated soy protein.

⚖ FYI 8.1   STEPS IN THE RESEARCH PROCESS

Making predictions. From empirical data within the clinical setting or from reading professional journals, the researcher notices patterns and then makes inferences and hypotheses about cause and effect or comes up with questions.

Defining the research study. The researcher outlines how best to ascertain the answers to the questions regarding observations.

Defining the population. From the questions, the researcher selects who or what can benefit from the research.

Selecting a sample. The researcher defines a representational model that will reflect the larger population being studied.

Making a data collection plan. The researcher determines the method by which data will be collected, including the tools, instruments, machines, and research design.

Checking reliability and validity. The researcher applies certain criteria to test whether instruments, tools, machines, and research designs will give accurate results to the questions or hypothesis being studied.

Collecting data. The researcher or designated assistants collect data.

Interpreting the results. With statistical programs that minimize the effects of variables beyond control, the researcher gives meaning to the data that have been collected.

Communicating the results. The information gained through the research is disseminated to those who can best utilize the findings.

Defining the Research Study

Research can be approached or conducted in several ways, which are formulated in the **research design.** Research can be either experimental, where the researcher actively participates by introducing an intervention, or nonexperimental, where the researcher observes a situation and collects data without introducing an intervention. **Experimental design** controls the independent variables and randomly assigns the subjects to study groups. The random assignment helps explain some of the variables not actually being manipulated by the researchers. **Quasi-experimental design** varies from experimental design in that the researcher does not attempt to randomize the subjects but does attempt to show a relationship between the dependent and independent variables.

Defining the Population

Once the research design is selected, the researcher defines the **population** to be studied. The population chosen is one that will potentially benefit from the study results. For example, the researcher may identify a need for a policy to make an automatic referral to a lactation consultant for all first-time mothers planning on breastfeeding. The researcher believes this will increase the number of successful breastfeeding attempts and would like to design a study to identify the cost-benefit relationship. The population would be defined to include first-time mothers who choose to breastfeed and agree to enter into the study and exclude subjects who are not first-time mothers. By defining the population in such a way, the researcher attempts to exclude variables that may influence the outcomes, such as previous experience with breastfeeding.

Selecting a Sample

Sample selection is the process of determining a representational model of the entire population on which data can be easily or realistically collected. For example, in a research study on the circulatory problems that lead to foot ulcers in diabetics, trying to look at the entire population of diabetics would be unrealistic. If a cross section of diabetic patients with various characteristics representative of the entire population could be studied, then the sample would be statistically strong. The **sample size** is determined through statistics that take into account general characteristics of the population in question and give a probability number that will closely account for the varied characteristics within the sample size. The sample size might be 50 or 100 subjects, or it could be 1000 or more subjects, but it needs to be within the resources of the researcher.

In addition, inferences may be made about how the variable relationships can be generalized to subjects not defined within the population. These generalizations tend to suggest areas for further study, which can assist in refining the original hypothesis and making research utilization applicable to greater numbers of subjects within the population.

Making a Data Collection Plan

The researcher develops a plan to collect data that includes the method, the necessary tools, the people designated to collect the data, and any training needed. A **quantitative study** asks the question who, what, why, where, when, or how and attempts to describe the relationship between one variable and another. A quantitative study plan is highly structured and controlled. A **qualitative study** attempts to clarify underlying assumptions that are vague or unclear by asking what the perceptions, beliefs, or tenets are within a particular setting. A qualitative study is loosely structured and allows more subjective input from both the researcher and the subjects. Often qualitative studies generate questions for quantitative study. Among the tools used to collect data are self-reports, surveys, questionnaires, graphs, and unique designs specifically developed to measure a variable.

Generally, the researcher conducts a pilot study to work out unforeseen problems with the main study or the study tools and determine whether the research is feasible. The pilot study may include a small part of the population and may include ways to determine whether the tools are measuring what they are expected to measure or whether any instrument that the researcher uses is impractical.

Checking Reliability and Validity

Reliability and validity are criteria that researchers use to test whether instruments, tools, machines, and research designs will give accurate results with the questions or hypotheses being studied. **Reliability** measures the device or technique, or the instrument, the researcher uses to collect data by asking how trustworthy it is at gathering the intended data. The researcher would not want to use an instrument with low reliability because it would skew the results of the study. The instrument could be a questionnaire, interview technique, observation, or test or machines, monitors, scales, or other devices or methods. Several tests for reliability, stability, consistency, and equivalence exist, and the results are reported as decimals, such as "0.89 internal consistency." An example of a test for reliability would be to use an external monitor to record venous oxygen saturation. If the external monitor consistently recorded venous oxygen saturation within 1% or 2% of venous blood draws or another machine with a proven record of reliability, then the research instrument would have a high degree of reliability.

Validity measures the degree to which an instrument is measuring what it is supposed to measure. Validity has various aspects, such as content validity, criterion-related validity, and construct validity. Validity can be difficult to measure with accuracy, and the researcher may settle for a specific level of validity. For example, a researcher may be testing whether a correlation exists between the Apgar scores of newborns and tachypnea of newborns. The researcher will document the tested validity report of the Apgar scoring instrument as an indication of the validity of the new study. Consistency in how the Apgar score is assigned must also be considered as part of the validity study.

Collecting Data

Once the sample has been defined and selected and the instrument proposed, the process of collecting data begins. Data collection within an institution needs to be approved by the research review committee of the health care organization. A research report will include the approval of the committee as well as any patient consent forms that may be needed. Ethical and legal issues raised by the research must be considered and addressed before the actual collection of the data. A research report generally mentions the ways subject rights were protected.

Interpreting the Results

Once the data have been collected, the researcher interprets the results, which requires providing information on how the data were analyzed, what limitations were identified, and how the results support the hypothesis. A formal statistical analysis is able to assist the researchers in identifying how close the data came to demonstrating a statistically significant relationship between the variables. In addition, the results are examined for how they may apply to the larger population as well as the study population. Often further research questions are asked due to the outcomes or to limitations that are discovered.

Communicating the Results

Communicating the results so nurses will be able to use the findings in their practice is the final step. Research summaries may be submitted for publication, including a section that demonstrates how the research will apply to nursing. This application may be implied, or it may be stated clearly. If implied, the interpretation of the results will need to be made by the reader of the research article. The use of the information by the RN will require thoughtful consideration.

RESEARCH UTILIZATION

The RN is expected to follow certain policies and procedures when acting as a manager of care. The standard of care expectation is that these policies and procedures be based on scientific research. The RN should recognize situations in which clinical judgment might be required, and in such situations research-based decisions will have better outcomes than decisions based on tradition. The RN should also be aware of how research can affect the nursing process, requiring the RN to read research articles critically. The RN can take a research course, attend continuing education classes on research, or read research textbooks to better understand the research process. Utilization of research does not necessarily require the RN to be proficient at conducting research. It does require RNs to make a sound judgment as to the reliability and validity of the research and ultimately make the decision as to whether to include the findings in one's practice.

Validating Research Results

Some basic steps should be followed in order to identify whether a research report is valid and can be used to make a change in thinking or support a clinical judgment regarding patient care. The first step is to understand the terminology of research. Familiarization with the definitions and examples allows the RN to read the research articles with more understanding. The second step is to conduct a literature search, identifying other research that has been done in the problem area. Ovid and MEDLINE provide access to nursing and allied health journals. Medical libraries in hospitals, as well as medical universities, have online access to both Ovid and MEDLINE.

Actual research reports contain all components of the research, reporting on the problem, variables, research design, population, and sample, as well as results, discussion, and the application to practice. A journal article may report on original research or on literature search findings. Articles reporting on literature searches do not give complete pictures of each research study but rather summarize the results of several studies. The RN should read the original research reports to decide whether the interpretations are accurate or useful. Generally, articles accepted by nursing or allied health journals that have a peer review or juried acceptance process will have credible research. Even so, the RN should still critically read in order to determine whether the research has applications to practice.

Applying Research to Practice

After reading research, the RN should put into practice what he or she has learned. Estabrooks (1999) suggests that an RN in the practice setting can utilize research in three main ways:

1. *Direct research utilization* is the use of research knowledge to actually change a practice habit or include a new intervention in your practice. Direct utilization of research by the RN would constitute a personal commitment to change for the betterment of the practice. The RN would actively and critically read research to find new ways to implement patient care that is safer and promotes positive patient outcomes. An example would be to find research on a particular nursing intervention, such as a new technique to start IVs in children that reduces pain and gains more trust. The RN who begins to use the intervention has directly utilized research to effect a change in practice.

2. *Indirect research utilization* is when the RN has a new conceptual understanding of situations or treatments based on knowledge of current research. Enhancing the

knowledge base is a direct result of indirect research utilization. If the RN is able to identify a new patient problem as a result of reading a research article, the RN is utilizing research to enhance assessment of the patient's response to the illness or treatment. The greater knowledge gained by the scientific approach has increased the RN's critical thinking abilities and should create positive outcomes as a result. The RN should be better able to plan patient care with clear rationales.

3. *Persuasive research utilization* is the process of advocating for a change in policy or procedure, behavioral change of an individual, or a change in the way things are normally done, based on research awareness. For example, working on a committee that is updating policies and procedures, the RN may advocate a specific policy change based on research. The RN must recognize the need to read and incorporate research into practice, which is becoming a practice standard. The RN should follow and understand policies and procedures but also know that even policies and procedures must be research-based. If the RN is aware of policies and procedures that are not current to practice standards, then it is time to advocate change. The RN can begin by giving the unit manager a written report summarizing the research findings and including a proposal for change. The RN can also propose to run a research study that will demonstrate the benefits of the change in policy. In this way the staff RN can play an important role in developing research.

Read the scenario in Exercise 8.2 and answer the questions concerning the three ways to utilize research.

Identifying Areas for Research

The staff nurse is aware of empirical data (i.e., objective evidence from clinical observations) gathered from patient care experiences. Such experiences are often the basis for research questions. Staff RNs may be recruited to take part in the study through data gathering or testing new procedures or products. Encouraging all nurses to bring research into their daily practice will ultimately help improve patient care.

---

⑦ EXERCISE 8.2

On a particular medical-surgical floor, many patients are being admitted who have decubitus ulcers, also known as pressure ulcers. The risk factors for developing pressure ulcers have been widely studied and disseminated in literature as well as in educational arenas.

In admission assessments, the RN decides to begin including assessing for pressure ulcer risk factors in each of the patients admitted to the unit. If the RN compiled assessment data that supported the research findings on risk factors for decubitus ulcer formation, it will also lend credence to the RN's original clinical judgment. Critical thinking skills are improved, and the RN is better able to plan care that meets the holistic needs of the patient. The RN then takes the information gathered during the assessment of several patients at risk for decubitus ulcers, along with research findings in the literature, and persuades management to change the admission forms to include a standard decubitus ulcer risk assessment.

1. In this scenario, which would be direct, indirect, and persuasive uses of research?
2. Give another example of direct, indirect, and persuasive uses of research that you would utilize within your practice.

KEY POINTS

After completion of this chapter, you have learned:

- Evidence-based practice requires a paradigm shift on the part of the RN and the health care institution.
- The current paradigm of traditional clinical practice based on intuition, clinical experience, and pathophysiological methods of treatment must be transformed to reflect clinical expertise that is integrated with the best scientific evidence, patient values and preferences, and clinical circumstances.
- The intent of EBP is to improve patient outcomes by evaluating and tracking outcomes, including qualitative reports by patients.
- The ANCC development of the Magnet Recognition Program is a positive step in challenging every health care practitioner to provide excellent patient outcomes through the application of excellent, proactive patient care.
- Research utilization is a practice standard, and the RN who knows how to read and interpret research will gain the knowledge needed to make better clinical judgments.
- Striving for excellence in nursing is a worthy goal, and gaining knowledge is one way to attain excellence.
- The RN must have a basic foundation in research utilization to best meet the needs of patients.
- Knowledge that has its foundation in scientific study will assist the RN in making optimal clinical judgments as well as formulating a sound plan of care.

CRITICAL THINKING QUESTIONS

1. Should it be mandatory for health care facilities to achieve and maintain credentialing by the American Nurses Credentialing Center (ANCC)? If so, what would be the advantages or disadvantages for the patient as well as the nursing staff?
2. What factors would need to be considered when utilizing the PICO format to develop a well-built clinical question for an elderly patient with heart failure and a normal heart rhythm, who is receiving Digoxin therapy with the possibility of a diuretic being added?
3. A 42-year-old woman presents in the emergency department with shortness of breath and diffuse chest pain. You suspect that she may have a clot in her lung (a pulmonary embolism). Which is more effective at ruling out pulmonary emboli: pulmonary angiography or a ventilation perfusion scan (V/Q scan)? Based on this scenario, write your own well-built clinical question.
4. A traditional nursing intervention has been to conduct daily weights on patients between the hours of 4:00 and 6:00 AM.
   a. If the nursing staff notices that patients with ordered daily weights showed less satisfaction compared with patients who did not have daily weights, what questions would need to be asked with regard to the relationship between the time of the daily weights and patient satisfaction?
   b. Conduct a literature search to see whether any research studies are related to the time of day when weights must be done; patient satisfaction and the traditional time for daily weights; and nurses' perceptions of the need for weights at a specific time.

5. Pick a policy or procedure in a health care agency and note whether research citations exist within its rationale statement. If no citation exists, conduct a literature search of research that would either support the policy or procedure or suggest the need for change. How would this information affect the standard of care as interpreted within the policy or procedure?

6. Medication A is ordered to be given to a pediatric patient with an acute asthma attack. The physician has ordered the dose to be 250 mg q6h around the clock. The recommended dosage for pediatric patients is to receive 50 mg/kg/24 hr in divided doses qid.
   a. For a patient who weighs 30 lb, what is the recommended dose?
   b. Is the ordered dose within safe limits?
   c. What type of research utilization would be best for advocating for a patient with a physician who consistently ignores recommended medication doses?
   d. How would you communicate your findings to the physician in a professional manner?

7. After reading the following scenarios, generate a PICO for each:
   a. On average, across the United States the childhood obesity rates are falling for the first time; however, in one large metropolitan school district the rates are found to be on the rise. The school district in question currently meets only minimum requirements for physical activity during the school day for elementary age children. The nurse believes that the children in her school would benefit from having a full hour of structured, physical play activities; after a year, she expects to see the obesity rate fall for the children of her school.
   b. Statistics demonstrate that new nurses leave the profession at an alarming rate after only the first 6 months after graduation, and in one specific acute care facility the nurse educator recognizes that the rate is quite high. In this facility, they offer only an 8-week precepted orientation, after which the new nurse functions independently with an assignment. The nurse educator believes that a new nurse residency that is graduated and structured, lasting 6 months, will decrease the attrition rate for new grad new hires after 1 year.
   c. The educators for a two-hospital system have historically educated the nurses on the use of new dressings for pressure ulcer treatment at one facility in a face to face format with a supervised hands-on practice, while at the other facilty, nurses watch the live presentation via web conference and have product samples available to examine, but without supervised practice. It was found that after the educational sessions use of the new dressings was consistent with best practice at the facility that got to see the demonstrations face to face and practice using the products with the educator physically present. Whereas at the other facility, the new products were rarely used or were used ineffectively.
   d. In a rural county, it was found that newly diagnosed type 2 diabetics were poorly managing their disease even though they were provided appropriate education at the clinic during their visits. The clinic educator believes that offering a community-based series of educational presentations for their clients would improve compliance with disease self-management.

WEB RESOURCES

http://ninr.nih.gov
http://ahrq.gov/about/nursing
http://nursingcenter.com/home/index.asp
http://cochrane.org
http://nursecredentialing.org/Magnet.aspx

REFERENCES

American Library Association. (2017). *Information literacy competency standards for higher education*. Retrieved from http://ala.org/acrl/standards/informationliteracycompetency.

American Nurses Credentialing Center. (2017). *Magnet recognition program overview*. Retrieved from http://www.nursecredentialing.org/Magnet/ProgramOverview.

American Nurses Credentialing Center. (2017). *Find a magnet hospital*. Retrieved from http://nursecredentialing.org/Magnet/FindaMagnetFacility.

Bingle, J. (2007). *Creating a culture for evidence-based nursing practice*. Community Health Network, Indiana. Retrieved from http://google.com/url?sa=t&rct=j&q=&esrc=s&frm=1&source=web&cd=3&ved=0CCwQFjAC&url=http%3A%2F%2Firhaweb.ehost-services159.com%2F3%2520-Jan%2520Bingle%2520Presentation%2520-%25202007%2520Plainfield%2520In.ppt&ei=cLh1UMbCD4mIqQGUkoCgAQ&usg=AFQjCNHS9HM237LL6GZOvCuc06w7-qIbpw.

Carroll, D. L., Greenwood, R., Lynch, K. E., Sullivan, J. K., Ready, C. H., & Fitzmaurice, J. B. (1997). Barriers and facilitators to the utilization of nursing research. *Clinical Nurse Specialist, 11*(5), 207–212.

Cassey, M. Z. (2007). Incorporating the National Guideline Clearinghouse into evidence-based nursing practice. *Nursing Economics, 25*(5). Retrieved from http://ncbi.nlm.nih.gov/pubmed/18080629.

Estabrooks, C. A. (1999). The conceptual structure of research utilization. *Research in Nursing & Health, 22*(3), 203–216.

Gilbert, R., Salanti, G., Harden, M., & See, S. (2005). Infant sleeping position and the sudden infant death syndrome: systematic review of observational studies and historical review of recommendations from 1940 to 2002. *International Journal of Epidemiology, 34*(4), 874–887.

Guyatt, G., Meade, M. O., Jaeschke, R., Cook, D., & Haynes, R. B. (2000). Practitioners of evidence based care. *British Medical Journal, 310*, 934–935. Retrieved from http://bmj.com/content/320/7240/954.

Mackay, M. H. (1998). Research utilization and the CNS: confronting the issues. *Clinical Nurse Specialist, 12*(6), 232–237.

Pipe, T. B., Wellik, K. E., Buchda, V. L., & Hansen, C. M. (2005). Implementing evidence-based practice. *Urology Nursing, 25*(5), 365–370. Retrieved from http://medscape.com/viewarticle/514532.

Sackett, D. L., Straus, S. E., Richardson, W. S., Rosenberg, W., & Haynes, R. B. (2000). Evidence-based medicine. In *How to practice and teach evidence-based medicine* (pp. 1–35). Edinburgh, Scotland: Churchill Livingstone.

Salmond, S. (2007). Advancing evidence based practice: a primer. *Orthopedic Nursing, 26*(2), 114–123. Retrieved from http://ncbi.nlm.nih.gov/pubmed/17414381.

The Oncology Nursing Society. (2008). *ONS evidence-based author guidelines*. Retrieved from http://ons.org/Publications/Books/AuthorGuidelines.

University of Alaska, Anchorage, Consortium Library. (n.d.). *Evidence based practice*. Retrieved from http://consortiumlibrary.org/aml/researchaids/ebp/.

CHAPTER 9

Communicating with Patients and Co-Workers

⊖volve WEBSITE

Additional resources are available online at:
http://evolve.elsevier.com/Claywell/transitions

OBJECTIVES

After completing this chapter, you will be prepared to:

1. Describe the principles of communication.
2. State the purpose of the therapeutic relationship and apply therapeutic communication to the clinical setting.
3. Compare and contrast facilitators and blockers of communication.
4. Conduct a patient interview in the clinical setting utilizing effective communication skills and active listening.
5. Respect the cultural diversity among individuals.
6. Appreciate the value of collaborative communication in the health care environment.
7. Utilize SBAR to assertively communicate with co-workers within the health care team to minimize risks associated with handoffs.
8. Discuss delegation in terms of effective communication.
9. Demonstrate effective communication skills to resolve conflict in the health care setting.

KEY TERMS

active listening
collaboration
communication blocker
communication facilitator
conflict
cultural competence
delegation

documentation
empathy
health literacy
nonverbal communication
nurse–patient
  relationship

nurse–physician
  relationship
SBAR
TeamSTEPPS
therapeutic
  communication

OVERVIEW

Communication is an integral part of the role of the registered nurse. The exchange and recording of essential information are fundamental and must be completed with clarity and precision. Competent communication is a professional standard of practice for the RN. As an RN, you will need to delegate duties, collaborate with members of the interdisciplinary team, and confer with individuals involved in patient care. As a patient advocate, you must be able to assess the patient's understanding of treatment options, assess the disease process and prognosis, assist the patient in understanding his or her own health concerns, and understand how to use therapeutic communication to assist the patient and others in coping with their concerns or problems. This chapter addresses ways to improve communication skills and provides opportunities to learn the importance of effective and culturally competent communication.

Communication, like any skill, has elements and principles. Good communication evolves by practicing correct principles and using the elements appropriately. Recognizing this, plan to refer to your past experiences in applying the new knowledge you will gain about communication.

COMMUNICATION BASICS

VERBAL AND NONVERBAL COMMUNICATION

Communication is the interaction between two or more individuals in which an exchange of information occurs. For communication to occur, an expression from one individual (sender) must be received by at least one other (receiver) (Varcarolis & Halter, 2010).

All interactions consist of both verbal (content) and **nonverbal** (process) messages. Verbal (or spoken) communication is the symbol by which we communicate our beliefs, values, perceptions, meanings, ideas, desires, feelings, and understanding. This is our primary means of expression.

How we communicate is as important as what we communicate. For instance, tone, pitch, inflection, and the intensity of how we speak all affect how messages are communicated. These are nonverbal behaviors. Other examples of **nonverbal communication** include body behaviors (posture, body movements), facial expressions (frowning, smiling), personal appearance (grooming, dress), eye contact (direct or indirect), eye cast (angry, suspicious), and physical characteristics (height, weight) (Varcarolis & Halter, 2010). Nonverbal behaviors also include how we listen and how we use silence, touch, and space. It has been estimated that approximately 10% of communication is verbal, whereas from 70% to 90% is nonverbal. As a general rule, we are more aware of our verbal messages than we are of nonverbal ones. When verbal communication agrees with nonverbal communication, the message is clearer. Take, for example, the patient you are assessing for pain. If the patient tells you he or she is having no pain while guarding an area and grimacing, the message is not congruent. If the patient is experiencing an impaired ability to communicate, such as in the case of intubation, aphasia, a voice problem, dysarthria, or a hearing problem, the RN should find an alternate means to communicate. Nonverbal behavior must be interpreted within the context of a patient's culture, gender, age, sexual orientation, and spiritual concerns.

✗ Know Def.

Therapeutic Communication

Hospitalization can be stressful and anxiety provoking for patients and families. When a nurse engages in a helping relationship with a patient and family, therapeutic communication is at the heart of the interaction. During the interviewing process, the patient may disclose a number of concerns. The RN should try to understand such concerns with sensitivity. **Therapeutic communication** and the establishment of the therapeutic relationship require empathy, genuineness, positive regard, and self-awareness. **Empathy** is the ability to accurately perceive the patient's needs, feelings, and situation. Sympathy, on the other hand, implies pity. Carl Rogers (1961), an American psychologist, said that real communication occurs when we listen with understanding, see the situation from the other person's point of view, and empathize and achieve their frame of reference; he believes the major barrier to interpersonal communication is our tendency to judge, evaluate, approve, or disapprove. Genuineness refers to having self-awareness of your feelings and the ability to meet person-to-person in a therapeutic relationship.

Positive regard implies respect and a willingness to work with the patient and communicate (through your actions) that the patient is a person worthy of caring about. Finally, you must be able to suspend value judgments. According to Varcarolis and Halter (2010), we can take the following steps to eliminate judgmental thinking and behaviors:

- Recognize its presence.
- Identify how or where we learned these responses to the patient's behavior.
- Construct alternative ways to view the patient's thinking and behavior.

An angry, hurting, or grieving patient may be confrontational, passive, highly emotional, or crying uncontrollably. Even though outward demonstrations of emotions may be directed at health care workers, the actual emotions may be a result of the patient's perception of how the health care concerns are affecting his or her life. In a situation where a patient is directing anger at the RN or other health care workers, maintaining silence, nodding in acknowledgment of the anger, and seeking clarification through careful questioning can bring about understanding of the reason behind the behavior. Health care workers must avoid taking negative patient behavior personally. Mastering therapeutic communication principles and techniques requires an awareness of the factors that can contribute to effective or ineffective therapeutic communication (FYI 9.1).

FYI 9.1 PHRASES THAT ILLUSTRATE THERAPEUTIC COMMUNICATION

- Tell me more about . . .
- I heard you say . . .
- You sound angry (sad, hurt, anxious). Can you tell me about it?
- I understand you want (need, feel) . . .
- It must be hard for you to tell me how you are feeling.
- Sometimes when I feel sad (angry, anxious, hurt), I find myself. . . . Is that how you see it as well?

Communication Facilitators

Communication facilitators are factors that enhance effective communication. The nurse must project warmth, acceptance, friendliness, openness, empathy, and respect in all interactions with the patient and family. Another communication facilitator is providing for the privacy, confidentiality, and comfort of the patient. Be mindful of the pace of your words and actions. In addition, appropriate humor and touch can help foster a closer nurse–patient relationship; however, remember that touching can be interpreted in a number of ways. The nurse should *always* ask permission before touching a patient.

Active Listening

One of the most important skills an RN can master is the skill of **active listening.** Active listening is attentive to the patient's verbal and nonverbal communication and establishes trust (Townsend, 2012). One of the most common errors we make when listening is thinking about what we are going to say next. The RN has many time constraints, duties, and decisions to make. These will often be on the nurse's mind when approaching a patient. Active listening requires an open mind and full concentration to hear what the patient is saying and requires clarification and verification of messages. Use questions that seek clarification: "You told the doctor about. . . . What more can you tell me?" "I'm not sure I understand. . . . Would you please explain a little more?" "You say your pain is in your chest. How would you describe the pain?"

Patients need to perceive that they are understood in order to feel connected. A strained posture, poor eye contact, or constant distracting movements or habits, such as chewing gum or jingling pocket change, would communicate lack of interest in what the patient is saying. Nodding your head, using empathy, and acknowledging the patient will demonstrate that you are interested in what the patient has to say. Using open-ended questions will elicit a more substantive response compared with a closed-ended question where the patient is likely to just answer "yes" or "no."

Communication Blockers

A **communication blocker** tends to stop conversation and build mistrust. Condescending language can also block conversation. Questioning a patient's reasons rather than accepting them will block therapeutic communication. "Why" questions or those that challenge the patient—such as "Why did you do that?" or "Did you really do that?"—are considered to be blockers. Instead, try saying, "I'm having a hard time understanding. Can you please clarify for me just how this happened?" Asking questions in this manner encourages the patient and family to share openly. Nonjudgmental acceptance of the information revealed is expected.

Other blocks to communication include a task-oriented approach to nursing care. The task-oriented nurse thinks of the patient in terms of what needs to be done. Referring to the patient using only a room and bed number does not convey a personal approach. Failing to listen attentively, offering unsolicited advice or false reassurances, using clichés, or engaging in gossip will all damage the nurse–patient relationship.

📌 FYI 9.2 **EXAMPLES OF BLOCKERS AND FACILITATORS TO THERAPEUTIC COMMUNICATION**

The following is a conversation with communication blockers:

Patient: "I feel as though I can't get my breath when I walk down the street."

RN: "What else makes you short of breath?" More like a detective, this RN gives a nontherapeutic response that does not acknowledge what is important to the patient. The RN who uses this type of question is generally trying to get through with the interviewing process.

Patient: "I don't know. I just can't walk very far, and I just have a hard time."

RN: "Tell me what other problems you have." As with the response above, the RN still seems primarily interested in finishing the interview, perhaps the health history. In this case, furthermore, the RN is ignoring the patient's concern.

Patient: "Well, umm, I just can't get to the corner store like I used to."

RN: "Well, okay, then. I will tell your doctor what you said to me. Is there anything else I can help you with?" In this response, the RN is deflecting responsibility to solve the problem. Rather than being understanding, the RN projects an unconcerned attitude.

The following is a conversation that facilitates trust.

Patient: "I feel as though I can't get my breath when I walk down the street."

RN: "You can't get your breath when you are walking outside? Is this the only time you feel you have trouble breathing?" In this response, the RN restates what the patient has said. This tells the patient that you heard him or her and allows you to probe further. It says to the patient that you want to know what he or she has to say and that you have time to listen.

Patient: "Well, no. I get short of breath whenever I walk any distance. I used to be able to go to the neighborhood store, and now I can't seem to walk to the end of my driveway before I have trouble."

RN: "So walking is getting harder for you lately. It sounds as though you are concerned that you are not able to do what you used to be able to do. What are you still able to do for yourself?" Empathy, a critical component of therapeutic conversation, projects understanding of the main concern of the patient. Here the nurse projects empathy by focusing on the main concern.

Patient: "Oh, I am able to get my mail, let the dog in and out, and I can get around the house all right, but I sit and rest more than I used to."

The RN and all health care workers should be aware of how their communication skills affect patients and patient care. Minimizing communication blockers while maximizing therapeutic interventions leads to greater patient satisfaction and positive patient outcomes. In FYI 9.2 and FYI 9.3, several facilitating and blocking communication techniques and examples are listed.

THE NURSE–PATIENT RELATIONSHIP

There are three types of relationships: intimate, social, and therapeutic. An intimate relationship occurs between two or more persons who are emotionally committed to each other and where mutual needs are met. In the social relationship, mutual needs

FYI 9.3   BLOCKERS AND FACILITATORS TO THERAPEUTIC COMMUNICATION

The following are blockers to therapeutic communication:

- Making value judgments
- Excessive questioning
- Giving approval or disapproval
- Advising
- Asking "why" questions
- Minimizing feelings
- Environmental factors
- Blurring boundaries
- Making irrelevant comments
- Making ambiguous comments
- Interrupting the patient
- Not responding when a response to the patient is called for
- Using too-familiar or impersonal language
- Changing the subject or otherwise shifting the focus away from the patient's concerns
- Turning away from the patient or becoming distracted
- Inappropriately kidding or joking
- Displaying annoying tics or habits, such as tapping a foot

The following are ways to facilitate therapeutic communication:

- Responding directly to the patient's statements
- Nodding one's head or leaning toward the patient (active listening)
- Staying on the topic at hand or directing the topic toward the major concerns
- Showing verbal and nonverbal interest in and awareness of what is being said
- Expressing understanding of what is being said or seeking clarification toward understanding
- Elaborating on the content; giving examples to broaden understanding
- Presenting hypotheses or assumptions; seeking clarification for validation
- Making eye contact
- Using silence
- Being nonjudgmental
- Giving unconditional positive regard
- Being genuine
- Demonstrating empathy
- Being self-aware
- Showing cultural awareness

are met and ideas, feelings, and experiences are shared and may include giving advice. In contrast, the therapeutic relationship between nurse and patient is a planned and goal-directed process that focuses on the patient's feelings, problems, and needs (Varcarolis & Holter, 2010). This relationship is a partnership between the patient and all members of the health care team and is termed *patient-centered care.*

The **nurse–patient relationship** moves through three phases: the orientation phase, the working phase, and the termination phase.

Orientation

The orientation (or introductory) phase begins with the initiation of the nurse–patient relationship and the development of a trusting relationship with the patient. During this phase, introductions take place and goals are set. The nurse must provide orientation to the patient regarding the entire facility, the unit, and the patient's room, making sure to point out devices such as the call bell and to explain any initial orders left by the physician. The nurse should also give the patient his or her name and discipline so the patient can read it and have it at hand. The nurse and the patient or family members should come to know one another by name (FYI 9.4).

> ## ⚖ FYI 9.4   **PREPARING FOR COMMUNICATION**
>
> - Establishing a nurse–patient contract facilitates a trusting relationship.
> - Patient concerns are to be respected, and the RN should plan questions that are sensitive to the patient's beliefs.
> - Assessing the patient's readiness and willingness to engage in communication is important to maintain positive outcomes.
> - The RN must establish a therapeutic environment for effective communication to take place.

Working

The working phase is considered the longest phase of the nurse–patient relationship. This phase begins with the nursing assessment, interview, and physical examination and continues until the relationship is terminated. Responding to patient cues, the RN develops a series of questions and completes an assessment that allows identification of patient concerns. As problems are identified, prioritize the list and collaborate with the patient to design a plan of care. All interactions during this phase are deliberately planned, implemented, and evaluated in concert with the patient to reach mutually agreed-upon goals.

Before beginning a conversation with a patient, review available information. Perhaps other health care team members have gathered information. Getting to know the patient's story begins with understanding the circumstances that led the patient to seek health care. The EMT report, the admission record, the physician's admitting notes, available diagnostic reports, and the report from the admitting RN are some of the resources for preparing for the initial contact with the patient. Establishing a caring relationship with a patient requires that you be engaged in understanding the patient's story. The RN should access preliminary information about the patient as a means to begin the process. From this preliminary knowledge, you will begin to formulate a sense of the patient's concerns.

The patient's family, if appropriate, can be a valuable source of information about the patient's history. The family can relate any changes they have seen, set time frames, and introduce the spiritual, emotional, and cultural concerns of the patient. The RN who is familiar with all available information gathered before entering the patient's room better understands the severity of the situation, can relate the condition to similar situations, and can better understand the specific individual nature of the patient's condition.

Note the questions already asked and answered by others. During the admission process, some questions will appear to be redundant, and a patient can become frustrated with many people asking the same or similar questions, perceiving that no one is really listening. The nursing admission form has questions that the physician or other health care professionals have already asked and documented. Review the chart before conducting the interview to save time and energy for both you and the patient. Let the patient know that any redundant questions are for the purpose of verifying information already documented.

> 🔨 | FYI 9.5   **UNDERSTANDING THE PATIENT'S STORY**
>
> The RN who begins the communication process prepared will have valuable informa-
> tion for formulating a sound understanding of the patient's story.
> - In understanding the patient's story, the RN is in the best position to recognize
>   subtle changes.
> - The RN engaged in understanding the patient's story is at the "heart of the caring
>   practice of nursing."
> - The RN must plan for sufficient time to understand the patient's story.

Perhaps you are the first to greet the patient and there is no history available. Preparation would then begin as you enter the room and survey the situation. This means paying attention to the verbal and nonverbal information the patient and family members offer to assist in preparing for the interview. Posture, facial expression, and general appearance can determine the patient's readiness to be interviewed.

Plan sufficient time to engage in conversations and allow for the patient's story to be told as completely as possible. Generally, a practiced interview process can take as short as 20 minutes or as long as 60 minutes. You may have to explain to the patient the need to break up the interview into shorter intervals intentionally rather than conducting it all at once. Inform the patient of your responsibilities while assuring the patient that his or her needs will be met. Delegate other responsibilities, as appropriate, to team members. Organization is important, and a relaxed, unhurried approach is most effective to obtain the needed data (FYI 9.5).

The patient's condition must also be considered. The patient may be so fatigued, weak, ill, sedated, in pain, in a state of agitation, or mentally incapable as to be unable to engage in a conversation. Before beginning a conversation, ask the patient whether he or she has any needs that should be taken care of first. Providing nourishment, allowing the patient to satisfy elimination needs, and adjusting the bed to a comfortable position will all help establish a therapeutic environment. As much privacy should be arranged as possible. Ask visitors to leave, turn off the television, eliminate all other distracting noise, and provide enough light. Lighting is important because it allows both parties to see each other clearly and respond to nonverbal communication, such as gestures, facial expressions, and posture, which contribute to the validity of the information exchange. Eyeglasses and any hearing-assistance devices should be in place. If possible, sit in a position so that you can be seen (preferably at eye level), but maintain the appropriate distance between you and the patient. Lean forward to demonstrate that you are interested in what the patient has to say. Respond to the patient's cues; watch for open gestures, such as palms up or eye contact, and closed gestures, such as arms crossed over the torso or lack of eye contact. Culture must be taken into consideration, however, to avoid misinterpreting a nonverbal behavior.

Be flexible when conducting the health history. Determining the chief complaint helps define the order in which to collect the rest of the health history data. Questions such as "What were you doing just before deciding to seek help?" and "What do you think caused you to feel this way?" will help clarify the patient's concerns. The patient may feel the need to talk about a problem with his feet while you are listening to his lungs. Take note, and explore the patient's concern without getting sidetracked. The patient will be more cooperative if he feels you are paying attention to this stated concern (FYI 9.6).

FYI 9.6 OPENING QUESTIONS

"Tell me what your concerns are." This is a broad opening statement that will allow the patient to begin to share concerns. Such a broad opening statement will allow the nurse to begin at the patient's level of understanding, but following questions must be more focused.

"I see that you told the doctor you were 'not feeling well.' Can you tell me more about how you are feeling? How is it different now from how you normally feel?" This type of question is useful if there is an identified chief concern, but clarification is needed. Again, follow-up questions will become more focused.

"You say you have been having 'this problem' for a while now. Tell me what changed that led you to seek help for the problem at this time?" This question is helpful if you feel a patient might have delayed getting medical help. It also may be helpful to identify a readiness on the part of the patient to make a significant life change that can assist in a healthier way of living.

EXERCISE 9.1

The father of a 3-year-old child hospitalized with complications of cystic fibrosis and pneumonia had been in the pediatric intensive care unit by the child's side for the first 48 hours. The last few days before the child was discharged from the unit, the father had left only to go to work, sleeping at the child's bedside each night. During the child's hospitalization, the mother had not been seen, although she had called several times. The RNs in the pediatric intensive care unit had assumed that the mother was not devoted to the child, and many of the RNs expressed anger that she had not come to visit.

The father was interviewed as part of a research project to determine the needs of family members of patients in intensive care units. During the interview process, it was discovered that this family also had an older child with cystic fibrosis. The father expressed that what he needed most was the assurance that his wife was taking care of this other child. This need for internal family support had developed over the years while they coped with having children with chronic illnesses. The couple decided that one parent would stay home to care for the older child, and the other would be with the hospitalized child. In this case, the mother would continue the older child's treatments at home. They reasoned that they could reduce the risk of giving the older child pneumonia if, for the duration of the younger child's illness, they gave separate care to each child, not risking carrying the pneumonia home to the older child (Corbin, 1990).
1. What could be the consequences of the nurses not knowing the whole story?
2. What questions could the nurses ask to help the staff understand the patient's story with more accuracy?

As you work with patients, be careful to avoid developing assumptions. Unconfirmed assumptions, or questions left unasked because of improper preparation, can lead to erroneous conclusions. You may run the risk for developing false or even prejudicial beliefs and misconceptions about the patient or situation, which may hinder developing a trusting relationship and impair your ability to deliver optimal patient care. Exercise 9.1 illustrates a scenario in which staff RNs *made erroneous assumptions as a result of an incomplete patient story.*

Understand the patient's point of view, and do not interject your own opinions, beliefs, or prejudices. The patient's personal beliefs may have an influence on his or her willingness or even ability to answer questions readily. Specific questions may embarrass or offend an individual. Pose questions in such a way that the importance of the information is sensitively communicated to the patient. The patient also needs to feel secure that the information will be confidential and communicated only to those with a need to know. The patient may also need permission to not share information that he or she is uncomfortable disclosing. However, if the patient feels secure and you have successfully established trust, then cooperation will be more forthcoming.

Another barrier that may hinder communication may not be the way a question is asked but who is asking the question. For instance, a male patient may have difficulty answering a female RN regarding problems with urination or erections. Equally awkward may be a female patient being asked questions by a male RN regarding problems with her breasts or reproductive organs. It may be necessary to defer these questions to a nurse whose gender is the same as the patient's. When this accommodation is not possible, assure the patient that as a nurse, your primary concern is his or her needs, and carry on in a matter-of-fact manner. Cultural or personal patient beliefs may also determine who should or should not be given intimate access to the patient.

Keep in mind that even though medical terminology is frequently seen and heard in the media, both in news reporting and in entertainment programs, we must not assume that the patient will understand questions that include medical terms and jargon. However, it is equally important not to "talk down" to the patient. In every interaction, you must assess the patient's knowledge level, educational background, and health care experiences to determine the appropriate orientation of the explanation. A patient may misunderstand even a fairly common word, such as *allergy*. If asked about whether he or she has any allergies, the patient may simply reply with a yes or a no. Often the patient who answers no might not consider food or environmental allergies as important or might not understand that the reactions to foods he or she eats may be allergic reactions. It is possible that when the patient reported being allergic to a medication, he or she might have equated medication side effects with an allergic reaction. Instead, the nurse might ask whether the patient has had any "problematic reactions" to medications or foods. Then the nurse can elicit more information and determine whether the reaction was an allergic response or a side effect.

Open, honest, and respectful dialogue with the patient and family is a standard of practice for the RN, who is to provide for the safety and security of the patient, while respecting rights to privacy and the integrity of the person. The RN must offer a clear explanation and sound rationale for a nursing action before conducting the action if he or she is to gain the patient's cooperation (FYI 9.7).

FYI 9.7   POSITIVE INTERVIEWING TECHNIQUES

- The RN who practices sound listening techniques demonstrates a caring attitude.
- The interview should expand the RN's knowledge of the patient's story.
- Strong communication is at the level of the patient's understanding, promoting accuracy in the patient's story.
- Open-ended questions allow patients the opportunity to voice their primary concerns.
- Focused questioning helps to establish patients' perception of how their health concerns are affecting their life.

Termination

The nurse–patient relationship terminates when the relationship is completed. Completion may be a result of patient discharge or transfer or because of the nurse's time off or change in employment. The RN should anticipate when this will occur and plan to conclude the relationship that has developed. The termination phase of the nurse–patient relationship needs sufficient planning for time to review goals and outcomes as well as patient teaching (FYI 9.8).

With any ending to a relationship, an individual may experience a sense of loss. One characteristic of loss is a feeling of apprehension over the possibility of losing the perceived safety net that has been provided. The patient will need to be supported through the communication efforts of the RN. Allow the patient to express fears, and gently point out the progress that has been made. Offer as much information as possible to smooth the course of the termination phase for both the patient and

---

📌 FYI 9.8   QUESTIONING TECHNIQUES TO ASSESS OUTCOMES

- "Do you remember how far you could walk before you got short of breath? How far can you walk now? What do you think has changed between now and then?" *This allows the patient to see where he or she is in relation to where he or she was. It also directs the patient to identify those things that might be helping, such as the medications and the medication schedule. Perhaps a question such as* "What do you think will happen if you forget to take your medication as the doctor has prescribed?" *might help the patient identify unacceptable outcomes that could help him or her understand the need for compliance.*
- "When I first met you, you were asking for pain medication just about every 2 hours. Tell me how you see your pain control now." *Remember that the patient's story is the most important indicator of how he or she is doing. Pain is subjective, and the nurse cannot assess the level of pain. By listening to the patient's description of his or her pain, the RN can also ask,* "What helps you best cope with the pain?" *or* "What works best to control the pain?"
- "I see that you are beginning to care for your ostomy, emptying and cleaning it. How do you see yourself differently now that you are able to care for yourself?" *The patient should express feelings when faced with a significant lifestyle change or image change. The RN who compassionately questions the patient with regard to feelings will gain a better understanding of the patient's progress.*
- "Most individuals who have just started giving themselves insulin and checking their blood sugar levels have a lot of questions. Now that you are giving yourself insulin and are able to do your blood sugar checks, you may still have some questions. What questions do you have?" *Acknowledging that it is okay to have questions, even when the patient is expected to be independent in his or her own care, gives the patient permission not to know everything about the process.*
- "Right now it must seem a bit puzzling to you, but with time, you will know your body's needs, and you will be adjusting your insulin within the guidelines that the doctor will give you with confidence. How might you get answers to questions you may have once you leave the hospital?" *A statement and a question like these can give reassurance that the patient is progressing as expected and still able to explore available support systems.*

the nurse. If care is to be ongoing, try to prepare the patient and family to establish a relationship with the new caregivers.

HEALTH LITERACY AND CULTURAL COMPETENCE

Health Literacy Can they read / hear / Speak english?

The World Health Organization (WHO, 2009) defines **health literacy** as "the cognitive and social skills which determine the motivation and ability of individuals to gain access to, understand, and use information in ways which promote and maintain good health." Health literacy is affected by education, culture, society, and the health system itself. Navigation through the health care system is challenging for well-educated individuals, and individuals with low health literacy have a more difficult time.

Some patient behaviors that may indicate low health literacy skills may include making excuses to read or fill out forms; pointing to the text with a finger while reading or wandering with their eyes over a page without focusing; missing appointments or making errors with their medication; answering questions incorrectly when asked what they have read; or showing signs of confusion, frustration, and nervousness (Cornett, 2009). Some effective strategies to use when communicating and teaching individuals with low health literacy include speaking slowly, being specific and concrete (rather than general), avoiding jargon and medical terminology, reinforcing information (use the "teach-back" technique), and using easy-to-read or visual materials (Cornett, 2009). Visual materials can include pictures, diagrams, videos, or printed material using a large typeface. Provide focused information, utilize interpreters when necessary, and evaluate the patient's understanding. The principles of teaching and learning should be applied to make an accurate assessment of learning needs and evaluate the effectiveness of teaching provided.

The ability to access health information and use it effectively empowers patients (WHO, 2009). The Joint Commission (2007) has stated that effective communication is a priority in protecting the safety of patients and recommends 35 strategies to address health literacy and patient safety. These recommendations can be found on The Joint Commission's website in its public policy white paper "What Did the Doctor Say?: Improving Health Literacy to Protect Patient Safety."

The Health Resources and Services Administration (HRSA) has an excellent website http://www.hrsa.gov/culturalcompetence/index.html that contains essential information for improving care for those of diverse cultures related to race and ethnicity, age, and gender and other special populations. HRSA states, "Effective health communication is as important to health care as clinical skill. To improve individual health and build healthy communities, health care providers need to recognize and address the unique culture, language and health literacy of diverse consumers and communities" (n.d., para 1).

Culture

In order for communication to be successful, the sender and receiver must share a common language or another means of communicating effectively. Culture refers to beliefs, values, and learned patterns of behavior, and these guide our thinking, actions, and decision making (Osborn, Wraa, & Watson, 2010). The meaning of our words is filtered through culture. **Cultural competence** refers to the ability to competently provide care to diverse cultures.

In a nationwide study conducted in 2003 by the National Center of Education Statistics, between 40% and 50% of individuals 16 years and older had literacy skills at basic or below basic levels, and about 5% of individuals sampled (or about 11 million American adults) could not be tested because of a language barrier, cognitive impairment, or literacy skills below the basic level. Additionally, some people may be ashamed that they cannot understand and will not ask for help (Markova & Broome, 2007). Compounding this dilemma is that the inability to speak English may make some individuals feel inferior and ashamed. According to the U.S. Census Bureau (2008), the Hispanic population is projected to reach 30% of the nation's total population by 2050, or nearly one in three U.S. residents. The Asian population is projected to increase to 9.2% of the total population. These figures emphasize the fact that you must be culturally knowledgeable and sensitive in order to provide holistic care that meets the physical, social, emotional, and spiritual needs of your patients.

In the course of your career, you will care for individuals from diverse cultures and backgrounds. Many of these patients will not be able to speak, read, or write English, and this has the potential to alter the care that your patients deserve. The care you provide to individuals from other cultures may be affected by your lack of knowledge, prejudice, bias, and stereotyping. Additionally, you may feel at odds with what patients from another culture might consider appropriate decisions regarding health care. In order to be culturally competent, you must first have self-awareness of these potential conflicting feelings. If your patient does not speak English, your ability to work past the language and communication barrier can prevent errors. At times, health care professionals may have underlying feelings of resentment to those who do not speak English. You may also believe that poor communication skills indicate a lack of intelligence.

Developing communication skills with people of different cultural backgrounds is especially challenging to the registered nurse. You must realize that people of different cultures have different views and meanings to their language that may differ greatly from English. Using an interpreter is vital so that misunderstandings do not occur. Culture and language also influence speaking and listening (Singleton & Krause, 2009). In addition, the nurse must understand that different cultures have different emotions as well as verbal and nonverbal behaviors that may be misunderstood by both the patient and the health care professional.

The Older Adult

The U.S. Census Bureau (2008) projects that by 2030, 19% of the U.S. population will be 65 and older. By 2050, this percentage is expected to increase to 20%, or 88.5 million people aged 65 and older. This will create additional challenges to nurses. Speros (2009) states, "Communicating in a manner in which the older adult can understand and use health information is a professional, ethical, and legal responsibility of the nurse." Special accommodations must be made for changes in hearing, vision, and physical challenges, as well as psychological factors such as depression, poor self-concept, mood, attitude, and loss of control (Speros, 2009). Normal changes in cognition as a result of aging include distractibility and a reduced ability to process new information (U.S. Department of Health and Human Services, 2012). Medication can also contribute to changes in cognition. You must avoid stereotyping older adults and realize that these are cognitive changes, not cognitive "impairments."

Speros (2009) states that communication must be purposeful and individualized to meet the needs of the elder patient and outlines a number of ways to improve communication with older adults, including age-appropriate teaching strategies. These include adjusting the pace of instructions and providing extra time, minimizing distractions, repeating information, avoiding the use of abstract terms, and avoiding negative messages. For example, tell the patient to check her blood sugar in the morning and evening before meals rather than "twice a day." Face the patient directly, make sure there is adequate light, provide a magnifying glass if necessary, and avoid blue, green, or violet ink. To compensate for auditory changes, use a lower-pitch voice, eliminate background noise, provide a paper and pencil, and ask the patient to repeat your message back to you.

In addition to these recommendations, the U.S. Department of Health and Human Services (2012) emphasizes that health care providers must consider how illness, stress, and fatigue can temporarily reduce cognitive function. Finally, you must also consider health literacy, because this may present another challenge to effective communication.

COLLABORATIVE COMMUNICATION

Collaborative communication refers to the interactions and functioning among the patient and members of the health care team to provide safe, patient-centered, quality care. Pecukonis and colleagues (2008) discuss discipline-specific professional culture and state that health care workers in various disciplines (e.g., nurses, social workers, and physicians) must learn to see their colleagues as people with needs, vulnerabilities, and strengths. Thus, cultural competence extends not only to the recipients of health care but to the workplace as well, and this influences working relationships. Some examples of cultural diversity include values, beliefs, customs, practices, race, nationality, religious affiliation, language, physical size, gender, sexual orientation, and age (Campinha-Bacote, 2003). One of the most difficult cultural differences to overcome in the workplace is generational. Nurses are likely to work with individuals from four generations: military veterans, baby boomers, Generation Xers, and Millennials.

Individuals born between 1922 and 1945 are known as the Veteran generation (military veterans). Individuals from this generation were taught to respect and obey authority and learned that sacrifice and hard work are rewarded. They value loyalty, respect authority, and expect to reap the rewards for their hard work (Weston, 2006). Veterans value seniority and experience and are most comfortable with traditional one-on-one coaching as well as instruction on how to improve their performance. Veteran nurses bring wisdom and organizational history to nursing teams, and they can quickly shift back to traditional ways in the event of a technological failure (Sherman, 2006).

The Baby Boom generation (baby boomers) is made up of individuals born between 1946 and 1964. Born into the post–World War II economic prosperity, boomers view the future with optimism and promise and desire to prosper financially as well as to contribute meaningfully. Boomers experienced the Vietnam War, the limited role of women, racism, and Watergate and learned that people in positions of authority were not to be trusted (Weston, 2006). Boomers prefer to be coached in peer-to-peer situations and enjoy recognition for a job well done. Boomers are valued for their clinical and organizational experience and can be used to coach and mentor younger nurses. Boomers like to feel empowered and to be asked for their feedback (Sherman, 2006).

Individuals born between the mid 1960s and the early 1980s are known as Generation X (Gen Xers). They were generally raised in two-career households and often in single-parent households. This generation is also known as the "latchkey" generation, referring to the fact that many children born in this generation went home after school to empty houses as a result of working parents. This generation learned at an early age to manage on their own, to advocate for their own point of view, and to have the expectation that their opinions will be considered. Gen Xers tend to be loyal to their profession but unwilling to compromise their personal, professional, or family well-being and to sacrifice for an employer who may let them go at any time. Gen Xers are resourceful, independent, technically sophisticated, and adaptable to change (Weston, 2006). They believe that advancement should be based on merit. Gen Xers are valued for their innovation and creative approaches to issues and problems (Sherman, 2006).

The Millennial generation (Millennials) includes individuals born between 1980 and 2000. Even though 60% of Millennials were born into two-career homes, their experiences were different from Gen Xers because child care, preschool, and after-school programs flourished and supported families. This generation has grown up in a multicultural, multiethnic, and global world with biracial and multicultural marriages and tends to be open-minded, collaborating, and civic-minded (Weston, 2006). They expect more coaching and mentoring than any other generation and want structure, guidance, and extensive orientation (Sherman, 2006).

This generational diversity in the workplace can cause misunderstandings and **conflicts.** Differences in expectations, work habits, attitudes, and beliefs are challenging. Nursing has changed over the past 60 years, which has forced more interaction among generations (Sherman, 2006). Shared leadership (e.g., shared governance) or transformation to the information age (younger nurses rely less on their older peers) has led, in many ways, to misperceptions, prejudices, and judgmental attitudes. Each generation has its own strengths. Learning from the unique strengths of each generation can decrease tension, enhance personal and professional growth, and encourage exploration of new and different ways of thinking (Weston, 2006). In addition to generational differences, culture in the workplace also includes ethnicity, age, religion, gender, sexual differences, and socioeconomic status. In 2010, of every 100 workers, 30 were Hispanic, African American, Asian American, or other people of color, and 48 were women (U.S. Census Bureau, 2010). This diversity requires us to recognize, appreciate, value, and utilize the unique talents and contributions of all individuals and can affect how we communicate with the health care team.

Your words can be powerful, but how they are perceived depends on verbal and nonverbal congruence, your intention, and the manner in which you present your message. Three possible ways to communicate are assertive, aggressive, and passive-aggressive. Assertive communication refers to being direct and honest and not infringing on the rights of others, whereas aggressive communication is hostile and infringes on those rights (Marquis & Huston, 2012). In passive-aggressive communication, individuals are aggressive in a passive way; in other words, it is a way to manipulate the situation (Marquis & Huston, 2012). Assertive messages begin with "I" as opposed to "you." Let's say that Mary is frequently late for work. Consider the difference in how you may receive the message "You made me so angry when you were late!" as opposed to "I felt angry when you came in late." The former statement "blames" the other individual and likely will make that individual defensive, whereas the latter statement removes the blame. With passive-aggressive behavior, individual A may say "no problem" to individual B who apologizes for being late, but then individual A tells a co-worker, "I'm so sick of her coming in late." Cox (2007) recommends an assertive approach using the "DESC" mnemonic, which stands for describe, explain, state, and consequences. The first step is to describe the behavior succinctly; the second step is to explain how the behavior impacts you; and in step three you state the desired outcome. Using this method, an assertive approach to the example above might be "I notice you come in late. It's difficult for me to give report on time so that I and staff on my shift can go home. I expect you to be on time." Let's say that Mary is late again for the next shift. At that point, it is time to state consequences: "If you continue to be late, we will need to meet with our manager to discuss this issue." This approach can help you to communicate assertively, not aggressively.

The most difficult form of communication may be when co-workers need to pass information on to one another. The Joint Commission (TJC) has set improving the effectiveness of communication among caregivers as its second goal in the 2012 National Patient Safety Goals. This includes timeliness of reporting critical results of tests and diagnostic procedures (TJC, 2012). One technique that has been proven effective in improving communication is the **SBAR** system (situation, background, assessment, recommendation). SBAR was developed by the U.S. Navy to improve communication and has been further developed by Kaiser Permanente (2012) for use in health care systems. This process is helpful for both emergent patient situations and routine handoffs. Using this process, you state the issue, describe the background, state the problems, and make recommendations. FYI 9.9 provides an example of this technique.

In order to effectively collaborate in the health care setting, the RN must exercise strong communication skills. As an LPN/LVN, you have been told what to include in your shift reports and charts and what information is important to pass on to the RN, and you can anticipate information the physician wants to know. Although there are LPN/LVNs who have formal management roles, most will have been the delegated recipients of information from RNs in charge. Your new role as RN will require many new communication skills. Effective communication in delegation is paramount to achieving expected outcomes.

Delegation

The RN as care manager needs to delegate many aspects of patient care to a variety of individuals. **Delegation** is a key role of the professional RN and requires critical thinking. **Delegation** is differentiated from an assignment in that the delagatee is given the authority to complete a task that is outside the usual activities of the role of the delegatee

📌 FYI 9.9 GUIDELINES FOR COMMUNICATING USING THE SBAR PROCESS

1. Use the following modalities according to physician preference, if known. Wait no longer than 5 minutes between attempts.
   - Direct page (if known)
   - Physician's call service
   - During weekdays, the physician's office directly
   - On weekends and after hours during the week, physician's home phone
   - Cell phone

   Before assuming that the physician you are attempting to reach is not responding, utilize all modalities. For emergent situations, use appropriate resident service as needed to ensure safe patient care.

2. Prior to calling the physician, follow these steps:
   - Have I seen and assessed the patient myself before calling?
   - Has the situation been discussed with the resource nurse or preceptor?
   - Review the chart for appropriate physician to call.
   - Know the admitting diagnosis and date of admission.
   - Have I read the most recent MD progress notes and notes from the nurse who worked the shift ahead of me?
   - Have available the following when speaking with the physician:
     Patient's chart
     List of current medications, allergies, IV fluids, and lab results
     Most recent vital signs
     Reporting lab results: provide the date and time test was done and results of previous tests for comparison.
     Code status

3. When calling the physician, follow the SBAR process:
   (S) Situation: What is the situation you are calling about?
   - Identify self, unit, patient, and room number.
   - Briefly state the problem, what it is, when it happened or started, and how severe it is.

   (B) Background: Pertinent background information related to the situation could include the following:
   - The admitting diagnosis and date of admission
   - List of current medications, allergies, IV fluids, and lab results
   - Most recent vital signs
   - Lab results: provide the date and time test was done and results of previous tests for comparison.
   - Other clinical information
   - Code status

   (A) Assessment: What is the nurse's assessment of the situation?

   (R) Recommendation: What is the nurse's recommendation, or what does he/she want?
   Examples:
   - Notification that patient has been admitted
   - Patient needs to be seen now
   - Order change

4. Document the change in the patient's condition and physician notification.

This SBAR tool was developed by Kaiser Permanente. Please feel free to use and reproduce these materials in the spirit of patient safety, and please retain this credit in the spirit of appropriate recognition.

(NCSBN, 2016). Importantly, delegation must be made to another who is qualified *(via education, training and validated competence)* and who has demonstrated competent ability to carry out the task. A task that can be delegated is one that is within the scope of practice of the person to whom it has been assigned based on the state nurse practice act. Tasks that cannot be delegated are those that require assessment, planning, evaluation, nursing judgment, or critical decision-making (NCSBN, 2016). Remember that the RN delegator retains accountability for tasks delegated. It is the responsibility of the RN to not only assess that the other health care worker has the knowledge and skills to perform a task, but the RN must also provide an opportunity for the individual to ask questions or clarify expectations (NCSBN, 2016). You should already be familiar with the five rights of delegation that the NCSBN issued in 1995: right task, right circumstance, right person, right direction/communication, and right supervision/evaluation. The Joint Statement on Delegation from the ANA and the NCSBN (Fig. 9.1) remains applicable and is a valuable tool in determining appropriateness of a delgation decision. The NCSBN updated the Delegation Model in 2015 (see Chapter 14), which clearly identifies the responsibilities of each of those involved in delegation including the nurse leader/organization, the licensed nurse (as delegator) and the delegate You must understand your state's laws and regulations concerning delegation as well as the policies of your organization.

Recall that the health care environment is culturally diverse, so you must communicate clearly and concisely while considering cultural or ethical barriers. Successful delegation requires sensitive but assertive communication on the part of the RN who assumes a fair-handed and considerate approach, as well as knowing the capabilities and scopes of practice of other staff members. No single simple way exists to ask for cooperation from everyone because each of us is unique and responds to direction in a singular way. The RN who learns to be fair but firm, however, will have greater success in gaining cooperation from more individuals. Consider which of the following requests would more likely be followed:

- Request 1: "You need to take that blood pressure and get the reading to me now."
- Request 2: "I need for you to take the blood pressure right away because I am trying to get through to the physician to get the medication order. The blood pressure will help him decide what's needed, and I expect that he will get back to me quickly."

Both speakers need the requests completed quickly. Request 1 is more likely to foster resentment because it may be considered aggressive. Request 2 is more respectful, yet assertive, and it offers a reason for its urgency. It is important to communicate frequently and clearly because the meaning of your communication could be interpreted in several ways (Anthony & Vidal, 2010).

At times a request may need to be especially firm and exacting, such as when a team member has not been following directions. This might have been going on for a while. For whatever reason, the LPN/LVN, nurse aide, or another RN does not want to follow an important direction or request. In such an instance, the RN in charge eventually needs to find the reason for the resistance, but at the time the request is needed, especially after an explanation has been given, it may be necessary to make the request stronger and more to the point. For example, the RN may say, "I expect the blood pressure to be obtained and the results given to me before the physician calls back."

Once the urgency of the medical situation has passed and as soon as possible after the incident, the RN needs to ascertain the reason for the resistance. This will take tact as well as assertive communication, which includes being respectful and allowing

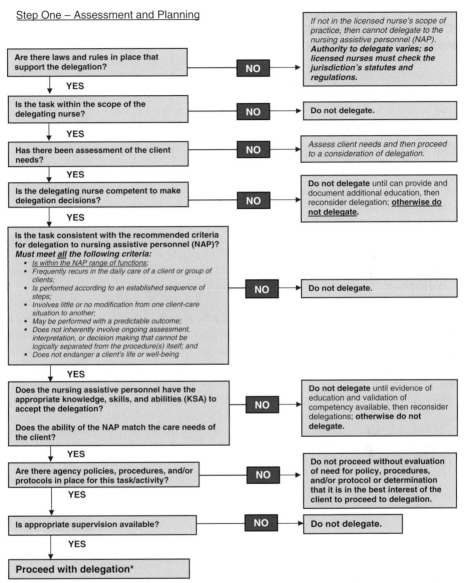

Step One – Assessment and Planning

FIG. 9.1 NCSBN Decision Tree: delegation to nursing assistive personnel. (NCSBN and ANA Joint Statement on Delegation.)

an explanation to be given. One approach initially is to ask for the seemingly insubordinate individual's own view of the situation: "What was your perception of my request when I first asked you to get a blood pressure on Mr. Smith?" Once this co-worker begins the explanation, the RN should use the same listening skills as would be afforded to a patient's concerns. The nurse should also leave his or her emotions behind, no matter how powerful.

Once you have listened attentively, then you can point out how the behavior is getting in the way of giving safe and effective care. If the individual becomes aggressive, then you must recognize the need to stop the conversation and enlist the help of the unit manager or supervisor, who should be trained to act as a neutral party, to arbitrate the situation.

Effective communication in delegation requires respect, honesty, and trust. Building effective interpersonal relationships with co-workers will facilitate teamwork, create synergy, and improve patient care. The more you are able to effectively communicate your expectations, the more your co-workers will come to trust you and rely on you for clear direction.

The Nurse–Physician Relationship

Professional **collaboration** refers to an exchange of ideas and opinions and requires mutual respect and trust. Effective collaboration creates effective teams and improves the work environment. Power-gender issues and generational differences can cause conflict in the health care environment, and **nurse–physician relationships** are among the most problematic that nurses encounter. Some of the problems identified by nurses include inappropriate, disruptive, or abusive behavior; dismissive attitudes; and belittling or intimidating behavior by physicians. The Joint Commission has called for zero tolerance of abusive physicians in the workplace and has found that failure to communicate among health care professionals caused 70% of 2455 reported sentinel events (TJC, 2004). Stein-Parbury and Liaschenko (2007) analyzed collaboration between nurses and physicians in an ICU and concluded that there was a breakdown in collaboration when physicians dismissed nurses' clinical assessment and concerns. Physicians take a task-oriented, curative approach to health care, while nurses focus on care. These differences can cause communication breakdown and conflict.

Conflict can occur in any practice setting between peers, nurses and management, staff and patient and/or family, and nurses and physicians. Conflict can be positive and can contribute to personal growth and development, but we must be willing to resolve conflict constructively.

Two ways that nurses can work toward improving nurse–physician relationships are empowerment and improving communication (Sirota, 2007). Nurses are empowered when they feel secure in clinical knowledge and expertise. You can accomplish this through lifelong learning. Staying abreast of advances in health care, participating in committees, joining professional organizations, and obtaining specialty certification are some ways to empower yourself as a professional RN. In order to improve communication skills, you must first take responsibility for your relationship with physicians. In other words, you must act in a mature, professional manner no matter how badly a physician behaves toward you (Sirota, 2007).

In a study conducted by Robinson and colleagues (2010), nurses and physicians identified effective and ineffective communication themes. These participants felt that "effective communication was enhanced when they were confident that what was being heard or said was accurate" and that "accuracy seemed to rely on verification and confirmation" (p. 209). The participants identified the following effective communication techniques:

- Clarity and precision of message that relies on verification
- Collaborative problem solving

> **📌 FYI 9.10 LEVELS OF GRADED ASSERTIVENESS AND EXAMPLES**
>
> Level 1: express initial concern with an "I" statement.
>   "I am concerned about . . . ."
> Level 2: make an inquiry or offer a solution.
>   "Would you like me to . . . ."
> Level 3: ask for an explanation.
>   "It would help me to understand . . . ."
> Level 4: a definitive challenge demanding a response.
>   "For the safety of the patient, you must listen to me."

Curtis, Tzannes, and Rudge (2011)

- Calm and supportive demeanor under stress
- Maintenance of mutual respect
- Authentic understanding of the unique role

Emotional maturity is the ability to be self-aware of your moods, feelings, and behaviors. Recognizing how you react in difficult situations is key to developing emotional maturity. Lindeke and Sieckert (2005) state, "Emotional maturity is foundational to effective collaboration," and collaboration is influenced by self-confidence. Curtis and colleagues (2011) point out that unexpressed thoughts or emotions can surface in ways such as hostility (to other staff or patients), passive-aggressive behavior, and absenteeism. They suggest that you self-assess your own emotional state and try to understand the emotional state of the other person, be mentally prepared prior to contacting the physician, determine exactly with whom you want to speak, and anticipate the needs of the other person (for instance, will the physician need vital signs?). Nurses should frame their communication with physicians in medical terms whenever possible. Reading back, clarifying, and questioning physician orders will decrease the chances of compromised patient safety and enhance communication. Use a structured approach such as SBAR and be assertive (Curtis, Tzannes, & Rudge, 2011). Curtis and colleagues (2011) identify four levels of assertiveness, called graded assertiveness, that are intended to ensure that the concerns of each team member have been addressed and that each team member is satisfied. FYI 9.10 provides these levels of graded assertiveness and gives examples.

TeamSTEPPS

Teamwork is essential for optimal patient outcomes and safety. **TeamSTEPPS,** which stands for Team Strategies and Tools to Enhance Performance and Patient Safety, is an evidence-based toolkit developed by the Health Research and Educational Trust (HRET) composed of materials and educational programs intended to promote teamwork principles among health care professionals. Through training provided in the toolkit caregivers learn to better adapt to rapidly changing conditions, have a clear and common understanding of the care plans, and have a solid understanding of the benefits of teamwork in delivering safe, effective, and consistent patient care. TeamSTEPPS training covers four major areas of competencies including leadership, situation monitoring, mutual support, and communication. Developing competency in these four areas can reduce errors and improve patient outcomes (HRET, 2016). In addition, TeamSTEPPS can improve communication that takes place during crisis situations to ensure clear, coordinated action and reduced risk. When a crisis occurs, communication must be rapid and include all relevant information to improve decision making.

Documentation as Communication

The RN communicates in many different ways. The RN is responsible for effectively gathering information from the patient regarding current health concerns and documenting how the patient responds to interventions and the overall treatment plan. This information will be shared with physicians and other health care team members. This written communication becomes a legal record; it is used to measure outcomes and determine costs and may serve to defend the care given if litigation occurs. The nursing process forms the foundation for nursing **documentation.**

In the course of a day, nurses communicate verbally, in writing, or electronically. As an RN you will be asked to transmit instructions, write a plan of care, record interventions and outcomes, communicate assessment information, record and explain incidences, and pass on information. In addition to nursing histories and nursing notes, the RN often uses memoranda, emails, letters, interdepartmental and interinstitutional forms, and personal diaries or anecdotes to record important information. Each of these forms of communication must be complete, succinct, relevant, accurate, and factual.

As mentioned earlier, your words become powerful tools that not only contribute to quality patient care but also protect patients, nurses, and the health care agency. The patient's record is documentation establishing that standards of practice, policies, and procedures were followed and that standards of care were met. As a legal document, the patient's chart must be an accurate accounting of the patient's response to the illness and treatment. The nurse must treat the chart as though it will be read in court or at a deposition. Keep in mind that such proceedings often take place more than a few years from the event. Consistently using standard language and approved abbreviations in documentation ensures that if the nurse does need to refer to the charting and stand behind it at a later date, he or she will be better prepared in the event of legal matters.

One common error in charting is using a medical diagnosis rather than acceptable nursing language to communicate a patient condition. Using broad terms instead of specific signs and symptoms opens the nurse to error. For example, an infant with a feeding disorder is given the common medical diagnosis of "dehydration." Describing the infant as dehydrated implies that the nurse has the power to prescribe a medical treatment plan. Nursing documentation should reflect the signs and symptoms assessed that led the nurse to the conclusion that the infant is dehydrated. The nursing diagnosis of *Fluid volume deficit* is within the nursing realm.

When charting, record the patient's exact words verbatim as much as possible, rather than paraphrasing. For example, not many patients would describe their difficulty breathing as "dyspnea," but they may say, "I feel as though I can't catch my breath." Use quotation marks and write exactly what the patient (or family) said that you consider relevant. Always avoid charting your own opinions, thoughts, and feelings. Be truthful and stick to the facts.

A common saying is that if you do not chart the nursing or collaborative intervention or the patient response to a treatment, then it did not happen. This implies that all charting must reflect the total nursing process—assessment, diagnosis, planning, implementation, and evaluation—as well as revisions to the plan of care. Common omissions in charting include neglecting to record the patient's response to the intervention, such as whether the patient had pain relief after being given pain medication or whether the patient had a rhythm change after receiving a cardiac medication. Another common problem with charting is vague or ambiguous terms, such as "worse" and "better." Supplement such patient terms with measures or other quantifications. For example, use a numeric scale or other tool to help the patient describe the intensity of pain and document the pain scale that was used for your assessment. Use proper grammar and spelling, and write legibly. Credibility is maintained when the written word is legible, clear, and precise.

Technology can create additional issues in communicating. You may find yourself communicating through email, charting electronically, using handheld computers and smartphones, or providing care or collaborating with other professionals via telecommunication technologies (known as telehealth). Emails and memoranda communicate information regarding policy and procedural updates, in-service education, announcements, and patient care. The RN is often asked to respond to such emails and memoranda to give input or an opinion or to acknowledge having read and understood the message. When a need arises to request services or report patient care concerns to another department, email and memorandum responses will become a challenge for the RN, because the responses will become a record that may be used for or against the writer and are subject to confidentiality issues and federal regulation concerning electronic patient information. Remember that patient identification, such as name, Social Security number, age, or medical record number, should never be transmitted electronically unless you are charting in the official medical record.

In Exercise 9.1, read the scenario and answer the questions related to communication. Official written communications, like oral communication, must be clear and accurate. To ensure clarity and accuracy, include the following elements in your written communication:

- Purpose or need
- Problem or question at issue
- Information, data, observations, or experiences
- Conclusions or solutions
- Consequences or implications
- Perspective or frame of reference from which the reporting is being made

Each written or electronic communication, including occurrence and incident reports, must include an attempt to explain through illustration and examples the importance of the incident to patient safety. In addition, an attempt should be made

? EXERCISE 9.2

1. Is the nursing entry dated? _____ Timed? _____ Signed? _____
2. Is the nursing entry legible? _____
3. Are the parts of the nursing process present?
   a. Assessment _____
   b. Diagnosis _____
   c. Outcome identification _____
   d. Planning _____
   e. Implementation _____
   f. Evaluation _____
4. Was a pain medication given? _____
   a. Did the nurse document the patient's pain intensity? _____ Location? _____
   b. Did the nurse document the patient's response to pain? _____
5. Was a medication given that needed prior special assessment? _____
   a. Did the nurse document the assessment data? _____
   b. Was there a lab value, and was it documented? _____
   c. Was the patient's response to the medication documented? _____
6. Was there evidence of patient teaching? _____
   a. Did the nurse document the need for education? _____
   b. What method of education was used? Lecture _____ Video _____ Pamphlet _____ Other _____
   c. Did the nurse indicate if there were any special patient considerations? _____
   d. Did the nurse document patient understanding? _____
7. How many spelling and grammatical errors are there? _____

to maintain neutrality in the reporting, avoiding giving opinions, expressing feelings, or "labeling" patients. Unsafe practice must be reported to division supervisors, facility management, and ultimately the board of nursing. Documentation and correspondence to officials regarding incidences of unsafe practice must be accurate, truthful, and without personal opinion.

In Exercise 9.2, conduct a chart audit, looking at the charting of the nurses in different units. For each nursing entry for a 24-hour period, answer the questions provided. During clinical conference, share the responses with the students in your clinical setting. In Exercise 9.3, read the scenario and answer the questions related to communication.

A different level of exchanging and recording essential information is fundamental to your role change from LPN/LVN to RN. The RN is responsible for maintaining ethical and legal integrity with all forms of communication. Personal integrity as well as accountability for the advancement of nursing as a profession requires the RN to excel in all forms of communication. Among the consequences of poor communication are less effective care, low patient satisfaction levels, and unmet or deleterious patient outcomes. A team approach to health care requires the RN to be aware of how he or she communicates with the other team members. Sound communication skills are a professional standard of practice for the RN.

💡 EXERCISE 9.3

Consider a time when a request for more staff members is made to meet the needs on a specific shift. The data clearly show that acuity levels justify the request, yet the staffing department is unable to find additional staff. After conferring with the supervisor, who is also unable to provide assistance, you become concerned that not all of the care required for the patients will be completed safely and in a timely fashion.

As the RN charge nurse, you will write a memorandum to your unit manager, as well as to the department head, documenting the incidents of the shift. You need to be accurate as well as clear, without being incriminating, in your correspondence.

1. What information is important to include in the memorandum?
2. Use this information to create an outline.
3. How would you avoid demonstrating anger, frustration, or biases, while at the same time providing an explanation for specific patient care not being completed?

KEY POINTS

After completion of this chapter, you have learned:

- Communication is the exchange of information and can be either verbal or nonverbal. The majority of communication is nonverbal and includes body behaviors, facial expressions, personal appearance, eye contact, physical characteristics, touch, and voice. Cultural considerations must be taken into account.
- The purpose of the therapeutic relationship is to establish trust. It requires empathy rather than sympathy and requires an accepting, nonjudgmental attitude.
- Active listening is being fully attentive to verbal and nonverbal communication. Care must be taken to consider culturally appropriate nonverbal behaviors.
- Communication facilitators enhance communication, whereas communication blockers tend to stop communication.
- Health literacy refers to the ability of individuals to gain access to information and be able to understand and use that information to maintain good health, and it is affected by education, culture, society, and the health system.
- Cultural competence applies to patients, co-workers, physicians, and other members of the health care team. Diversity among these individuals includes generational differences, culture, ethnicity, language, socioeconomic status, religion, gender, age, and sexual differences. These differences can affect how we communicate with patients, co-workers, and members of the health care team.
- The aging adult may experience physiological and psychological changes that require special accommodations so that communication is received and understood. Communication must be individualized to meet specific needs.
- Collaborative communication is the ability to effectively collaborate and make decisions with patients and members of the health care team. This collaboration will enhance safety, improve quality care, minimize risks, and support effective teamwork.
- Delegation is a key role of the professional RN. You must be able to critically think about the needs of each of your patients and whether or not an LPN/LVN or nursing aide can perform tasks competently and safely. Whether or not to delegate will depend on your assessment of the patient and your professional judgment.

- The professional work environment is significantly influenced by the nurse–physician relationship. It is important to learn ways to effectively communicate vital information to physicians. SBAR is one method to use to assertively communicate information, concerns, and recommendations to physicians. It has been shown that clear and precise messages, collaborative problem solving, being calm and supportive, demonstrating mutual respect, and understanding discipline-specific roles are effective communication themes among nurses and physicians.
- Documentation allows you to communicate information to the health care team. Documentation must be factual, to the point, descriptive, relevant, accurate, legible, and clear. Include subjective statements as much as you can, and avoid documenting personal opinions, thoughts, or feelings concerning the patient. Your documentation will assist the members of the health care team in evaluating the effectiveness of interventions and whether outcomes have been met. Remember that your documentation is a legal document and can be used in litigation.

CRITICAL THINKING QUESTIONS

The answers to each of the following questions should use the elements of critical thinking: purpose, questions at issue, available information, basic concepts, assumptions, inferences and interpretations, implications and consequences, and point of view.

1. Take a recent clinical situation in which you had a conversation with a patient where there was a need for the patient to understand your point of view in relation to the plan of care. Write out the conversation, including at least ten exchanges between you and the patient. From the perspective of sound communication principles, critique your interaction line by line. For each of your statements, give one other way you might have said the same thing and cite a communication principle to back your decision.

2. At report for the beginning of your shift, you are short one staff RN and one nursing aide, according to census data and acuity markers. The staffing office refuses to even look at your request. Although you and your staff make it through the shift and your patients remain safe, you find yourself playing catch-up with charting, and not all the assigned care is complete. A physician is upset that at 7:00 AM his patient's morning weight is not available. Write a memorandum to your unit manager regarding the situation.

3. A new antibiotic medication is being used as part of a clinical trial and is under a strict protocol for administration. The dose for medication X is to be 1000 units/kg of body weight. The physician has ordered your patient to receive 100,000 units IVPB over 1 hour. Your patient weighs 125 lb.
   a. What should be the dosage according to the protocol?
   b. Write out what you would say to the physician to get the ordered dosage corrected.

4. You are working with a new doctor who recently began seeing patients on your unit. She has a very strong accent and has been abrasive to the nursing staff. You are taking orders for Humalin R sliding scale. As she is giving the orders, you

cannot understand the full sliding scale ranges due to her accent. You feel hesitant to clarify some of the sliding scale ranges because she has yelled at other nurses for asking her to write out her orders rather than give them verbally.

a. What are some cultural considerations that apply to health care workers such as doctors?

b. What is your duty to your patient's care?

c. What principles of communication are mandated by The Joint Commission?

d. How would you approach this situation?

5. Consider the following scenario and write out the appropriate SBAR communication: Upon entering the patient room, James, the RN on duty, noted that the patient, who was admitted this afternoon after an ORIF of the ulna this morning, had vomited the food he ate for dinner and was still complaining of nausea and that he was still in pain even after the Percocet you gave him just before dinner. He states he was not feeling nauseous before he took the Percocet. You find upon assessment that his bowel sounds are active in all quadrants, and vital signs are within normal limits though his BP and pulse are slightly higher than at the previous reading. Patient states that narcotic pain meds have made him nauseous in the past.

a. S:

b. B:

c. A:

d. R:

6. Consider the following scenario and write out the appropriate SBAR communication: Your patient, a 72-year-old female who is to have a portacath inserted in the morning has a BP of 180/92 and pulse of 96, both up from readings from 2 hours prior when they were 126/82 and 70. Patient is alert and oriented times three and states she is becoming very anxious about the procedure and feels like she needs "something" to help her calm down.

a. S:

b. B:

c. A:

d. R:

WEB RESOURCES

Southern Cross University, http://communicationskillsinfo.com

American Nurses Association, http://nursingworld.org

The Joint Commission, http://jointcommission.org

U.S. Department of Health and Human Services, http://hhs.gov/ocr/civilrights/resources/specialtopics/hospitalcommunication/

Institute for Healthcare Safety. (free) SBAR, http://ihi.org/knowledge/Pages/Tools/SBARTechniqueforCommunicationASituationalBriefingModel.aspx

Mind Tools. Communication, http://mindtools.com/page8.html

Transcultural Nursing, http://culturediversity.org/index.html

Centers for Disease Control and Prevention, http://cdc.gov

USDHHS, http://health.gov/communication/literacy/quickguide/

USDHHS, http://health.gov/communication/literacy/olderadults/default.htm
NCSBN Delegation Decision-Making Tree, http://ncsbn.org/delegationtree.pdf
The Health Resources and Services Administration (HRSA) Cultural Competence
http://www.hrsa.gov/culturalcompetence/index.html

REFERENCES

Anthony, M. K., & Vidal, K. (2010). Mindful communication: a novel approach to improving delegation and increasing patient safety. *Online Journal of Issues in Nursing, 15*(2). http://dx.doi.org/10.3912/OJIN.Vol15No2Man02.

Campinha-Bacote, J. C. (2003). Many faces: addressing diversity in health care. *Online Journal of Issues in Nursing, 8*(1). Retrieved from http://nursingworld.org.

Corbin, B. (1990). *Identification of family members' self-care knowledge: qualitative study. MSN thesis.* Allendale, MI: Grand Valley State University.

Cornett, S. (2009). Assessing and addressing health literacy. *Online Journal of Issues in Nursing, 4*(3). http://dx.doi.org/10.3912/OJIN.Vol14No03Man02.

Cox, S. (2007). Good communication: finding the middle ground. *Nursing, 37*(1), 57.

Curtis, K., Tzannes, A., & Rudge, T. (2011). How to talk to doctors–a guide for effective communication. *International Nursing Review, 58*, 13–20.

Health Research & Educational Trust. (2016). TeamSTEPPS. Retrieved from www.teamsteppsportal.org.

Kaiser Permanente. (2012). Guidelines for communicating with physicians using the SBAR process. Retrieved from http://ihi.org/knowledge/Pages/Tools/SBARTechniqueforCommunicationASituationalBriefingModel.aspx.

Lindeke, L. L., & Sieckert, A. M. (2005). Nurse–physician workplace collaboration. *Online Journal of Issues in Nursing, 10*(1), Manuscript 4. Retrieved from http://nursingworld.org/MainMenuCategories/ANAMarketplace/ANAPeriodicals/OJIN/TableofContents/Volume102005/No1Jan05/tpc26_416011.html.

Markova, T., & Broome, B. (2007). Effective communication and delivery of culturally competent care. *Urologic Nursing, 27*(3), 239–242.

Marquis, B. L., & Huston, C. J. (2012). *Leadership roles and management functions in nursing: theory and application* (7th ed.). Philadelphia, PA: Lippincott Williams & Wilkins.

National Council of State Boards of Nursing. (2016). *National guidelines for nursing delegation. Journal of Nursing Regulation, 7*(1), 5–14.

Osborn, K. S., Wraa, C. E., & Watson, A. B. (2010). *Medical–surgical nursing: preparation for practice.* Upper Saddle River, NJ: Pearson.

Pecukonis, E., Doyle, O., & Bliss, D. L. (2008). Reducing barriers to interprofessional training? Promoting, interprofessional cultural competence. *Journal of Interprofessional Care, 22*(4), 417–428.

Robinson, F. P., Gorman, G., Slimmer, L. W., & Yudkowsky, R. (2010). Perceptions of effective and ineffective nurse–physician communication in hospitals. *Nursing Forum, 45*(3), 206–216.

Rogers, C. (1961). *On becoming a person.* New York, NY: Houghton Mifflin.

Sherman, R. O. (2006). Leading a multigenerational nursing workforce: issues, challenges, and strategies. *Online Journal of Issues in Nursing, 11*(2). Retrieved from http://nursingworld.org.

Singleton, K., & Krause, E. M. (2009). Understanding cultural and linguistic barriers to health literacy. *Online Journal of Issues in Nursing.* http://dx.doi.org/10.3912/OJIN.Vol14No03Man04.

Sirota, T. (2007). Nurse/physician relationships: improving or not? *Nursing, 37*, 52–55.

Speros, C. I. (2009). More than words: promoting health literacy in older adults. *Online Journal of Issues in Nursing, 14*(3). http://www.nursingworld.org/MainMenuCategories/ANAMarketplace/ANAPeriodicals/OJIN/TableofContents/Vol142009/No3Sept09/Health-Literacy-in-Older-Adults.html.

Stein-Parbury, J., & Liaschenko, J. (2007). Understanding collaboration between nurses and physicians as knowledge at work. *American Journal of Critical Care, 16*(5), 470–477.

The Joint Commission. (2007). *What did the doctor say? Improving health literacy to protect patient safety.* Retrieved from http://jointcommission.org/What_Did_the_Doctor_Say/.

The Joint Commission on Accreditation of Healthcare Organizations. (2004). *Sentinel Event Statistics.* Retrieved from http://JCAHO.org.

The Joint Commission. (2008). *Low health literacy puts patients at risk.* Retrieved from http://jointcommission.org/NewsRoom/PressKits/Health_Literacy/hl_020607.htm.

The Joint Commission. (2012). *National patient safety goals.* Retrieved from http://jointcommission.org/assets/1/6/2012_NPSG_HAP.pdf.

Townsend, M. C. (2012). *Psychiatric mental health nursing* (7th ed.). Philadelphia, PA: F. A. Davis Company.

U. S. Census Bureau. (2008). *An older and more diverse nation by midcentury.* Retrieved from http://census.gov/newsroom/releases/archives/population/cb08-123.html.

U. S. Census Bureau. (2010). *2010 census briefs.* Retrieved from http://2010.census.gov/news/press-kits/briefs/briefs.html.

U. S. Department of Health & Human Services. (2012). *National action plan to improve health literacy.* Retrieved from http://health.gov/communication/HLActionPlan/.

Varcarolis, E. M., & Halter, M. J. (2010). *Foundations of psychiatric and mental health nursing: a clinical approach* (6th ed.). St. Louis, MO: Elsevier.

Weston, M. J. (2006). Integrating generational perspectives in nursing. *Online Journal of Issues in Nursing, 11*(2). Retrieved from http://nursingworld.org.

World Health Organization. (2009). *Health literacy and health behaviour.* Retrieved from http://who.int/healthpromotion/conferences/7gchp/track2/en/.

CHAPTER

10

Teaching Patients and Their Families

evolve WEBSITE

Additional resources are available online at:
http://evolve.elsevier.com/Claywell/transitions

OBJECTIVES

After completing this chapter, the student will be prepared to:
1. Understand the requirements for patient education.
2. Compare motivators, facilitators, and barriers to learning.
3. Explain the unique qualities of adult learning.
4. Describe the impact of readiness on learning.
5. Identify factors conducive to learning.
6. Identify ways to evaluate learning.
7. Describe characteristics of a successful teacher.

KEY TERMS

adult learning	learning	readiness for learning
advocacy	motivation to learn	teaching plan
credibility	principles of learning	
demonstration of learning	principles of effective teaching	

OVERVIEW

An important role of the registered nurse, and one defined within state Nurse Practice Acts, is the role of teacher. Additionally, a standard of practice expectation is that patient teaching is ultimately the RN's responsibility. The Joint Commission (formerly The Joint Commission on Accreditation of Healthcare Organizations [JCAHO]) (2001) defines the patient education standards to which health care agencies are held accountable. Evidence of performance must demonstrate compliance with these standards for Joint Commission accreditation. The implication is that patients have a right to information about their treatment and that a coordinated interdisciplinary effort with patient education is consistently implemented.

The policy of the Centers for Medicare and Medicaid Services (CMS) is that reimbursement to hospitals will be limited for patient readmits for the same conditions within a certain time period after discharge. Transitional care is considered a requirement for preventing needless readmissions. Education is a critical part of transitional care, and nurses are key to providing adequate patient and family/caregiver education. The RN is constantly engaging in both formal and informal patient teaching about some part of care. Education empowers the patient to become active in his or her own health care. Therefore, the RN needs to understand basic principles of teaching and learning in order to provide the best environment for the patient and family to learn.

This chapter lays a foundation of sound teaching standards for the student in transition from LPN/LVN to RN to develop a teaching plan of care that will empower the patient to be an informed health care consumer and steward of his or her own health. It introduces the student to the principles of learning and the traits of the adult learner. The chapter presents content related to the process of teaching and learning and theoretical underpinnings of teaching adults, tools for assessing a patient's readiness to learn, for evaluating the effectiveness of patient education, and documenting that the education and learning have taken place.

THE PATIENT AS A LEARNER

The health care consumer is becoming more informed about health and health care. The consumer is expecting to be educated as to the particular plan of care and to take part in creating that plan. Recent laws and regulations protect consumers by requiring that they receive certain information so that they will be able to make informed choices about their care. The Joint Commission (TJC) standards state, "The patient receives education and training specific to the patient's assessed needs, abilities, learning preferences, and readiness to learn as appropriate to the care and services provided by the hospital" (TJC, 2001). There must be evidence of the education through clear documentation in the patient record, and TJC requires patient education to be interdisciplinary. Furthermore, health care facilities must audit patient education to ensure consistency of teaching and that the health care team members are evaluating the effectiveness of the patient education they give. Just because a consumer received information does not necessarily mean that he or she can demonstrate understanding it. The nurse must assess the patient's level of understanding and be prepared to deliver information in a clear and proficient manner.

PRINCIPLES OF TEACHING AND LEARNING

Learning is said to have occurred when a subsequent change in behavior occurs. An informed patient is better able to manage health care, is more compliant with the plan of care, and, as a result, experiences more positive outcomes. The role of the teacher is important, and mastery of the role is essential to professional practice. As a teacher, you will advocate for the patient by giving the information needed to make decisions.

Advocacy means to promote an idea, a belief, or a person or to put someone in the best possible position to assist himself or herself. As a patient advocate, you will use your teaching skills as a means to empower patients toward healthier lifestyles.

Basic Assumptions of Learning

You have chosen to return to school to learn what is needed to become an RN. You have chosen the opportunity to learn by enrolling in and attending classes. Interestingly, although students recognize the need for additional knowledge and experience, they often question the necessity of some of the readings and other material presented in class or clinical. You may question the need to study particular assigned material and choose to concentrate on material that seems more important for a test. Given this, two basic assumptions for learning are important for the individual to understand:

1. Individuals choose to learn or not to learn.
2. What the individual perceives as important is more readily learned.

In the health care setting, patients are seldom given a choice about whether they need to learn. RNs, LPN/LVNs, physicians, and other health care providers generally dictate what each patient needs to know. They will either direct the teaching or present the teaching material without consulting the patient. Often this includes little or no assessment of the patient's learning needs. For example, patients with newly diagnosed insulin-dependent diabetes mellitus will be given lessons on how to monitor their glucose levels and to give themselves insulin. Even so, many patients return to the acute care setting with complications related to "noncompliance" with their new regimens. When questioned, the patients often do not remember anyone telling them how to deal with their new diagnosis in great detail.

Much of what is presented as patient education ignores basic principles of learning. Patients may not be in a condition to learn. Furthermore, unless the patient clearly states it, he or she may not understand the relevance of the information to the condition. In general, where patient education is concerned, more is better than less, and multiple methods of presenting information will increase the likelihood that your patient will retain it.

BASIC PRINCIPLES OF LEARNING

According to Carnegie Mellon (2015), the following principles are present in all learners. The same can be applied whether the learners are students, patients, or caregivers.

1. A student's prior learning will either positively or negatively impact new learning.
2. How students bring together information will influence how they are able to apply that knowledge.
3. Students' motivation to learn is paramount in the process.
4. To develop mastery, students must understand each part of the skill, be able to practice the skill in part and as a whole, and understand when the skill in necessary.
5. Practice paired with concurrent feedback is critical to the quality of the learning process.
6. Students' current levels of psychosocial development interacting with environmental factors impact learning.

7. Becoming self-directed as a learner is a process that requires the ability to self-monitor and adjust one's approach to learning.

Integration of the **principles of learning** into the routine of patient teaching will help to guide the process and ensure that the best opportunity for learning has been established. These principles are incorporated throughout the following major areas applicable in the health care setting.

Motivation to Learn

Individuals inherently hold to their own values and beliefs as truths until they have significant motivation to change. The **motivation to learn** often results from a life-changing event, such as childbirth or illness. A patient may perceive learning as an opportunity to improve the condition or make a difference in another significant way. The RN who recognizes the significance of the event can seize the opportunity to explore the patient's motivation to learn.

Barriers to Learning

Myths and misconceptions about health, illness, and health care are often perpetuated by the experiences of the individual. The patient who has had knowledge of someone dying from a particular disorder is more likely to see that disorder in a dismal light and be willing to accept statistics that support a bleak picture. The nurse may have difficulty convincing the patient that his or her particular prognosis is actually more optimistic. The opposite may also be true. A patient with the same disorder but who has known someone who got better and lived a long and healthy life may not be as willing to accept statistics showing that the disorder may have a bleak outcome. For example, despite the amount of hard evidence showing a positive relationship between cigarette smoking and a multitude of health problems, many people are not willing to believe it. This way of thinking is known as *denial*.

Patient values influence the willingness to accept the need to change and therefore the need to learn. Patients whose values are contrary to the evidence will need to have time to understand the relevance of the information that you are giving them. The smoker will need time to understand that a relationship exists between his or her symptoms and smoking. Therefore, the RN must use rational thought and convey that logic in the presentation of the facts. The patient must decide that the change is necessary. The RN can only act as a conduit of knowledge and for rational thought, leaving prejudices, feelings, and frustrations behind. You may need to set up a referral for further assistance. In any case, you must understand the patient's decision and show acceptance of it.

Facilitation of Learning

Other general principles of learning should be considered when engaging patients in the learning process. FYI 10.1 outlines some of the principles that facilitate learning. The RN must understand that learning takes place in segments and that a patient can absorb only so much, or reach a plateau, before the learning process becomes ineffective. These plateaus often do not correspond with the goals and outcomes set by the nurse. When a patient has reached a plateau, the behavior may be labeled as lazy, noncompliant, or difficult to manage. The RN must remember that true learning is a life-changing event,

---

⚡ FYI 10.1   FACILITATORS TO LEARNING

A learner:
- Is motivated to make a change in life.
- Believes that the information to be learned will be beneficial.
- Believes that it is possible to learn what is needed.
- Has clear and reasonable outcome objectives.
- Has a low to moderate level of stress.
- Has had other immediate needs met.
- Believes that the changes related to learning will have a positive influence on his or her life.

---

and change is stressful. A patient being asked, or forced by necessity, to go through a lot of change at one time can resist. Positive reinforcement for the change that has taken place, rather than negative feedback as to what the patient still needs to learn, will maintain a trusting relationship, which will foster continued learning.

Understanding how the learning process occurs will help the RN plan teaching sessions. If the patient is involved in the process of planning and active in learning, a better patient outcome is inevitable.

Adult Learners

Adult patients are adult learners. Adults bring to the health care setting a lifetime of experiences that will influence how they perceive formal and informal learning. Assessment of a patient's life experiences will help you plan learning activities. The closer the learning can be applied to the patient's experiences, the easier it is for the patient to accept the need to learn and thus to change behavior.

Eduard Lindeman (1926), one of the founding fathers of the theory of **adult learning,** made five important assumptions about adult learners that may serve to guide the nurse's efforts at patient education:
1. Adults will learn as they develop needs that they believe learning will fulfill.
2. Adults use their lives as the point of reference for all learning.
3. Adults learn best from and in relation to their experiences.
4. Adults prefer to be self-directed in learning or at the very least have a say in it.
5. Differences between individuals broaden with age and experience.

Relating to the Learner's Level of Understanding

Adults need new information to be related to something they already know. This creates a link so that the information can be readily recalled. For example, compliance with fluid restriction may be easier if you, as a nurse, create an analogy or familiar frame of reference. Most adults will be able to relate to the heart and blood vessels in household plumbing terms. Compare the heart to a sump pump that must run in order for a basement not to fill up with water. When this concept is applied to the need for the heart to pump effectively so the lungs will not fill up with water, the patient may better understand congestive heart failure. Additionally, the individual will understand the need not to add to the water in the basement and that this concept applies to not adding to the water in the lungs.

In many cases, institutions provide written instructions to patients in the hope that they will use them as references. Studies have shown that a lower-than-expected level of literacy may exist in patient populations seeking health care within the United States, as reported in a study by Fisher (1999). A report from the Ad Hoc Committee on Health Literacy for the Council on Scientific Affairs, American Medical Association (1999), concluded that "patients with the greatest health care needs may have the least ability to read and comprehend information needed to function successfully as patients" (p. 552). The implication of this for nursing and other studies is that the RN should recognize that patients may not have the comprehension of material needed to manage their own care. Simply asking patients whether they understand may not be enough to ensure that understanding is adequate. Patients who experience difficulty with reading or understanding written instructions may be too embarrassed to say so. In regard to English as a second language (ESL) learners, be aware that just because a person can speak enough English to get by, that does not necessarily mean he or she can read and understand written English.

A need exists to design further research that will include literacy and comprehension assessment tools. Providing written instructions or brochures without knowing the level of the patient's ability to understand may put the patient at risk for further health complications. A review of current patient education literature, consent forms, and discharge instruction sheets may be necessary to assess the reading level. Consider that the recommended reading level for patient education materials is at the sixth-grade level, and then think of the consent forms and other materials we often ask patients to understand. Can you think of instances where the reading level may have been much too high? Recommendations may need to be made to adjust material to ensure that as many patients as possible are served. FYI 10.2 provides general learning principles for adult patients.

FYI 10.2 GENERAL PRINCIPLES OF LEARNING

- Individuals will learn in response to perceived needs. A sound teaching plan is designed from the assessed learning needs of the patient.
- Active learning (being able to direct and assist in assessing and planning learning) facilitates the learning process. An RN who recognizes the need for the patient to be an active learner will gain trust and empower the patient to take charge of health care concerns.
- If the material to be learned has meaning to the individual, learning is easier. Concepts or ideas form the foundation for learning facts, procedures, and rules.
- Learning that has direct application or use for the individual will be retained longer. Assessment of the patient's understanding of the health concerns in relation to his or her experiences will help you design a teaching plan that is empathetic to the patient's individual needs.
- A patient who can see progress is motivated to learn more.
- Mild anxiety enhances learning, but moderate to severe anxiety detracts from the learning process.
- Patients come to the health care setting with a lifetime of learning experiences. If learning can be associated with relevant real-life experiences, then the patient has a greater chance for retention of the material.

In Exercise 10.1, read the scenario and answer the questions concerning an adult learner's level of understanding.

ASSESSMENT OF READINESS TO LEARN

Two assumptions we often make when educating is that the patient has benefited from the experience and that learning has taken place. The reality is often the opposite because the patient will be under stress from the medical problem as well as the environment, and the addition of a learning experience would add to the stress. The patient may be motivated to learn, yet not ready to learn. **Readiness for learning** must be assessed before beginning the teaching process (FYI 10.3).

Understanding Stressors

The number of stresses on the patient will influence the patient's ability to understand and remember new information. Take, for example, a patient entering a same-day surgery center. The time frame before the surgery, or for any procedure, is typically

---

❓ EXERCISE 10.1

RN: "It must be difficult for you to quit smoking."

Patient: "I have been smoking all my life, and I don't plan to stop just because my doctor has told me to."

RN: "What has the doctor told you about smoking and the problems you are having?"

Patient: "He said that my breathing will get better if I stop smoking. I find that hard to believe, because when I have a cigarette, I tend to feel more relaxed, and my breathing becomes easier. I have the hardest time in the morning when I haven't had a cigarette all night."

RN: "Are there other times when you have difficulty breathing?"

Patient: "Yes, but only when I exert myself more than normal, like walking up a flight of stairs. I just use elevators when I can."

RN: "So, you find the times you have the most difficulty are when you awaken and when you exert yourself. When was the last time you can remember not having difficulty with your breathing in the morning?"

Patient: "Oh, I suppose it was when I was younger, maybe in my twenties. I was in good shape then. I have gotten older, I guess less fit."

RN: "So, you were more fit when you were in your twenties, and now that you are in your fifties, you feel less fit?"

Patient: "Yes, I guess so. I get around all right. This blasted pneumonia was unexpected."

RN: "Do you think you are having more or less difficulty than other men your age have with their breathing?"

Patient: "Oh, I know a few people who are like me, and I know some who are in better shape. I think I am like my father. He had lung problems and died of them."

What type of prejudicial thinking does this patient have that the RN will need to overcome?

What further questions could be asked of the patient to assist him toward a better understanding of his problem?

What would the nursing diagnosis KNOWLEDGE deficit be related to in this scenario?

What would the nursing diagnosis DENIAL be related to in this scenario?

FYI 10.3 FACTORS CONDUCIVE TO SUCCESSFUL LEARNING

- Learning takes place when behavior has changed. Change is stressful, and if the patient is experiencing additional stress, learning will be compromised.
- An RN must assess a patient's readiness to learn.
- The patient must be in the best possible condition before a teaching session.
- The family can assist the patient in the learning process.
- The patient's environment must be prepared before a teaching session.
- The patient who becomes an expert in his or her own care is empowered to maintain physical and psychological well-being.

---

short, yet the standard of care requires the RN to teach the patients about the care. The patient should understand several elements of the impending surgery. The RN will also need to teach the patient about his or her active participation in the recovery process (e.g., coughing and deep-breathing exercises or pain control methods). In many instances, after the procedure, the patient forgets what was said because true learning did not occur.

How can such a situation be avoided? In an outpatient surgical setting, teaching is typically done at the physician's office sometime before the procedure. Providing written material in advance of the day of surgery will give the patient time to read and understand the information.

Need to Include Family in the Learning Process

Family members and close friends can be assets to the RN during a patient teaching session. They will be able to reinforce the patient's education. Family members may advocate for loved ones, seek clarification, and act as coaches to encourage compliance with health care teaching. Often their need for information will be met as a result of their inclusion in the education sessions. Be certain, however, to assess the accuracy of the family's understanding of what you present.

Assess the Patient's Current Level of Knowledge

Some patients are experts in regard to their ailment. A lot of information is available about illnesses and treatments, and with the advent of the Internet, this information is even more readily available. This means that the patient entering the health care system may be well informed and have expectations for care. Such a patient has taken control of his or her life by learning as much as possible and incorporating it into elements of daily care. Hutchings (1999) described, through a case study, the importance of developing a health-promoting plan of care for a chronic illness by recognizing patients as experts. According to Hutchings, getting all patients to this expert position is important as a means of empowering them to better master their environment by maintaining both physical and psychological well-being.

To avoid or correct errors, determine the accuracy of information the patient provides about the condition. Not only are many reliable resources of medical information available but many unreliable, untested sources are as well. Ask the patient where the information came from.

✎ FYI 10.4   EVALUATION OF LEARNING

- The RN must be able to demonstrate that learning has taken place.
- The RN must take into consideration the literacy levels of the patient when evaluating learning and the patient's level of knowledge.
- More research needs to take place regarding the effectiveness of patient teaching.

？ EXERCISE 10.2

Two patients have been taught about their dietary restrictions with regard to their newly diagnosed diabetes mellitus. Each is being assessed for understanding of the limitations to diet.

Patient One: When I take my DiaBeta in the morning, I am free to eat what I want during the day. I will be glad not to have to be on the diet I was on before. It's okay for me to keep some hard candies in case the DiaBeta causes my blood sugar to go too low. In fact, I think I should eat one every now and then just to keep it from getting too low.

Patient Two: I know that the DiaBeta will help me keep my blood sugar down if I stay with my diet. I am concerned about the times that I might get low blood sugar levels. Should I carry some sort of candy with me for those times, or should I use something else instead? It is hard for me to know just what to do.

Which patient would need further teaching?

EVALUATION OF EFFECTIVENESS OF LEARNING

The RN must verify that learning, not just teaching, has taken place (FYI 10.4 and Exercise 10.2). For learning to have occurred, the patient must incorporate the learned behavior into his or her life. Assessment of the patient's learning is often completed at the time the teaching is done, yet in reality, an assessment done a day or two later may be a better indicator of the retention and incorporation of new information or behavior changes.

Legal Implications

While the standard of care is for the RN to be aware of the learning needs of the patient and provide a plan of care that will meet those needs, the RN often has difficulty demonstrating that learning has taken place. The standard of care dictates that patient teaching should include information regarding both the disorder and the treatment plan. The legal and ethical consequences of not providing and/or documenting that learning has occurred may place the RN in a position of being accused of inability to provide safe patient care.

Demonstration of Learning

Demonstration of learning or evaluating that learning has occurred can take place when a patient is observed completing a task without complications or consequences. The skill of a patient or family member who must do dressing changes at home can be observed and evaluated for effectiveness. The patient's understanding of the concept of sterility or of hypoglycemia, for example, is more difficult for the RN to assess. The RN may need to request an order for home health visits to follow up on patient teaching. A home health nurse can reassess the patient's knowledge and determine the need for further teaching.

A return demonstration of a procedure one time does not mean the patient has achieved understanding. Health care providers have a way of coaching patients through a procedure and then documenting that the patients "demonstrated understanding." Documentation of patient education is more important now than ever. Avoid words that cannot be measured, such as "understanding." While it is imperative that your documentation explain that a patient understands the material, use of the word alone is not enough. When you are documenting, all that you can record is that the patient both started and completed the educational session and was able to answer questions and demonstrate procedures correctly at the time of observation. You'll also need to demonstrate how much time it took to complete the educational sessions. To state that the patient demonstrated understanding as a result of one observation would be incorrect because many factors are present at the time of the observation that may influence the patient's ability to understand. However, you can document what you did, what the patient did, how, and when.

Following Up After Discharge

Another method to evaluate effectiveness of patient learning may be a call system, where the patient receives a telephone call from the RN 2 or 3 days after discharge. The RN will assess the patient's condition and need for further instruction. Careful assessment questions can identify problems and uncover teaching needs that have not been met. The RN will then revise the teaching plan to include areas of patient need and provide for follow-up if an assessed need exists.

BASIC PRINCIPLES OF TEACHING

Carnegie Mellon (2015) has also listed the following **principles** as standard to **effective teaching,** and these have been applied to the health care situation:

1. As teachers, we must gather relevant information about our patients and their families and allow that information to guide the development of all aspects of the experience.
2. For teaching to be effective, we must start with determining the learning objectives, figure the appropriate assessments that will evaluate associated learning, and choose instructional activities that best suit the need and the learner characteristics.
3. We need to be clear with patients about why the teaching is required.
4. Prioritization is critical, especially in the fast-paced health care environment. Patients can only absorb so much at one time, and there is usually precious little time, so it is absolutely imperative that we carefully prioritize what gets taught and when.
5. Remember that as experts (as opposed to the lay population) our understanding is automatic, and when we teach patients and families about their conditions, we can have a tendency to skip steps that may be critical to their understanding. Patients and families do not have the background or knowledge to intuitively know minute

details, so all processes need to be broken down into the minute steps that make up the whole.

6. Effective teachers take on multiple roles depending on the need of the student, and these are determined based on the outcomes desired.

7. We must consistently ask for an evaluation of our teaching and the experience as a whole in order to improve the quality of the learning experience for the patient and families.

CHARACTERISTICS OF A TEACHER

You may have had teachers who made an impression on you as either motivating and skilled or boring and dictatorial. You have perhaps attended conferences where one of the speakers was so inspiring that you may have made a change. Among several important characteristics of successful teachers are credibility, confidence, and the ability to communicate effectively.

Nurse Credibility

Credibility implies that the nurse has credentials or licensure and is honest enough to fulfill duties to the fullest and best of his or her ability. The RN has basic and advanced knowledge of how to decrease the risk factors for many diseases as well as how to promote a wellness state. A fundamental concept of the role of teacher is the maintenance of current knowledge of all aspects of patient care within the specialty. Knowledge must be practiced as well and taught by example. Many nurses do not practice wellness habits themselves and thus have difficulty promoting wellness habits in their patients. The nurse who is a smoker, yet teaches patients about smoking cessation, for example, will not be as credible as one who has quit smoking or never smoked.

Confidence

The RN must communicate effectively with confidence and be well prepared with the material to be presented. The RN must have knowledge and skill and present it as a credible source. A teacher needs to speak clearly and precisely for the patient to gain from the learning experience. Practice is important for patient teaching to be effective. Because the teacher role is one that the RN assumes on a daily basis, he or she should make the effort to hone this skill. Knowing the basics of adult learning and ensuring the patient's readiness to learn will assist in preparation for teaching, but to deliver a message effectively, you should practice interpersonal communication skills.

To improve at teaching, you should critique yourself. A self-evaluation journal is one way to look at what worked and what you could have done differently. A self-evaluation should take place as soon as you exit the teaching experience or as soon as possible before the end of the day.

Clear and Effective Communication

Clear, precise communication skills are fundamental to teaching. Terminology that is well defined and understood by the patient is a major consideration. For example, an RN may explain about the patient's heart failure, talking about how sodium intake causes osmosis to occur in the kidneys, resulting in pulmonary edema. In this scenario, at least four or five terms would be difficult for the patient to comprehend. When asked to comply with the dietary restrictions, the patient may then be too confused to understand what is needed. Adjust your explanations such that your patient education is delivered clearly, accurately, and in understandable terms.

PROCESSES OF TEACHING PATIENTS AND FAMILIES

Preparing the Environment

To ensure that the patient and family are ready to learn, the RN must prepare the learning environment. Providing as much privacy as possible can help ensure that the patient and family are comfortable discussing the treatment plan. Minimize distractions and noise by asking that the television be turned off. Provide privacy by selecting a private location or excusing roommates or certain family members. Ensure that the patient has received medications that help him or her feel well, and delay (if advisable) medication that may cause distracting side effects, such as nausea or drowsiness. The RN should be positioned to deliver teaching comfortably, while looking relaxed and interested in the process rather than stressed or hurried. Teaching can often take place while the RN is seated next to the patient.

Teaching Plan

For the teaching session to be most efficient, the RN should develop an individualized **teaching plan** that identifies the purpose, goals, and objectives of the teaching. The teaching plan also identifies the content outline, method of instruction that works best for the patient, the time that is required to deliver the teaching, the resources the RN will need, and the method of evaluation. If all of these things are clearly planned and in written form, then any nurse who takes care of the patient can deliver the education and reinforce the learning in a consistent manner, leading to improved outcomes (Bastable, 2014). Many evidence-based resources are available for inclusion in teaching plans. It is important that resources are current and from authoritative references. In general, a key to a successful teaching plan is to individualize it for the patient regarding culture, learning style, developmental stage, and level of literacy. See Fig. 10.1 for an example of a teaching plan.

Resources

As noted in the teaching plan example, to assist in the learning process, the RN should have appropriate teaching aids ready. A model of the baby, heart, kidney, or central line, for example, will help the patient picture the position, procedure, or condition. The patient can also view a video or a PowerPoint slide show on a tablet, and the RN will then be available to answer questions and clarify the content. Discussion with hand-outs and note pages and hands-on practice are all good choices of resources that can be customized for your patient. Pamphlets can be good resources for the patient, again leaving the RN to clarify or expand on the content. An obvious determination to make before offering reading material is whether the patient is able to read it, so the RN must assess the patient's reading level. Most health-related reading material is at the sixth- through eighth-grade levels, but not all patients will read even

Purpose: To provide mother of newborn with information necessary to promote successful and sustained breastfeeding

Goal: The mother will independently manage breastfeeding of infant.

Objectives	Content Outline	Method of Instruction	Time Allotted	Resources	Method of Evaluation
Following a 20-minute teaching session, the mother will be able to: 1.) State two benefits for both baby and mother of breastfeeding	1.) Passive immunity Infant brain development Improved health later in life (diabetes, cancer) Maternal hormonal change	PPT and discussion	10 minutes	1.) http://www.cdc.gov/breastfeeding/	Teach back
2.) Demonstrate positions for breastfeeding	2.) Belly to belly, Football hold, Cradle hold	Demonstration	10 minutes	PowerPoint via tablet demonstration With doll, poster, and pamphlet	Return demonstration

FIG. 10.1 Example teaching plan.

that well. Including family members by offering them the pamphlets may be helpful because they may be able to assist the patient in reading comprehension. Some patients may have a learning disability that decreases their ability to read or understand written words, so other methods will need to be devised in these instances. Special needs should be assessed and addressed individually and in a sensitive manner. Reading material must also be in the appropriate language for the patient; a patient who reads only Spanish will not be able to learn much from a pamphlet in English. Your patient may require pamphlets or other materials written in Braille or provided in audio recordings.

Culture and Learning

Assessment for and sensitivity to differences between cultures are imperative in preparing the appropriate teaching for your patient. Cultural beliefs influence how teaching is received by each individual and his or her family. In some cases, it may not be the patient who must receive the teaching, but a family member. There may be instances where what you need to teach may be in disagreement with a culturally held belief or cultural health practice. In these cases it is critical that you have a clear understanding of how the patient's culture influences his or her learning or readiness to learn. The RN should build on the patient's knowledge and beliefs (where possible), which will encourage learning and improve the patient's response to health teaching (Bastable, 2014).

One model, by Cordell and Price (1994), as presented by Bastable (2014), that will help you to provide culturally appropriate teaching for your patient includes a four-step process. First, examining your own personal culture provides a foundation and perspective. Second, familiarize yourself with your patient's culture. Next, it is important to identify any adaptations that your patient has already made, and finally modify your teaching plan based on information gathered in the three earlier steps (Bastable, 2014).

Learning Styles

You should also consider the learning style of the individual patient. Learning styles are indicators of how a person prefers to learn, that is the way a person most effectively takes in, processes, remembers, and is able to recall and apply what is learned (Bastable, 2014). For example, some people learn best by practice or hands-on experiences. Others learn by reading, watching a video, looking at diagrams and pictures, or by listening to a lecture. Determining how your patient prefers to learn must be done quickly, and there are a few ways this to do this, including observation, interview, and having the patient complete a learning styles inventory. Several instruments or inventories can be administered that will also help to determine learning style. In the patient care situation, you may not have the time or opportunity to implement the tools. However, you can certainly ask your patients what works best for them and, alternatively, planning to include multiple methods of instruction will help to address the various styles. Providing a variety of ways to deliver the information—by video, demonstrations, posters, pictures, pamphlets, discussions, hands-on practice, and more—will assist each learner in understanding and retaining the information.

KEY POINTS

After completion of this chapter, you have learned:

- The RN is constantly engaging in formal and informal patient teaching.
- The RN must practice basic principles of teaching and understand the fundamentals of adult learning.
- A standard of care is for the RN to engage in patient teaching.
- Effective teaching can empower the patient to better manage his or her own health care, become more compliant with the plan of care, and have more positive outcomes.
- Teaching plans should be customized to accommodate the patient's culture, literacy level, readiness to learn, and learning style.

CRITICAL THINKING QUESTIONS

1. Identify a teaching need in a patient for whom you are to care. Design a simple teaching plan that includes the following:
   - How you will assess the patient for a teaching need
   - The identified teaching need
   - Relevant information about the patient requiring accommodation that will guide your teaching, such as culture and readiness to learn
   - Information you will need to gather to teach the topic, including references from at least two sources
   - Where the teaching will take place
   - Props, audiovisuals, or reading material you will need
   - How you will prepare the environment to optimize learning
   - How much time you will need to teach
   - Data that support the patient's readiness to learn
   - Measures you will take to evaluate whether learning has taken place
   - Evaluation of the teaching and a self-evaluation of your ability as a teacher
2. A patient is to receive an experimental treatment. The physician has been in to explain the procedure, and the patient has signed the consent form. In doing an assessment before the procedure, the patient states, "I really didn't understand what the doctor told me, except he said I should get better. I hope I do get better."
   a. What is your responsibility as an RN at this point?
   b. What questions would you ask the patient at this time?
   c. What questions would you ask your supervisor or manager if the patient had significant unease about the impending procedure?

WEB RESOURCES

Carnegie Mellon University, http://cmu.edu/teaching/principles/index.html
The Joint Commission, http://jointcommission.org/topics/default.aspx?k=683
Centers for Disease Control and Prevention, http://cdc.gov/
The National Library of Medicine and The National Institutes of Health, http://nlm.nih.gov/medlineplus/tutorial.html

REFERENCES

American Medical Association Ad Hoc Committee on Health Literacy for the Council on Scientific Affairs. (1999). Health literacy: report of the Council on Scientific Affairs. *Journal of the American Medical Association, 281*(6), 552–557.

Bastable, S. B. (2014). *Nurse as educator.* Burlington, MA: Jones & Bartlett Learning.

Carnegie Mellon University. (2015). *Principles of Teaching & Learning.* Retrieved from http://www.cmu.edu/teaching/principles/index.html.

Fisher, E. (1999). Low literacy levels in adults: implications for patient education. *Journal of Continuing Education in Nursing, 30*(2), 56–61.

Hutchings, D. (1999). Partnership in education: an example of client and educator collaboration. *Journal of Continuing Education in Nursing, 30*(3), 128–131.

Lindeman, E. C. (1926). *The meaning of adult education.* New York, NY: New Republic.

The Joint Commission. (2001). *2001 Hospital accreditation standards.* Oakbrook Terrace, IL: Author.

11

The Nurses, Ideas, and Forces That Define the Profession

⊖volve WEBSITE

Additional resources are available online at:
http://evolve.elsevier.com/Claywell/transitions

OBJECTIVES

After completing this chapter, the student will be prepared to:
1. Discuss historical contributions to modern nursing.
2. Describe the impact of managed care and merging health care services on the nursing profession.
3. Discuss the role of nursing in quality improvement of patient care.
4. Describe at least three ways in which trends in health care will affect nursing practice.

KEY TERMS

Alexian Brothers	Dock, Lavinia	Montag, Mildred
Barton, Clara	Hotel Dieu	Nightingale, Florence
Breckenridge, Mary	Knights Hospitalers of St. John of Jerusalem	Nutting, Mary Adelaide
continuous quality improvement	Knights of Saint Lazarus	Richards, Linda
Dix, Dorothea	managed care	Robb, Isabel Hampton
		Wald, Lillian

OVERVIEW

From the time of the ancient folk healers to that of the present-day nurse practitioner, nursing's history is rich with change (Fig. 11.1). The earliest documented nursing organization was formed in 1099 during the First Crusade (1095–1099). Known as the **Knights Hospitalers of St. John of Jerusalem,** this organization's members

188

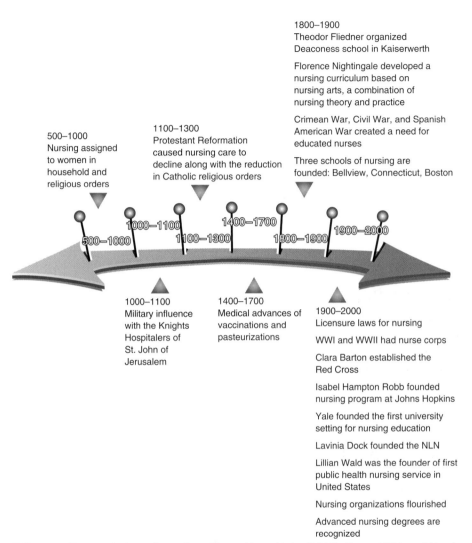

FIG. 11.1 The evolution of nursing. (From Ham K. L. (2002) *From LPN to RN role transitions.* St Louis: Mosby.)

provided hospitality and care to thousands of pilgrims and crusaders in the Holy Land (Kalisch & Kalisch, 1995).

During the Middle Ages, most nursing care was performed by religious orders. Later, nursing care became more secular and more structured. Formal training programs were begun, such as that at the Deaconess Institute at Kaiserwerth, Germany, established in 1836.

Influenced by social and political forces and driven by inadequate health care for the hospitalized, **Florence Nightingale,** a graduate of the Kaiserwerth program, revolutionized the manner in which nurses cared for patients. She instituted changes that affected patient survival rates, made nursing more appealing as a profession to young women, and profoundly affected modern-day nursing.

During the early 1980s, the nature of health care began changing dramatically as cost reduction and quality improvement issues surfaced. Shorter hospital stays have forced patients back to the community for completion of care, and nurses have refocused nursing care planning on meeting patient-expected outcomes as quickly as possible. Managed care has become a reality, and it has affected the way in which patients can access the health care system.

As you obtain registered nurse licensure and take on greater responsibilities, you will be facing increasingly difficult challenges. Now, in the 21st century, we are again experiencing a nursing shortage. Fewer young people are seeking careers in nursing, largely because of increasingly attractive jobs in high-tech areas, which promise better benefits and less stress. In addition, there are fewer nursing faculty, so the numbers of students who can be admitted into prelicensure nursing programs is limited.

As a new graduate entering the registered nursing workforce, you need to be aware of past influences that have shaped nursing, as well as the nature of the present health care environment. This chapter takes you through a brief history of nursing, emphasizing religious, social, and political aspects of nursing's development as a profession. Factors affecting nursing practice in today's world are explored.

HISTORICAL FOUNDATIONS

The history of nursing can be traced to the modern day by examining societal influences that shaped the development of the profession. Religious, social, and political factors have all contributed to nursing's history.

Religious

In the West, the establishment of Christianity coincided with the development of groups organized to help care for the sick, orphans, widows, the elderly, and the poor in the name of charity (Kalisch & Kalisch, 1995). Throughout history, nursing has been considered a calling by many—a special vocation in which an individual gives selflessly to others. Hard work, dedication to duty, and benevolence are basic religious values that many denominations honor, and these are the principles upon which nursing began.

Despite the fact that nursing has been a predominantly female profession, males in religious orders took an active part in early care of the sick. The **Knights of Saint Lazarus** (established about 1200) dedicated themselves to caring for people with leprosy, syphilis, and other socially unacceptable diseases (Donahue, 1996). The Knights Hospitalers of Saint John of Jerusalem were members of a male organization that provided care to travelers pursuing spiritual goals. During the bubonic plague epidemic of 1348, another male nursing group, the **Alexian Brothers,** was founded and continues to exist today in dual spiritual/nursing roles.

Benedictine monasteries organized medical schools, some of which afforded female deaconesses the opportunity to pursue a program of study in caring for the sick. In this way, women were able to satisfy intellectual and spiritual aspirations while contributing to the needs of others (Nutting & Dock, 1935). By joining a religious order, unmarried women were given the freedom to provide a service to others outside their own families.

Apart from formal religious orders, some groups of women joined together to care for the sick outside the bounds of the cloister or convent. One such group was the Beguines of Flanders, Belgium. This group was a religious association established in the 12th century, but its members took no monastic vows. Members, or "sisters," received their preparation to care for others as apprentices under the guidance of more experienced Beguines. They devoted themselves to the needs of widows and orphans of the Crusaders. One of the most famous Beguine hospitals is the **Hotel Dieu** in Paris. Besides working in the hospital, the Beguine sisters also cared for people in their homes (Dolan, Fitzpatrick, & Herrmann, 1983).

The Renaissance, which began in the 14th and 15th centuries and peaked in the 16th and 17th centuries, saw a decline in the influence of religious orders, helped along by the emergence of the Protestant Reformation in Europe. With these transformations, nursing care, too, saw significant secularizing changes. It has continued to move more fully into the general population, and it is no longer primarily the province of religious orders. In our own era, however, we have seen a renewed interest in returning nursing care to the church. During the past several years, parish nursing has achieved a certain popularity. Many churches have instituted parish nursing as a service for their parishioners. The duties of the parish nurse vary with each church organization but may include visiting the ill, health teaching, and wellness screening for members. Parish nurses provide holistic health care to a faith community (Bergquist & King, 1994).

Social

Perhaps the major social factor affecting the development of nursing is society's attitude toward the role of women. Traditionally, women have been expected to assume the role of wife and mother, tending primarily to their immediate family's needs. Following the Reformation, hospital nursing was often carried out by the "undesirables" of society, such as criminals and prostitutes (Donahue, 1996). They were poorly educated and were described as being drunken and abusive to patients.

With the establishment of the first real school of nursing at Kaiserwerth, Germany, many young women were better educated and more fully prepared to improve nursing care. Perhaps the most famous graduate of this school was Florence Nightingale (Fig. 11.2). Born into a wealthy family, Florence Nightingale (1820–1910) was highly educated and had social standing in England. Victorian English attitudes of the time supported the belief that gentlewomen should not work outside the home. But rebelling against her parents' wishes, she received training to become a nurse.

When she learned of the lack of medical and nursing care for British troops during the Crimean War (1853–1856), Nightingale organized a group of 38 nurses to travel to the Crimea in southern Russia. Despite societal opposition, she and her team reached the Crimean battlefields in 1854. They found overcrowding in the hospitals, no medical supplies, and limited space for the sick and injured. Using her own funds, Nightingale obtained supplies, cleaned up the unsanitary conditions, and established laundries to wash linens.

At the end of 6 months, Nightingale and her nurses had decreased the death rate from 42% to 2% (Dolan et al., 1983). Working long hours to care for casualties of the war, Florence Nightingale was observed many nights making rounds through the battlefields with a lighted lantern, earning her the nickname "the Lady with the

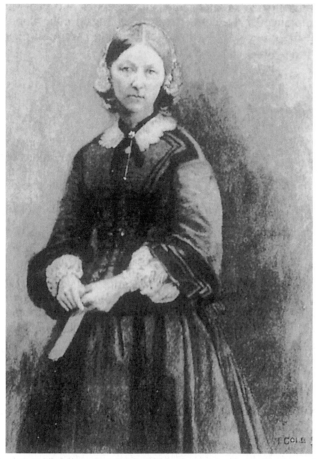

FIG. 11.2 Florence Nightingale, 1820–1910, founder of modern nursing. (Cole, T. *Wood engraving*. National Library of Medicine, Bethesda, Maryland.)

Lamp." For her tireless efforts, she was recognized and praised by her countrymen both in the Crimea and in England.

Upon her return home, Florence Nightingale was given a monetary award by the British people. With this money, she established a school of nursing at London's St. Thomas's Hospital in 1860. Again, she was met with opposition from members of society who believed women should remain in the home to care for their own family members (Kalisch & Kalisch, 1995). Nevertheless, the school prospered, largely because of Nightingale's reputation. She was the first woman to be awarded the British Order of Merit, which she received in 1907.

Florence Nightingale's school of nursing emphasized health of both body and soul (Dolan et al., 1983). Nightingale believed that nursing was an art—one that required organized, practical, and scientific training. She resisted the idea that nurses were to be servants of physicians or any other health care professionals. Florence Nightingale supported the idea that nurses should be educated to possess a unique body of knowledge that is nursing.

In her book *Notes on Nursing*, published in 1860, Nightingale defined nursing as "that care which puts a person in the best possible condition for nature to restore or to preserve health, and to prevent or to cure disease or injury." Upon her death, she left contributions in the areas of nursing process, education, theory, and research. Through Nightingale's efforts, nursing gradually came to be viewed as a profession for women of all social levels.

Nineteenth-century attitudes toward women in America were similar to those in Europe. But throughout that century, characterized by the Industrial Revolution, women continued to push past societal boundaries to improve nursing education and patient care. In 1900, **Clara Barton** (1821–1912)—the "Angel of the Battlefield" during the American Civil War (1861–1865)—organized the American Red Cross, which she headed until 1904. In the early 20th century, two other women were of particular importance: **Lillian Wald** (1867–1940), who established a visiting nursing service for poor tenement families in New York City, and **Mary Breckenridge** (1881–1965), who organized a frontier nurses' organization in rural Kentucky, which is still in operation today.

As the public began to recognize the benefits of better-trained nurses, courtesy of Florence Nightingale's efforts in England, nursing schools began to spring up in the United States. Nursing was becoming more attractive as a vocation for young women. **Linda Richards** (1841–1930), known as America's first trained nurse, worked many years to help improve nursing education. Other contributors to nursing education in America were **Isabel Hampton Robb** (1860–1910), who reduced working hours of students and promoted licensure exams, and **Mary Adelaide Nutting** (1858–1948), who wrote a book on the history of nursing.

The transition to the 20th century in the United States brought new rights and freedoms for women, together with more recognition of their place in the working world. **Lavinia Dock** (1858–1956) was a well-known nurse who fought for women's rights issues and for the right to vote. Education for nurses became established at universities, and **Mildred Montag** (1908–2004) promoted creation of the associate degree as a shorter route into nursing. Medical advances created new ethical concerns, and nurses developed professional organizations.

Political

Religious orders, laypeople, and soldiers all have been called upon to provide assistance during times of political conflict throughout history. Whatever the reason, from territorial advancement to the preservation of personal freedoms, societies have waged wars in which nurses have been needed to care for the injured and their families. In fact, many important contributions to the development of professional nursing have been made during times of conflict.

While Florence Nightingale struggled to improve health care in England, Americans, North and South, were fighting the Civil War. Care of the injured was just as disorganized and unsanitary on Union and Confederate battlefields as it was in Europe. Several religious orders responded to the call for efficient, effective nursing care, yet more nurses were needed. Many women who had no formal nursing education volunteered to help.

One such woman was **Dorothea Dix** (1802–1887), a Boston schoolteacher who had been crusading to improve care of the mentally ill in institutions. Appointed superintendent of the Female Nurses of the [Union] Army, Dix organized a training program for women volunteers who met strict criteria, both in moral character and looks. (Dix insisted that nurses should be "plain"—i.e., unattractive.) At the end of a month-long training program, the women qualified to supervise care of the wounded during the Civil War. In the South, however, society continued to frown on women who worked outside the home. Therefore, the wounded were cared for by women in their own homes or by volunteers in hospitals.

The Spanish-American War of 1898 marked the first time trained nurses were accepted in military hospitals. By the outbreak of World War I (1914–1918), both the Army and the Navy had implemented a nurse corps. The Army School of Nursing was formed in 1918 to meet the rising need for nurses to care for battle casualties (Dolan et al., 1983).

During World War II (1939–1945), significant treatment advances helped to bring about a higher level of patient care. Antibiotics, blood transfusions, and immunizations improved survival rates. Trauma care and rehabilitation became a means of saving and restoring lives. Nurses were involved in all aspects of care, whether in military hospitals, on battleships, or flying on medical evacuation planes.

In the last half of the 20th century, nurses continued to assist the sick and wounded during the Korean conflict, the Vietnam War, Operation Desert Storm, and in the War on Terror. Today, nurses serve in various branches of the military as staff nurses, educators, and administrators.

NURSING TODAY: FACTORS INFLUENCING PRACTICE

The health care system in the United States has undergone many changes since the founding of the initial 13 colonies. Health care has moved from the home to the hospital and most recently back to the home again. As health education for the public has improved and technology has provided better medications and treatments for most diseases, Americans have enjoyed longer, healthier lives.

Until the early 1980s, most Americans were content to be passive recipients of care in a system that poured millions of dollars into acute care and rehabilitation, with little attention to cost containment and health promotion. As health care costs began to rise to uncontrollable levels, it became apparent that millions of Americans were either uninsured or were rapidly losing the ability to pay for health care (Catalano, 1996).

As you enter the health care environment of today as a registered nurse, you will encounter challenges created by several factors. Patient care of the present and future will be affected by (1) an aging population; (2) an emphasis on health maintenance and disease prevention; (3) outcomes-oriented, patient-centered care; (4) cost containment; and (5) quality improvement.

Aging Population

It is estimated that by 2030, there will be about 65 million older Americans (Campbell, 2001). With this "graying of America" will come an increase in patients with multisystem health care problems and chronic illnesses. The elderly currently utilize more health care dollars per person than do younger members of the American population. They typically have fewer years of schooling, rely heavily on Social Security for financial support, have chronic illnesses, and are widowed. These factors add up to more use of health care resources at a greater cost.

Nurses must respond to a shift in demographics by becoming more knowledgeable about geriatric and home health care. More research is needed, for example, in the areas of Alzheimer's disease and other forms of dementia so nurses are better equipped to care for the aged and their families. In the past, the elderly were placed in nursing homes when they were no longer able to care for themselves. Nursing education programs have emphasized care of hospitalized patients and have provided most of the clinical experiences for students in such settings rather than in long-term care facilities. As a result, many of today's practicing nurses have not received education specific to geriatric care, but in today's nursing education programs, specific content regarding geriatric care is included.

Because hospital stays have been reduced, future nursing education will need to be in settings where the elderly require assistance—the home, neighborhood clinics, churches, and community centers. Psychosocial aspects of aging need to be addressed, as does helping the elderly obtain access to needed resources.

Emphasis on Health Promotion and Disease Prevention

As the general population becomes more involved in maintaining a healthy lifestyle, nurses are taking an active part in patient teaching about health promotion and disease prevention. In the past, nurses usually had contact with patients only during an episode of illness or injury. At present, nurses counsel patients about health screening, dietary needs, exercise programs, and treatment regimens for various medical problems. Besides providing care during acute illnesses, nurses are instrumental in teaching patients self-care strategies for discharge home.

An integrative review of 40 research studies sought to define the health promotion roles of nurses and further identify the health promotion skills and expertise important in carrying out health promotion activities. What the authors found was that nurses carry out a wide variety of health promotion activities across care settings but that the most common form of health promotion activity was health education. It was identified that nurses who successfully implement health promotion are proficient in local, regional, and national health care and social care policies and programs and are able to use these in providing health promotion information and activities, helping their patients to navigate the complex and myriad systems associated with health care. In addition, nurses who engaged in health promotion did so in a patient-centered approach in that they saw the patient, family, or community as having individual traits such as age, developmental stage, gender, gender identity, culture, ethnicity, socioeconomic and literacy levels, and lifestyle and would tailor the activities to meet the specific need. Nurses must possess a number of competencies in order to successfully carry out health promotion activities. These include four major categories: multidisciplinary knowledge, skills, attitudes, and particular personal characteristics. Multidisciplinary knowledge includes a broad understanding of determinants of health and a theoretical background broad enough to facilitate learning, change, and healthy lifestyles. Required skills include collaboration, communication, and assessment. Attitudes that facilitate health promotion include a proactive stance and advocacy. Finally, being a healthy role model is a strong characteristic of a nurse engaged in health promotion (Kemppainen et al., 2013).

With an increased level of knowledge about their own health needs, consumers have become more involved in health care decision making. This has eased the transition into an outcomes-based system of care that is patient-centered, as patient participation is necessary to meet desired goals. As health care costs rise and insurance companies tighten restrictions on services provided, health care professionals are working very closely with patients to set goals that can be achieved as quickly as possible. In some cases, noncompliant patients are being discharged from care settings and provider practices; nurses can address this issue of widening access to care by helping patients engage more fully and successfully in health promotion activities. Through the nursing process, nurses help patients to develop expected outcomes and plan interventions to achieve the desired results (see Chapter 6).

Outcomes-Oriented Patient-Centered Care

Nurses are working with population groups, as well as individual patients, to develop health-related goals. For example, community health nurses participate in multidisciplinary planning meetings to set outcomes for patients. No matter where the patient is within the health care system, nurses are playing an important role in helping achieve positive experiences for patients with minimal complications.

Cost Containment

The dominant focus of patient care in the current health care environment is to contain rising costs. Hospitals, faced with financial difficulties, are merging into large health care systems. **Managed care,** an insurance-based approach to reducing costs, has invaded patient care in every setting. Case managers (see Chapter 14) coordinate patient care activities as the patient moves through the health care system.

Terms such as *diagnosis related groups* (DRGs), *preferred provider organizations* (PPOs), and *health maintenance organizations* (HMOs) (Box 11.1) have become commonplace. Consumers, once responsible for paying for their own health care, have become dependent on third parties to be able to afford treatment. Nurses are challenged to deliver quality nursing care in an environment that limits consumers' options.

Consider the Following Questions

1. Based on personal experience as a nurse, have you cared for a patient for whom you believe the type and amount of provided health care were influenced by his or her ability to pay for services? If so, please describe the circumstances and the outcome for the patient:

_____

_____

_____

BOX 11.1 HEALTH CARE PAYMENT SOURCES

- **Medicare:** National and state health insurance program for older adults.
- **Medicaid:** Federal public assistance program to assist those with financial needs.
- **Prospective Payment System:** Limits the amount paid to hospitals that are reimbursed by Medicare; uses diagnosis related groups (DRGs) to establish pretreatment diagnosis billing categories.
- **Private Insurance:** A form of third-party reimbursement. Carried as individual or group coverage through a job; the company pays either a portion or the entire cost.
- **Health Maintenance Organizations (HMOs):** A group health care agency. A prepaid fee is set without regard to type of treatment. The emphasis is on health maintenance and disease prevention; patients are limited in use of providers and services.
- **Preferred Provider Organizations (PPOs):** A group of physicians and agencies provide services to employees of a company through an insurance company. In return for using the specified physicians and agencies, patients receive a discounted rate for services.

---

2. What, if any, actions were taken by nursing personnel to ensure the best possible care for this patient? What do you think could or should have been done differently for this patient?

_____

_____

_____

Quality Improvement

Despite these restrictions, health care systems and patients share a common expectation: quality care. Nurses, who spend more time with patients than other health care professionals, are instrumental in ensuring appropriate, viable care (Malloch & Porter-O'Grady, 1999). What was once called *quality assurance* in patient care is now termed **continuous quality improvement.** This is a process in which the quality of patient care is continuously monitored for effectiveness.

The quality of care may be assessed from the time a patient enters the health care system through discharge and beyond to include transitional care. At each step of the way, all disciplines should be involved in measuring patient outcomes against a set of standards that promotes excellence. Many organizations utilize clinical care pathways, or care paths, as a format for ensuring that patients are "on track" to accomplish set goals (see Chapter 16). As problems are identified, action should be taken to prevent complications and increased length of stay within the system and avoid readmission for the same condition. In fact, "the Affordable Care Act added section 1886(q) to the Social Security Act establishing the Hospital Readmissions Reduction Program, which requires CMS [Centers for Medicare & Medicaid Services] to reduce payments to… hospitals with excess readmissions, effective for discharges beginning on October 1, 2012" (CMS.gov, 2016, para 1).

Hospitals and community agencies are employing nurses as outcomes managers, case managers, and quality improvement managers to monitor the quality of patient care. By maximizing a patient's chances of achieving expected outcomes, costs will be reduced, patients will have fewer complications, and customer satisfaction will be improved.

In 2002, The Joint Commission (TJC) established a set of core measures upon which hospitals report, including treatment of acute myocardial infarction, heart failure, ventilator-assisted pneumonia, surgical care, pregnancy and related conditions, and pediatric asthma. In 2003, the CMS created the Hospital Quality Initiatives (HCI) that included 20 measures or indicators as evidence of best practice. Leaping forward a decade, and now as organizations and providers prepare for national health reform, the emphasis on quality and safety is greater than ever. The National Quality Strategy has three aims: Better Care, Healthy People/Healthy Communities, and Affordable Care (U.S. Department of Health and Human Services, 2012). "Achieving these aims will require a concerted effort in four measurable focus areas: care coordination and patient safety; increased access to and use of preventive health services; better care for at risk populations; and enhanced patient & caregiver experience of care. The CMS measures achievement of these four areas through the formation and monitoring of accountable care organizations (ACOs) that measure and report 33 quality measures" (Weston & Roberts, 2013, para. 1). These measures are made public in order to inform consumers and payors. While the program is voluntary, the Medicare Prescription Drug, Improvement and Modernization Act (MMA) of 2003 required facilities to participate or receive a reduction in federal payments under CMS. "Quality and performance improvement initiatives are driving significant changes in the United States (U.S) healthcare system" (Weston & Roberts, 2013, para. 1).

Many other groups, such as the Leapfrog Group, collect and report patient safety and quality data to the public and payors. All of these systems create financial incentives for facilities to engage in formal quality improvement activities, and nurses are at the heart of that effort (Draper et al., 2008). Because nursing care is the major reason people come to hospitals, it is the nurses who are in a position to improve practice and outcomes.

According to Mary Wakefield, PhD, RN (2010), administrator of the U.S. Health Resources and Services Administration (HRSA), the passage of the Patient Protection and Affordable Care Act (2010) increases opportunities for grants to nurses in master's and doctoral studies. The Act increases the amount of funds student nurses may borrow and even offers partial loan cancellation. These programs are meant to encourage students from disadvantaged backgrounds to enter or stay in nursing. Another part of the Act provides for the Nurse Education, Practice and Retention grant program aimed at increasing nursing knowledge in quality standards, assessment, and improvement. The Act expanded the National Health Service Corps, and APRNs who agree to work in underserved areas receive up to $145,000 in loan repayments. Further, the Act created a grant program that can be funded up to $1.5 billion for Maternal and Child Programs for at-risk populations. More grant funding is now available for the Nurse Managed Health Centers, thus dramatically increasing access to care. All of this means that more nurses are needed now than ever and in roles with increasing responsibility. Truly the health of the nation rests in the hands of nurses.

As we consider nursing in the future, we must be aware of the number of social, economic, and political forces that will influence health care and, ultimately, the type of nursing care needed. The ANA's Social Policy statement for nursing has clearly evolved from a contract to a social covenant between nursing and society. Last updated in 2015, Fowler describes what is now known as the "16 elements of the social contract: reciprocal expectations between nursing and society" (p. 19). Listed here is an abridged version of "the obligations that nursing must meet as a profession" (p. 19), and each of these can be seen as seated firmly in and developing from our understanding of quality of care and trust:

- "Caring Service: That nursing care will be given with compassion and will preserve the dignity and recognize the worth of patients without prejudice.
- Primacy of the Patient: That the patient's needs and interests supersede those of the institution or the nurse.
- Knowledge, Skill, and Competence: That the professions will ensure the knowledge, skill, and competence of those newly entering the profession, and those in practice, at every level and in every role.
- Hazardous Service: That members of the profession will provide nursing care under conditions not customarily expected to those outside of the profession.
- Responsibility and Accountability: That nursing and nurses will be accountable and responsible for practice…
- Progress and Development: That the profession will incorporate knowledge development from the humanities and scientific advances…
- Ethical Practice: That the professional will promulgate, affirm, and uphold a code of ethics, to which individual nurses are expected to adhere.
- Collaboration: That nursing will contribute its distinctive perspective and voice to the wider healthcare conversation…
- Promotion of the Health of the Public: It is expected that nurses will address the problems faced by individual patients including issues of health disparities and… lead in health-related issues important to society.
- Autonomy of Practice: That society will authorize nursing to practice within its scope and standards…
- Self-Governance: That society will extend the authority to professional self-regulation of practice in accord with state nurse practice acts.
- Title and Practice Protection: That society will promulgate law that governs nursing…granting licensure that is mandatory…[and] protect the title 'registered Nurse'
- Respect and Just Remuneration: That society will accord the nursing profession respect…just wage and humane work conditions…
- Freedom to Practice: That nurses will have the authority and freedom to practice nursing to the full extent of their education and preparation…
- Workforce Sustainability: That society will develop, implement, and support a strategic plan to address workforce shortages…
- Protection in Hazardous Service: That society will provide legislative and other means to require organizations to minimize risk to nurses in the face of hazardous service…" (Fowler, 2015, pp. 20–22).

Nurses will be increasingly called upon to assume leadership roles in designing care for vulnerable population groups, in demonstrating quality care, and in cost containment (O'Neil & Coffman, 1998). We have indeed come a long way from the days of folk healers and untrained volunteers on the battlefield. Nurses have had a colorful, productive history. Let us look eagerly to the future by understanding our past, fully engaging with our professional covenant, and taking advantage of the opportunities for growth that are within our reach.

KEY POINTS

Much has transpired throughout the development of nursing to this point. Following is a quick look back at what you learned in this chapter:

- The earliest documented nursing organization, the Knights Hospitalers of St. John of Jerusalem, was formed in 1099 during the First Crusade (1095–1099).
- During the Middle Ages, the majority of nursing care was performed by religious orders.
- Later, nursing care became more secular and more structured. Formal training programs were begun, such as that at the Deaconess Institute at Kaiserwerth, Germany, established in 1836.
- Influenced by social and political forces and driven by inadequate health care for the hospitalized, Florence Nightingale, a graduate of the Kaiserwerth program, revolutionized the manner in which nurses cared for patients.
- During the early 1980s, the nature of health care began changing dramatically as cost reduction and quality improvement issues surfaced.
- Throughout history, nursing has been considered a calling by many—a special vocation in which an individual gives selflessly to others.
- Despite the fact that nursing has been a predominantly female profession, males in religious orders took an active part in early care of the sick. The Knights of Saint Lazarus (established about 1200) dedicated themselves to caring for people with leprosy, syphilis, and other socially unacceptable diseases.
- Apart from formal religious orders, some groups of women joined together to care for the sick outside the bounds of the cloister or convent.
- The Renaissance, which began in the 14th and 15th centuries and peaked in the 16th and 17th centuries, saw a decline in the influence of religious orders, helped along by the emergence of the Protestant Reformation in Europe. With these transformations, nursing care, too, saw significant secularizing changes. It has continued to move more fully into the general population and is no longer primarily the province of religious orders.
- Perhaps the major social factor affecting the development of nursing is society's attitude toward the role of women.
- Nightingale believed that nursing was an art—one that required organized, practical, and scientific training.
- Throughout the 19th century, characterized by the Industrial Revolution, women continued to push past societal boundaries to improve nursing education and patient care.
- As the public began to recognize the benefits of better-trained nurses, courtesy of Florence Nightingale's efforts in England, nursing schools began to spring up in the United States.
- Linda Richards (1841–1930), known as America's first trained nurse, worked many years to help improve nursing education.
- The transition to the 20th century in the United States brought new rights and freedoms for women, together with more recognition of their place in the working world.
- Many important contributions to the development of professional nursing have been made during times of conflict.

- Appointed superintendent of the Female Nurses of the [Union] Army, Dorothea Dix organized a training program for women volunteers who met strict criteria, both in moral character and looks.
- The Spanish-American War of 1898 marked the first time trained nurses were accepted in military hospitals.
- By the outbreak of World War I (1914–1918), both the Army and the Navy had implemented a nurse corps.
- During World War II (1939–1945), nurses were involved in all aspects of care, whether in military hospitals, on battleships, or flying on medical evacuation planes.
- Today, nurses serve in various branches of the military as staff nurses, educators, and administrators.
- Patient care of the present and future will be affected by an aging population; an emphasis on health promotion and disease prevention; outcomes-oriented, patient-centered care; cost containment; and quality improvement.
- Nursing's Social Policy Statement has evolved to a social contract and covenant with society based on honesty, ethics, competence, quality, and trust.

CRITICAL THINKING QUESTIONS

1. How have Florence Nightingale's contributions to nursing affected your practice? List three of her beliefs about nursing that you apply to patient care.
2. Explain the importance of understanding trends in health care to everyday nursing practice.
3. Consider the Patient Protection and Affordable Care Act and its provisions. How do you perceive that the Act will benefit you as a nursing professional? How do you perceive it will influence your practice? Your pursuit of advanced degrees? What do think it means to those we serve?

WEB RESOURCES

http://aahn.org/primer.html
http://ahrq.gov/qual/nurseshdbk/nurseshdbk.pdf
http://historians.org/
http://homeoint.org/books2/ww1/48nurses.htm
http://historians.org/
http://clendening.kumc.edu/dc/fn/
http://healthcare.gov
https://www.cms.gov/Medicare/Quality-Initiatives-Patient-Assessment-Instruments/QualityInitiativesGenInfo/index.html
http://www.pressganey.com/solutions/clinical-quality/nursing-quality

REFERENCES

Bergquist, S., & King, J. (1994). Parish nursing: a conceptual framework. *Journal of Holistic Nursing, 12*(2), 155–170.

Campbell, C. (2001). The social context of nursing. In K. Chitty (Ed.), *Professional nursing: concepts and challenges* (pp. 36–50). Philadelphia, PA: Saunders.

Catalano, J. (1996). *Contemporary professional nursing.* Philadelphia, PA: FA Davis.

Centers for Medicare & Medicaid Services. (2016). Readmissions Reduction Program (HRRP). Retrieved from https://www.cms.gov/Medicare/Medicare-Fee-for-Service-Payment/AcuteInpatientPPS/Readmissions-Reduction-Program.html.

Dolan, J., Fitzpatrick, M., & Herrmann, E. (1983). *Nursing in society: a historical perspective* (15th ed.). Philadelphia, PA: Saunders.

Donahue, M. (1996). *Nursing: the finest art, an illustrated history* (2nd ed.). St. Louis, MO: Mosby-Yearbook.

Draper, R. G., Fellend, L. E., & Melichar, L. (2008). *The role of nurses in hospital quality improvement.* HSC Research Brief No. 3.

Kalisch, P., & Kalisch, B. (1995). *The advance of American nursing* (3rd ed.). Philadelphia, PA: Lippincott.

Kemppainen, V., Tossavainen, K., & Turunen, H. (2013). Nurses' roles in health promotion practice: an integrative review. *Health Promotion International, 28*(4), 490–501.

Malloch, K., & Porter-O'Grady, T. (1999). Partnership economics: nursing's challenge in a quantum age. *Nursing Economics, 17*(6), 299–307.

Nutting, M., & Dock, L. (1935). *A history of nursing.* New York, NY: GP Putnam.

O'Neil, E., & Coffman, J. (1998). *Strategies for the future of nursing: changing roles, responsibilities, and employment patterns of registered nurses.* San Francisco, CA: Jossey-Bass.

U.S. Department of Health and Human Services. (2012). *2012 annual progress report to congress national strategy for quality improvement in health care.* Washington, DC: Government Printing Office.

Wakefield, M. K. (2010). Nurses and the affordable care act. *American Journal of Nursing, 110*(9), 11. http://dx.doi.org/10.1097/01.NAJ.0000388242.06365.4f.

Weston, M., & Roberts, D. (September 30, 2013). "The influence of quality improvement efforts on patient outcomes and nursing work: a perspective from chief nursing officers at three large health systems." *OJIN: The Online Journal of Issues in Nursing, Vol. 18.* No. 3, Manuscript 2.

Upholding Legal and Ethical Principles

⊖volve WEBSITE

Additional resources are available online at:
http://evolve.elsevier.com/Claywell/transitions

OBJECTIVES

1. Identify the three major types of law and explain how they apply to nursing.
2. Define professional negligence and malpractice.
3. Identify issues in nursing and health care that can constitute malpractice.
4. Discuss the meaning of accountability of the professional registered nurse.
5. Demonstrate effective use of technology and practices that support safe practice.
6. Define ethical principles and the *Code of Ethics for Nurses.*
7. Elicit the cultural values and preferences of patients in the health care setting as part of a clinical interview and include these in your plan of care.
8. Recognize your personal attitudes about working with patients from different ethnic and cultural backgrounds.
9. Value the need for registered nurses to demonstrate the ethical duties owed to self and others.
10. Identify an ethical dilemma in the clinical setting and outline a framework for ethical decision making.

KEY TERMS

abuse	*Code of Ethics for Nurses*	Ethic of Care
administrative law	*with Interpretive*	ethics
assault	*Statements*	failure to rescue
autonomy	common law	false imprisonment
battery	confidentiality	fidelity
beliefs	duty	informed consent
beneficence	ethical dilemma	integrity

Continued

KEY TERMS—cont'd

justice	morals	statutory law
legal nurse consultant	negligence	values
malpractice	nonmaleficence	veracity
mandatory reporting	patient rights	

OVERVIEW

Nurses grapple daily with legal and ethical responsibilities, though they are not necessarily aware of it. But how many nurses can say *why* they do what they do? We tend to make better decisions when we are fully informed, able to think critically, and articulate our reasoning. This chapter reviews basic legal and biomedical ethical principles and issues that affect the practice of the registered nurse. Law and ethics overlap in many cases. Changes in health care and practicing effectively as a professional registered nurse require that the RN understand and follow legal and ethical principles and responsibilities. Hall (2003) states that while law mandates how we *must* behave toward one another, **ethics** establishes how we *should* behave.

ISSUES IN LAW

Every day, nurses face issues such as staffing shortages, assault and battery, **patient rights, informed consent,** and confidentiality. Changes in health care, such as legislation regarding use of fetal tissue, right to die, right to life, staffing patterns, health care rationing, patient abandonment, and technological advances, all carry potential legal and ethical concerns. For instance, the failure of health care organizations to provide adequate staff can not only result in the denial of reimbursement under federal guidelines, but it also raises legal and ethical concerns related to safe practice. Of special concern to nurses is malpractice, which can be emotionally and financially devastating.

SOURCES OF LAW

The three major types of laws that govern our society are statutory law, administrative law, and common law (including case law). Law can be further categorized into civil and criminal law. Criminal law refers to crimes against the general welfare of the public; a crime may be either a misdemeanor (punishable by a fine or imprisonment of less than 1 year) or a felony (a heavier fine and longer period of imprisonment and even death).

Statutory laws are laws enacted by a legislative body. They are passed by Congress and signed into law by the president or a state governor. Statutory law includes constitutional law and enacted law (Ellis & Hartley, 2012). Examples of federal laws that impact and provide standards for your nursing care include Emergency Medical Treatment and Active Labor Act (EMTALA); the Americans with Disabilities Act (ADA); the Patient Self-Determination Act (PSDA); the Occupational Safety and Health Act (OSHA); and the Patient Safety and Quality Improvement Act (PSQI). Violations of federal laws are prosecuted as criminal offenses (Cherry & Jacob, 2017). Constitutional law has a major impact on our society and legal system. The U.S. Constitution is the foundation of American law and is considered the supreme law of the land. Each state also has its own constitution, but a state constitution cannot limit or remove rights protected or granted by the U.S. Constitution. An example of statutory law is a state Nurse Practice Act and state reporting statutes such as child or elder abuse and domestic violence (Cherry & Jacob, 2017).

Administrative law controls the administrative operations of government. Congress delegates certain agencies the duty to oversee federal and state governments. An example of administrative law at the federal level is the Centers for Medicare and Medicaid Services (CMS) or the National Labor Relations Board (Ellis & Hartley, 2012). At the state level, boards of nursing enforce the rules and regulations that govern the practice of nursing in that state (Ellis & Hartley, 2012).

Common law is law that has arisen from judicial decisions. You may think of common law as "judge-made" decisions, or laws that are created by judges when deciding cases. These decisions are binding on future decisions of lower courts. As new decisions are made, or decisions are overturned, upheld, or modified, common law changes. The judiciary in the United States is made up of the federal judicial system, the state judicial system, appeals courts, state supreme courts, and the U.S. Supreme Court.

LEGAL PRINCIPLES

The registered nurse will need, at a minimum, to be familiar with the legal principles of confidentiality and the right to privacy, patient rights, informed consent, assault and battery, false imprisonment, and failure to rescue.

Confidentiality and the Right to Privacy

The right to privacy is implied in the Bill of Rights of the U.S. Constitution. The Health Insurance Portability and Accountability Act of 1996 (HIPAA) that was fully implemented in 2003 was enacted for many reasons, including guaranteeing the security and privacy of medical records and other personal health information. Civil and criminal penalties can result from failure to comply with the requirements of HIPAA. There are exceptions to these laws such as the duty to warn to protect third parties from harm where there are threats of harm to others.

Patient Rights

Health care facilities and professional associations have issued patient bills of rights that generally include the right to be treated with dignity and respect, privacy, decision making, confidentiality, access to health records, and the right to refuse treatment. The Joint Commission (TJC) is a nonprofit independent organization dedicated to improving the quality of health care in organized health care settings. Its major functions include developing organizational standards, awarding accreditation decisions, and providing education and consultation to health care organizations. Noncompliance with applicable standards could result in loss of accreditation.

Informed Consent

The patient has the right to be free from unwanted medical treatment and has the right to know the potential risks, benefits, and alternatives. A patient must fully understand what he or she has consented to in order for the consent to be valid. The Patient Self-Determination Act enacted in 1991 made significant advancement in the patient's right to make decisions concerning treatment of end-of-life issues (Marquis & Huston, 2015). Autonomy, discussed later, is the ethical principle of the freedom to choose and make one's own decisions regarding health care.

Assault and Battery

An **assault**, a deliberate threat to physically harm another, is a crime. The two conditions that must be met for assault are that the offender must have the ability to commit a battery and the person must be aware of the immediate threat and must be fearful of it. **Battery** is the actual and intentional act of touching another without the person's consent. For example, the nurse tells the patient, "If you don't let me give you this injection, I'll have to put you in restraints" (assault). Battery occurs if the nurse gives the injection without the patient's consent.

False imprisonment is verbally or physically forcing an individual to stay in a place against his or her wishes and is an intentional tort. Prohibiting a competent patient from leaving the hospital or the unnecessary application of restraints or application of restraints without proper authorization is considered false imprisonment.

Read the following case study. As you read, think about how and why the following principles might apply to this case.

Negligence + Prudent Nurse

CASE STUDY

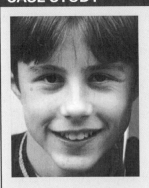

On November 2, 2000, Lewis Blackman, a healthy 15-year-old, entered a teaching hospital for elective surgery for *pectus excavatum*, a deformity of the anterior wall of the chest. The surgery was successful. Lewis was prescribed a full adult course of ketorolac (Toradol) for pain by a young senior resident who was following the postoperative protocols for that procedure. On the morning of the third postoperative day, Lewis began to experience severe pain in his upper abdomen, and his abdomen grew hard and distended. A nurse told him it was gas. By afternoon, his temperature was dropping, his skin was pale, and he was diaphoretic; his pulse was increasing. Lewis's parents were becoming increasingly alarmed at his rapid decline and asked nurses to call the attending physician. The physician who arrived, however, was a resident; despite repeated requests, nurses had not summoned the attending physician. Lewis was developing peritonitis and was also bleeding internally. Over 30 hours of alarming clinical decline were going unnoticed. Prescribed IV fluids were inadequate. Lewis went more than 24 hours with virtually no urine output and 4 hours

> ## CASE STUDY—cont'd
>
> of completely undetectable blood pressure, which nurses attributed to malfunctioning equipment. On day 4, the staff spent 2.5 hours looking for a blood pressure cuff to detect his blood pressure. Twelve attempts were made to take his blood pressure using seven different cuffs. On November 6, 2000, Lewis died of an NSAID-induced duodenal ulcer.
>
> Now that you have learned about legal and ethical issues surrounding health care, consider the following questions:
>
> 1. What legal and ethical duties were breached? Why?
> 2. What do you think were the factors involved in the health care providers' failure to rescue?
> 3. Assume you were Lewis's primary care nurse over the weekend. How would you have explained your rationale for your failure to contact a supervisor or the attending physician as Lewis's condition deteriorated?
> 4. Who should be held accountable for this tragic outcome?
> 5. What would you have done differently, and why?

Courtesy of Helen Haskell and LaBarre Blackman.

NEGLIGENCE AND MALPRACTICE

The Institute of Medicine, 1999 estimated that between 44,000 and 98,000 people a year died in U.S. hospitals due to medical errors. In 2013, a literature review of studies published from 2008 to 2011 estimates that the number is now approximately 210,000 "premature deaths associated with preventable harm to patients" each year and could, when figuring for data collection error, be as high as 400,000 (James, 2013, p. 20). Despite the safety measures that have been put in place in hospitals and health care facilities throughout the United States, preventable injuries and deaths continue to occur. Nurses are key to improving patient safety and improving outcomes.

Negligence has been defined by TJC (2011) as a "failure to use such care as a reasonable prudent and careful person would use under similar circumstances." **Malpractice** is defined as "improper or unethical conduct or unreasonable lack of skill by a holder of a professional or official position" (TJC, 2011). Professional negligence (also called medical malpractice or professional malpractice) is the omission or commission of an act that departs from the standard of care that a reasonably prudent person would provide in the same or similar circumstances. For example, commission of an act would be the administration of too much oxygen, while omission would be the failure to administer oxygen. The likelihood of professional negligence has increased with nursing authority, autonomy, accountability, and an increased scope of practice (Marquis & Huston, 2015). Accountability refers to the willingness to assume responsibility and accept the consequences for your actions. As a professional registered nurse, you are expected to practice competently and be accountable for your actions. As health care becomes increasingly complex, nurses are expected to practice autonomously—the ability of a nurse to act independently. The American Nurses Association (ANA, 2010b) states that "competence is foundational to autonomy; the public has a right to expect nurses to demonstrate professional competence."

Medical malpractice is professional misconduct, failure to perform professional duties, or failure to meet the professional standards of care that results in harm to another. A legal wrong committed against a person or property is called a tort and can be intentional or unintentional. Professional negligence is also called *professional malpractice* and is considered a tort. Intentional torts include assault and battery, false imprisonment, fraud, invasion of privacy, slander, and defamation (Marquis & Huston, 2015). Unintentional torts include professional negligence. In a malpractice suit, the burden of proof is on the plaintiff (the person who brings the lawsuit). (This is different from a criminal case, where the prosecutor must prove guilt beyond a reasonable doubt.) The plaintiff must prove by a preponderance of evidence that the following four elements are present in order for a person to recover damages:

- *Duty to care*: An obligation exists to conform to a recognized standard of care.
- *Breach of duty*: There must be a failure to adhere to an obligation and a deviation from a recognized standard of care.
- *Injury*: Actual damages have occurred.
- *Causation*: The injury was foreseeable and was caused by a breach of duty, and the conduct was the cause of the injury.

One of the high-risk areas in nursing practice is the administration of medication, and the avoidance of medication errors is of primary concern to the nurse. The Institute of Medicine (IOM) (2006) estimates that medication errors injure 1.5 million Americans each year. Following the six rights (right patient, right drug, right dose, right route, right time, and right documentation) of medication administration is crucial. Most nursing errors have been attributed to wrong dose, wrong technique, and wrong drug. Some threats to safe medication administration include miscommunication, confusing directions, poor technique, lack of safety checks, and others (Hughes & Blegen, 2008). Other factors include distractions and interruptions, work environment, patient acuity, staffing, workload, shift length, and lack of appropriate policies, procedures, and protocols (Hughes & Blegen, 2008). Your duty as a patient advocate includes challenging physician orders.

Specialty nursing areas have concerns that occur more frequently in those settings. For instance, in the emergency department setting, nurses must be familiar with the duty to treat, and the Emergency Medical Treatment and Active Labor Act (EMTALA) is a federal law that prohibits facilities that receive Medicare and Medicaid reimbursements from refusing to treat patients who cannot pay, as well as the duty to report certain patient conditions such as sexual assaults, food poisoning, communicable diseases, child abuse and neglect, industrial accidents, and wounds obtained by violent acts. Another example is the nurse practicing in the psychiatric mental health setting who must also understand state laws concerning the types of psychiatric admissions, seclusion and restraints, duty to warn, medication administration, and suicide precautions. Croke (2003) outlines factors that have been found to contribute to malpractice cases against nurses. These include delegation, early discharge, the nursing shortage and hospital downsizing, advances in technology, increased autonomy and responsibility of hospital nurses, better-informed consumers, and expanded legal definitions of liability. Delegation can also lead to malpractice claims if you delegate improperly (Reising & Allen, 2007).

According to Croke (2003) and Reising and Allen (2007), the most common malpractice claims against nurses include:

- Failure to follow standards of care
- Failure to use equipment in a responsible manner
- Failure to communicate
- Failure to document
- Failure to assess and monitor
- Failure to act as a patient advocate

FAILURE TO RESCUE

Failure to rescue is the lack of a timely and appropriate response to changes in a patient's condition and is strongly linked to nursing care. Failure to rescue is defined by the Agency for Health Research and Quality (AHRQ, 2009) as the failure to prevent a clinically important deterioration, such as death or permanent disability. It is critical to carefully monitor patients to identify deteriorations and intervene appropriately. One example is the failure to seek medical care for a patient; it is not enough that you notify the physician of your concern. You must make sure your concern is addressed. If it is not, it is your duty to contact the emergency room, notify your supervisor, or go up the chain of command until your concerns are properly addressed. Many factors are involved in incidences of failure to rescue, including nurse-to-patient ratios, increased responsibilities, fatigue, experience, and education. Nurses can be found to have breached a duty for failing to rescue a deteriorating patient; failure to rescue also has significant ethical considerations.

TJC has implemented a policy that requires health care organizations to self-report sentinel events such as patient suicide, unexpected deaths, medication errors, wrong site surgery, and deaths caused by delay in treatment, among others. When a sentinel event occurs, organizations are expected to conduct what is called a *root cause analysis* in order to determine the cause of the event and implement steps to improve performance outcomes (TJC, 2011). More information on the root cause analysis can be found on The Joint Commission website.

The ANA has published *Standards of Care* related to nursing in general as well as specialty practice. These standards of care, facility policies and procedures, protocols, job descriptions, professional literature, expert options, your state Nurse Practice Act, and the reasonable person standard will all be used to prove negligence and malpractice. The ANA (2010a) in its *Nursing's Social Policy Statement* states that "all nurses are responsible for practicing in accordance with recognized standards of professional nursing practice and the recognized professional code of ethics." It is imperative that you familiarize yourself with these standards.

Common sense and an awareness of your legal responsibilities will help you avoid liability. Box 12.1 lists some of the actions you can take to reduce your risks.

> ### BOX 12.1   TIPS FOR AVOIDING LIABILITY
>
> - Perform only skills that are within your scope of practice.
> - Stay current in your field or specialty area of practice.
> - Make a favorable first impression and maintain rapport.
> - Establish your baseline. (Know your patient!)
> - Be aware of your own strengths and weaknesses.
> - Evaluate your assignment.
> - Delegate carefully and legally.
> - Carry out orders cautiously.
> - Administer drugs carefully according to the six rights.
> - Think before you speak.
> - Document care accurately.
> - Exercise caution when assisting in procedures.
> - Attend equipment in-services.
> - Document the use of restraints.
> - Take steps to prevent patient falls.
> - Comply with laws about advance directives.
> - Adhere to your facility's policies, procedures, and protocols.
> - Provide a safe environment at all times.

Follin, S.A. (ed.). (2004). *Nurse's legal handbook* (5th ed.). Ambler, PA: Lippincott Williams & Wilkins.

DOCUMENTATION

The weight of the medical record in a legal proceeding cannot be overemphasized. According to Brous (2009):

> *The patient's chart is used to demonstrate accreditation and regulatory compliance, and to make reimbursement determination. It is also examined by licensing boards in deciding disciplinary action. For these reasons, it is imperative that nurses consistently use acceptable documentation practices. (p. 40)*

Some documentation errors include faulty record keeping, the failure to include information, charting after the fact, misplacing records, and failure to follow standards of care when charting by exception. The failure to document implies failure to provide care, and the prevailing rule is that if it wasn't documented, it wasn't done. Charting by exception can be problematic because it requires the nurse to document only deviations. Well-known guidelines to effective documentation include:

- Write legibly using black, permanent ink.
- Date and time all entries.
- Sign your name and credentials. Never document for another person, and *never* sign another nurse's name.
- Do not leave any blank spaces, and do not use white-out, obliterate, or erase any portion of the medical record.
- Entries should be factual without opinions, assumptions, or meaningless words; use subjective statements made by the patient as much as possible.
- Abbreviations must correspond to the ones adopted by your facility or health care system.

- Document as soon as possible after the care is given, and do not document care before it has been given.
- Document consent for or refusal of treatment.
- Document patient responses to medication, treatments, patient teaching, and other interventions.
- Do not add omitted information to an entry that has already been signed. Instead, add a "late entry."
- Document patient teaching and discharge planning. It is especially important to document that the patient has understood the information. Record how you assessed this (e.g., verbalization or return demonstration).
- Document when a patient leaves the nurse's care or the nurse leaves the patient's care (for instance, in home health).

Certain accrediting and licensing agencies, as well as national and organizational standards of care, have certain requirements for documentation (e.g., Medicare and TJC). No matter which method of charting and documentation of patient care your health care organization uses, use common sense and ask yourself how you would prove and justify your actions in the event of a lawsuit. Accurate documentation will provide your best defense to a lawsuit or claim for damages.

MANDATORY REPORTING

Mandatory reporting laws include two specific types: child abuse and neglect and elder abuse and neglect. Mandated reporters have certain protections that include not requiring "hard evidence" but rather a good-faith belief or a reasonable suspicion that **abuse** has taken place; immunity from civil and criminal liability and licensing actions; a presumption of good faith; nullifying any confidentiality, privilege, and privacy requirement of the health care provider; and making confidential any report made under the law. If a mandated reporter does not perform his or her reporting duties required by law, he or she may face various penalties, including criminal prosecution or proceedings under the state's licensing laws. Nurses have an unquestionable responsibility to advocate for victims of abuse and/or neglect.

LEGAL NURSE CONSULTANT

An important role for registered nurses with specialized training and education that has evolved since the 1980s is that of the **legal nurse consultant**. These nurses serve as experts in medical litigation in a variety of practice areas. They also provide consulting services related to malpractice, personal injury, worker's compensation cases, risk management, forensics, regulatory compliance, and more. While no degrees are required beyond the registered nursing designation and relevant experience, there are continuing education programs designed to comprehensively prepare the RN as a legal nurse consultant and provide certification of the preparation.

NURSING ETHICS

The term *ethics* comes from the Greek term *ethos*, which means "habits" or "customs" (Black, 2014). It is a branch of philosophy that offers a way of examining moral life and studies how we make decisions regarding right and wrong (Ellis & Hartley, 2012). Bioethics (or biomedical ethics) applies ethical theories and principles to moral issues or problems in the practice of medicine (Ellis & Hartley, 2012). Ethics requires a critical analysis of our actions or potential actions and helps us answer the question "What should I do in this situation?" Thus, ethics looks at how we decide between right and wrong and offers a way of examining how we live and how we practice.

Practicing as an RN requires that you practice according to your morals, values, and **beliefs**, which will guide you in your practice. **Morals** are what we believe to be right and wrong; these are often based on religious beliefs, culture, social influences, and life experiences (Ellis & Hartley, 2012). **Values** are enduring beliefs or ideals and are largely shaped by one's culture (Ellis & Hartley, 2012). Sometimes we must choose between two things that are important to us; this is known as a values conflict (Ellis & Hartley, 2012).

Moral development refers to how an individual learns to handle moral or ethical dilemmas. Lawrence Kohlberg and Carol Gilligan are the two most cited theorists in moral development (the basis for ethical reasoning). Kohlberg's theory of moral development focused on three levels and six stages of moral development. These three levels are known as preconventional, conventional, and postconventional and are based on experiences. These experiences include how individuals understand concepts such as justice, rights, equality, and human welfare. These stages are sequential; how quickly humans progress through these stages depends on psychological and environmental factors.

Carol Gilligan challenged Kohlberg's theory of moral development. She believed that Kohlberg's theory did not recognize the experiences of women because his theories were largely generated from research with men and boys and that morality does not develop by looking at justice alone. She believed that a difference existed in how men and women view moral problems and believed that one who responds to need and demonstrates care and responsibility in relationships is a moral person (Black, 2014).

Respect for the inherent worth, dignity, and human rights of every individual is a fundamental principle that underlies all nursing practice. Nurses "[affirm] and [preserve] the human dignity of all those with whom [they] have contact, in all nursing roles and settings" (ANA, 2015, p. 7). Universal principles of biomedical ethics include autonomy, veracity, beneficence, nonmaleficence, confidentiality, justice, and fidelity. Each will be discussed briefly. Recall the story of Lewis Blackman, and think of how these ethical principles might apply as you read the next few sections.

Autonomy

Autonomy is the freedom to choose and make one's own decisions regarding health care. Autonomy, the right of self-determination, includes respect for an individual, even when we do not agree with patients' decisions (Ellis & Hartley, 2012). This ethical principle is closely related to informed consent because informed consent requires that we provide the information sufficient for patients to make decisions for themselves (Ellis & Hartley, 2012). There are limitations, however, when one person's autonomy interferes with another individual's rights, health, or well-being (Ellis & Hartley, 2012).

Veracity

Veracity is the principle of truth telling and not intentionally deceiving or misleading patients (Ellis & Hartley, 2012). An example of veracity is the expectation that the nurse will be truthful with the patient (within the health care system's limits on what a nurse can tell a patient). But in some situations, could the truth cause more harm than good? Some cultures believe that an ill family member should not be told the truth about his or her illness; this can cause a values conflict. Veracity also includes the duty to report errors.

Fidelity

Fidelity refers to practicing faithfully within the boundaries of the nurse's roles as defined by state law and regulations. It is mandated that the nurse accept certain responsibilities as part of his or her contract with society when he or she accepts licensure as a nurse. This is the foundation of accountability.

Beneficence

Beneficence emphasizes preventing or removing harm or doing or promoting good. In other words, it is stated in terms of positive outcomes and is often thought of as the most critical ethical principle in health care (Black, 2014). It is our duty to promote the health and welfare of the patient while honoring personal autonomy. An example of beneficence is following the nursing process to develop a plan of care agreed upon by the nurse and patient.

Nonmaleficence

Nonmaleficence refers to doing no harm and is stated in terms of negative actions. Nonmaleficence is the foundation of the Hippocratic Oath of the medical profession (Black, 2014). An example of the violation of the ethical principles of nonmaleficence is the nurse who intentionally administers a lethal dose of a medication to a patient or the doctor who fails to rescue or respond to a deteriorating patient condition.

Confidentiality

Confidentiality, a legal and ethical term, refers to the protection of private health information gathered during the provision of health care services (Black, 2014). The nurse must safeguard a patient's right to privacy. An example of the violation of this principle is the nurse who discusses a patient's condition in the elevator with a co-worker. Recall your legal duty to comply with HIPAA laws.

Justice

The principle of **justice** is concerned with the concept of fairness: the quality of being just or fair, conforming to truth, or treating like cases similarly. Should we treat all people the same? In health care, it asks the question "Who should be entitled to and receive health care?" How do we measure fairness? What happens when one person's rights oppose the rights of another? This is one of the most important principles today as the United States grapples with the dilemma of the right to health care.

ETHICS AND CULTURE

Because beliefs influence ethical decision making, cultural differences must be recognized and respected. Culturally competent nursing care is the integration of knowledge, attitudes, and skills, and it means the nurse is able to work within the specific cultural context of an individual, family, or community. It is impossible to know the health-related beliefs and practices of the hundreds of different cultures that exist. A cultural self-assessment will provide insight into one's own cultural beliefs. The more insight you have into your own values, attitudes, beliefs, and practices, the more you are prepared to overcome prejudices, discrimination, judgmentalness, and preconceived beliefs. You may realize, for instance, that you have strong feelings against certain cultures. An awareness of these feelings will help you overcome them and stimulate an interest in learning more about a particular culture. The autonomy of culturally diverse individuals must be respected regardless of your personal beliefs.

Cultural competence also extends to the workplace. Within the health care work environments, multicultural groups can cause conflicts in the workplace when employees are unable to recognize and respect their differences. The workplace is made up of individuals from many cultures and generations, and those differences can cause staff conflicts that, in turn, compromise patient care.

ETHICAL DILEMMAS

An **ethical dilemma** exists when a conflict arises between health care professionals, patients, families, and health care organizations (Black, 2014). For example, ethical dilemmas can exist in issues involving patient self-determination, patient rights, safety, allocation of health care resources, loyalty, and truthfulness. Decision making, especially in health care settings, is rarely black or white. Think about a time when you encountered a situation that presented you with an ethical dilemma. For instance, you may have struggled with whether to report a physician or an impaired co-worker. How did you arrive at your decided course of action, and how did you feel about your action(s)? If you have not encountered this type of situation, how do you think you would act? What are the alternatives? What would happen to you if you reported the individual? Whose rights do you protect? Whistleblowing embraces the concepts of veracity (truth telling), nonmaleficence (to do no harm), and fidelity (keeping promises), but it carries with it significant risks. Provision 2 of the ANA's *Code of Ethics for Nurses* (2010, p. 11), discussed later in this chapter, states, "The nurse's primary commitment is to the patient, whether an individual, family, group, or community." This commitment calls for a great deal of courage. A recent example is the 2009 case of two registered nurses in Texas—Galle and Mitchell—who "blew the whistle" on a physician for improper surgical procedures and improper prescribing. They sent an anonymous letter expressing their concerns to the state's medical board. Their identity was discovered, and both were charged with a felony (misuse of official information); they were both fired. The ANA, the Texas Nurses Association, and nurses from around the country rallied to advocate for these two nurses. The charge against Galle was ultimately dropped, leaving Mitchell to stand trial. On February 8, 2010, after a 4-day jury trial and only 1 hour of deliberation, the jury acquitted Ms. Mitchell of the felony charges. Later, the hospital and government officials who accused the nurses of wrongdoing were indicted. "Nurses play a critical, duty-bound role in acting as patient safety watch-guards in the nation's health care system" ("Justice served," 2011). The actions of these two nurses took a great deal of courage. Murray (2010) states, "Moral courage is considered to be the pinnacle of ethical behavior; it requires a steadfast commitment to fundamental ethical principles despite potential risks, such as threats to reputation, shame, emotional anxiety, isolation from colleagues, retaliation, and loss of employment." Moral courage is seen in individuals who decide on a right course of action regardless of the possible consequences (Murray, 2010). *Moral distress* is the term used to describe situations where an individual knows the right action to take but feels powerless to take that action (Epstein & Delgado, 2010).

There are many types of ethical dilemmas. Dilemmas involving beneficence occur, for example, when health care providers, patients, or family members disagree about what is in the patient's best interest. Dilemmas of nonmaleficence may involve the nurse's responsibility to report unsafe or illegal practices. Autonomy, closely related to beneficence, involves decisions that maximize a patient's right to decide on his or her own treatment. Dilemmas that involve dividing limited health care resources fairly are dilemmas of justice, and dilemmas of fidelity are those involving honoring promises.

BIOETHICS

As mentioned earlier, biomedical ethics (or bioethics) deals with ethical considerations in medical practice. In addition to what has been discussed previously, bioethics is also applied to such issues as research, reproduction, abortion, family planning, the right to life, sterilization, and dilemmas surrounding death, including euthanasia, assisted suicide, advance directives, withdrawing and withholding treatment, and the right to die. The Human Genome Project, which mapped the entire human genome, began in 1990 and was completed in 2003 (Ellis & Hartley, 2012). Other ethical questions might arise from genetic screening, gene therapy, and stem cell research. A discussion of each of these is beyond the scope of this book, but you are likely to encounter one or more of these issues in your practice; therefore, it is important for you to develop self-awareness of your personal beliefs concerning these issues.

ETHICS COMMITTEES

Ethics committees are multidisciplinary and can include physicians, nurses, patients, families, social workers, and clergy, and they serve as a resource for staff, patients, and families. The goal of bioethical committees is to assist staff, patients, and caregivers in resolving ethical dilemmas. Frequent dilemmas include informed consent, the right to life, medical futility, the definition of death, and the right to die. Ethics committees began in 1976 with the Karen Ann Quinlan case where the New Jersey Supreme Court granted permission to her parents to remove her from a ventilator. Since then, they have become an integral part of health care organizations. Ethics committees promote, advocate, and protect patient rights; establish a moral care standard; and enhance the quality of patient care (Marquis & Huston, 2015). They have many functions, including policy and procedure development, staff and community education, conflict resolution, case reviews, support, and political advocacy. Cultural factors must be considered because values and beliefs are strongly influenced by culture. The role that nurses play on ethics committees varies among health care organizations and situations. The RN can be called upon to discuss his or her observations (such as patient responses to interventions) and patient statements.

ETHICAL THEORIES

As mentioned earlier, many of our decisions are made without thinking—an action is either right or wrong, black or white. But when we are dealing with health care ethics, we are dealing with many individuals involved in the provision of health care and many gray areas. Much of your responsibility with regard to ethics is to accept that individuals also feel strongly about their personal values and beliefs—just as you do. Individuals have differing opinions, so you must consider all sides of an argument. There are no easy answers for every ethical dilemma involving ethical questions, and many have more than one potential answer.

There are many value systems—or worldviews—that allow for the assessment of ethical problems and provide a decision-making framework. These are beyond the scope of this book, but we will review the four most common theories for ethical decision making: deontology, utilitarianism, virtue ethics, and the Ethic of Care.

Deontology

Deontology is a duty-oriented theory for ethical decision making derived from the Greek term *deon*, meaning "duty" and is also called Kantian ethics, named after Immanuel Kant, a German philosopher. Kant believed that the morality of an action should be judged based on the motive or intent behind the action (Black, 2014). Therefore, consequences or outcomes should not be used to judge the morality of actions, even if the consequence is negative. From this ethical perspective, one should not treat others only as a means to an end. This principle is especially important within the field of research.

Utilitarianism

Utilitarianism, on the other hand, is a theory that states that actions must be judged based on whether they produce the greatest good (or more happiness than unhappiness). Because this theory judges actions based on their consequences, it is sometimes called "consequentialism." David Hume, Jeremy Bentham, and John Stuart Mill are generally credited with the development of this theory. In this method, ethical decisions are usually made through a risk-to-benefit analysis (discussing, for instance, treatment options with a patient). Utilitarianism is used in many professional health care situations today, including issues that involve which patients to treat first and how health care dollars should be spent (Black, 2014).

Virtue Ethics

The theory of virtue ethics was first seen in the works of Plato, Aristotle, and early Christians (Black, 2014). The emphasis of virtue ethics is on the characteristics, traits, or virtues that a person should have, such as courage, **integrity**, magnanimity, honesty, justice, and temperament. Characteristics, traits, or virtues shape behaviors but do not guarantee that individuals will act in an ethical manner. The hope is that if an individual develops morally desirable virtues, moral decisions and actions are more likely.

The Ethic of Care

The **Ethic of Care** emphasizes the caring aspect of the nurse–patient relationship, intuition, minimizing or avoiding harm, and fairness. Jean Watson (1979), Carol Gilligan (1982), and Nel Noddings (1984) emphasized the aspect of caring in the nurse–patient relationship as the cornerstone for ethical decision making (Black, 2014). This ethical theory is discussed extensively in the nursing literature. Gilligan theorized that women usually exhibit a relationally based ethic (with a focus on feelings and relationships), while men prefer a rule-based ethic (with a focus on justice and rights) (Bennett-Woods, 2006). Primary attention is paid to preserving relationships and generating options through better communication and cooperation and finding solutions that avoid or minimize harm to all involved, while promoting caring (Bennett-Woods, 2006).

YOUR PROFESSIONAL COMMITMENT

A hallmark of the professions such as law, medicine, and nursing is the creation of a code of ethics. The American Nurses Association's *Code of Ethics for Nurses with Interpretive Statements* (2015) is nursing's expression of the ethical duties owed to ourselves and to the public, and it is how nursing informs society of the guiding principles and rules that the profession follows.

The *Code of Ethics for Nurses* (2015) evolved from Florence Nightingale's "Nightingale Pledge" in 1893. It was not until 1950 that the Code for Professional Nurses was unanimously accepted by the ANA House of Delegates. The current version is the product of ANA staff, a Code of Ethics Project Task Force, an advisory board, and state liaisons. There is also a Guide to the Code of Ethics for Nurses (Fowler, 2015) that can help you "reflect on the nine provisions for what they mean in your daily life as a nurse. ...they are what give voice to who we as professional nurses are at our very core" (p. xi-xii).

The ANA Code of Ethics for Nurses is "nonnegotiable in any setting" (2015, p. vii) and is clear on the **duty** and commitments of the professional nurse within the complexities of modern nursing practice. The *Code* is composed of the following nine provisions within which are seen the nurse's "fundamental values," "boundaries of duty and loyalty," and "aspects of duties beyond individual patient encounters" (p. xiii):

- "The nurse practices with compassion and respect for the inherent dignity, worth, and unique attributes of every person" (p. 1).
- "The nurse's primary commitment is to the patient whether an individual, family, group, community, or population" (p. 5).
- "The nurse promotes, advocates for, and protects the rights, health, and safety of the patient" (p. 9).

- "The nurse has authority, accountability, and responsibility for nursing practice; makes decisions; and takes action consistent with the obligation to promote health and to provide optimal care" (p. 15).
- "The nurse owes the same duties to self as to others, including the responsibility to promote health and safety, preserve wholeness of character and integrity, maintain competence, and continue personal and professional growth" (p. 19).
- "The nurse through individual and collective effort, establishes, maintains, and improves the ethical environment of the work setting and conditions of employment that are conducive to safe, quality health care" (p. 23).
- "The nurse in all roles and settings, advances the profession through research and scholarly inquiry, professional standards development, and the generation of both nursing and health policy" (p. 27).
- "The nurse collaborates with other health professionals and the public to protect human rights, promote health diplomacy, and reduce health disparities" (p. 31).
- "The profession of nursing, collectively through its professional organizations, must articulate nursing values, maintain the integrity of the profession, and integrate the principles of social justice into nursing and health policy" (p. 35).

ETHICAL DECISION MAKING

In our personal and professional lives, we are faced with ethical decision making every day. Most of the time, we make these decisions based on our own worldview and definitions of right and wrong. During those times, however, when we are not sure of what action to take, if any at all, it is helpful to understand the process of ethical decision making. A decision model will provide you with a step-by-step framework for ethical decision making.

Several models can be used for ethical decision making. One is an eight-step model: gathering relevant information; stating the practical problem; identifying the ethical issues and questions; selecting the ethical principles and/or theoretical frameworks to be considered; conducting an analysis and preparing a justification; considering one or more counterarguments; exploring the options for action; and selecting, completing, and evaluating the action (Bennett-Woods, 2006). As we review these steps, you will see how this process is similar to the nursing process.

In step 1, relevant information is identified and gathered. This information should consist of factual elements of the ethical dilemma and should be completely and concisely stated. What internal and external sources should be considered? For instance, internal constraints may include fear of losing one's job, anxiety about creating conflict, self-doubt, or lack of confidence (Epstein & Delgado, 2010). Power imbalances among members of the health care team, poor communication among team members, fear of legal action, and lack of administrative support are some external constraints that may contribute to moral distress (Epstein & Delgado, 2010).

In step 2, the practical problem is identified, and the problem is stated in terms of the decisions that must be made in order to take action. The focus here is on what specific action should be taken rather than the justification for a specific course of action. Step 3 involves identifying the most significant ethical issues. Once this occurs, primary and secondary ethical questions are identified. In step 4, the ethical principles and frameworks need to be considered, because these become the basis for our argument for taking a particular action or position. An argument is intended to prove that a particular action or position is right or wrong. A counterargument challenges the assumptions of that argument. In step 5, possible answers are formulated and justified using the principles and theoretical perspectives selected, and in step 6, one or more counterarguments are to be considered. In step 7, options are explored, and in step 8, the action will be selected, completed, and evaluated (Bennett-Woods, 2006). Evaluating the action means considering whether the action was justified. The final question should be "Would I make the same decision again based on the outcome of my action?" Note that based on the results of an evaluation, you may change your ways of thinking and doing. The ethical decision-making process may seem cumbersome and time-consuming, but with practice, you will find that it becomes much easier.

Legal and ethical considerations in patient care cannot be overemphasized. Knowledge of these principles will guide your provision of safe and effective care, reduce liability, and ensure that the expectations of your patients and society as a whole are met.

According to Fowler (2015), the nursing process model can also be used as a way to work through an ethical decision. In the assessment and data collection step, the nurse defines the type of problem at hand, such as ethical or moral, and begins to collect the pertinent data, facts, and values. In the second step of analysis, the data, facts, and values are examined within the context of the applicable theory or principles. The third step is diagnosis, or making a judgment about the issues that arise upon examination of the situation. The fourth step of outcomes/planning includes considering alternate arguments and approaches to the situation. Fifth, implementation requires a choice of a fitting and right answer to the situation. Finally, the last step in the process is evaluation of what can be learned from the circumstances and how the decision actually worked.

KEY POINTS

After completion of this chapter, you have learned:
- Law and ethics are virtually inseparable.
- Sources of law include statutory law, administrative law, and common law. The consequences for violation of these laws include civil or criminal action or both. Nurse Practice Acts are statutory laws.
- It is imperative that you understand the legal principles of confidentiality and the right to privacy, patient rights, informed consent, assault and battery, and failure to rescue.
- Negligence is based on the reasonable person standard. *Malpractice* is the term applied to professional misconduct, failure to perform professional duties, or failure to follow professional standards of care that results in harm to another. Medical malpractice applies to health care providers.
- Nurse Practice Acts, standards of care, facility policies and procedures, protocols, job descriptions, professional literature, expert opinions, and the reasonable person standard will be used to prove negligence and malpractice.

- Accountability refers to the willingness to assume responsibility for your actions and accepting the consequences for your actions. The most common claims against nurses include failure (1) to follow standards of care, (2) to use equipment in a responsible manner, (3) to communicate, (4) to document, (5) to assess and monitor, (6) to act as a patient advocate, (7) failure to rescue, and (8) medication errors.

- Some things you can do to avoid liability include performing only those skills that are within your scope of practice, staying current in your field of practice, delegating carefully and legally, administering drugs using the six rights, being aware of your own strengths and weaknesses, and advocating for your patients.

- Ethics is a branch of philosophy that studies how we make decisions regarding right and wrong and requires a critical analysis of our actions or potential actions.

- Ethical principles include autonomy (self-determination), veracity (truth telling), fidelity (keeping promises), beneficence (preventing harm or promoting good), nonmaleficence (do no harm), confidentiality (the right to privacy), and justice (fairness).

- The *Code of Ethics for Nurses* expresses the ethical duties owed to ourselves, our patients, society, our employers, and our colleagues and provides a framework for ethical analysis.

- Ethical dilemmas are conflicts among health care professionals, patients, families, and health care organizations and can involve autonomy, patient rights, withholding and withdrawing life support, the allocation of health care resources, loyalty, and truthfulness.

- The eight-step ethical decision-making model is one tool to guide you when you are faced with an ethical dilemma. These steps include gathering relevant information; stating the practical problem; identifying the ethical issues and questions; selecting the ethical principles to be considered; conducting an analysis and preparing a justification; considering one or more counterarguments; exploring the options; and selecting, completing, and evaluating the action.

- Knowledge of ethical and legal obligations of the professional registered nurse will guide the provision of safe and effective care, reduce liability, and ensure that the expectations of patients and society as a whole are met.

▌ CRITICAL THINKING QUESTIONS

Applying the biomedical ethical principles you learned in this chapter, reflect on and answer the following critical thinking questions:

1. Choose two of the biomedical ethical principles reviewed in this chapter, and give an example of the violation of each of those principles.
2. Under what circumstances would you feel justified in violating one or more of the ethical and legal principles discussed in this chapter?
3. You finally have your dream job working as a nurse in a large teaching hospital on a cardiology floor. One morning you arrive on the unit only to discover that two nurses have called in sick and are not being replaced. Acuity is high among the

20 patients on the unit, and as a result of the call-ins, you and another nurse each have 10 patients. What action do you take, and why? Consider your ethical and legal responsibilities.
4. Search the Internet for a recent ethical dilemma of interest to you. Apply the eight-step decision-making model you learned to the dilemma in order to come to resolution. Be prepared to support your decisions.
5. Use the nursing process model of decision making to resolve an ethical dilemma scenario you find by searching YouTube.

WEB RESOURCES

American Association of Legal Nurse Consultants at http://www.aalnc.org/page/what-is-an-lnc
American Nurses Association at http://nursingworld.org
Bioethics at http://bioethics.net
Ethics at a Glance at http://rhchp.regis.edu/HCE/EthicsAtAGlance/
EthicsWeb.ca at http://ethicsweb.ca/resources/bioethics
FindLaw at http://findlaw.com
Institute of Medicine at http://iom.edu/Reports/2006/Preventing-Medication-Errors-Quality-Chasm-Series.aspx
Library of Congress at http://thomas.loc.gov
National Institutes of Health, Bioethics Resources at http://bioethics.od.nih.gov/
Nurses Service Organization at http://nso.com/case-studies/index.jsf
Supreme Court of the United States at http://www.supremecourtus.gov
The Center for Ethics and Advocacy in Healthcare at http://healthcare-ethics.org/resources/links.asp
The Joint Commission at http://jointcommission.org

REFERENCES

Agency for Healthcare Quality and Research. (2009). *Failure to rescue.* Retrieved from http://psnet.ahrq.gov/popup_glossary.aspx?name=failuretorescue.
American Nurses Association. (2015). *Code of Ethics for Nurses with Interpretive Statements.* Silver Spring, MD: American Nurses Association.
American Nurses Association. (2010a). *Nursing's social policy statement: the essence of the profession.* Washington, D.C. Nursebooks.org.
American Nurses Association. (2010b). *Scope and standards of nursing practice.* Washington, D.C. Nursebooks.org.
Bennett-Woods, D. (2006). *Models and processes of ethical decision-making.* Denver, CO: Regis University.
Black, B. P. (2014). *Professional nursing: concepts & challenges* (7th ed.). St. Louis, MO: Saunders.
Brous, E. (2009). Documentation & litigation RN. *72*(2), 40–43.
Cherry, B., & Jacob, S. R. (2017). *Contemporary nursing: issues, trends, & management* (7th ed.). St. Louis: Elsevier.
Croke, E. M. (2003). Nurses, negligence, and malpractice. *American Journal of Nursing*, *103*(9), 54–63.

Ellis, J. R., & Hartley, C. L. (2012). *Nursing in today's world: trends, issues, and management* (10th ed.). Philadelphia, PA: Lippincott Williams & Wilkins.

Epstein, E. G., & Delgado, S. (Sept. 30, 2010). Understanding and addressing moral distress. *The Online Journal of Issues in Nursing, 15*(3), 31–34.

Fowler, M. D. M. (2015). *Guide to the Code of Ethics for Nurses with Interpretive Statements* (2nd ed.). Silver Spring, MD: American Nurses Association.

Hall, J. K. (2003). Legal consequences of the moral duty to report errors. *JONA's Healthcare Law, Ethics, and Regulations, 5*(3), 60–64.

Hughes, R. G., & Blegan, M. A. (2008). Patient safety and quality: an evidence-based handbook for nurses. Retrieved from http://ahrq.gov/qual/nurseshdbk/.

Institute of Medicine. (1999). To err is human: building a safer health system. Retrieved from http://iom.edu/~/media/Files/Report%20Files/1999/To-Err-is-Human/To%20Err%20is%20Human%201999%20%20report%20brief.pdf.

Institute of Medicine. (2006). Preventing medication errors: quality chasm series. Retrieved from http://iom.edu/Reports/2006/Preventing-Medication-Errors-Quality-Chasm-Series.aspx.

James, J. T. (2013). A new, evidence-based estimate of patient harms associated with hospital care. *Journal of Patient Safety, 9*(3), 122–128. http://dx.doi.org/10.1097/PTS.0b013e3182948a69.

Justice served in Winkler case. (2011). *The American Nurse.* Retrieved from http://theamericannurse.org/index.php/2011/12/05/justice-served-in-winkler-case/.

Marquis, B. L., & Huston, C. J. (2015). *Leadership roles and management functions in nursing: theory and application* (8th ed.). Philadelphia, PA: Lippincott Williams & Wilkins.

Murray, J. S. (2010). Moral courage in healthcare: acting ethically even in the presence of risk. *The Online Journal of Issues in Nursing, 15*(3), manuscript 2.

Reisling, D. L., & Allen, P. N. (2007). Protecting yourself from malpractice claims. *American Nurse Today, 2*(2). Retrieved from http://americannursetoday.com/article.aspx?id=4186.

The Joint Commission. (2011). Sentinel events. Retrieved from http://jointcommission.org/assets/1/6/2011_CAMBHC_SE.pdf.

Care and Safety Standards, Competence, and Nurse Accountability

⊖volve WEBSITE

Additional resources are available online at:
http://evolve.elsevier.com/Claywell/transitions

OBJECTIVES

After completing this chapter, the student will be prepared to:
1. Compare the theoretical classifications of nursing skill.
2. Identify the benchmarks for judging nursing care.
3. Describe accountability as it applies to nursing practice.
4. Identify the RN's role in managing care aberrances.
5. Describe how using the chain of command to resolve issues supports accountability.

KEY TERMS

accountability	expert nurse	root-cause analysis
advanced beginner	informatics	safety
chain of command	novice nurse	standards of care
competent nurse	occurrence report	standards of practice
culture of safety	patient-centered care	systems thinking
evidence-based practice (EBP)	proficient nurse	teamwork and collaboration
	quality improvement (QI)	

OVERVIEW

At the completion of your RN educational program, you are expected to be capable of safely managing the care of a variety of patients. Knowledge and skill acquisition are lifelong endeavors providing growth. This chapter assists you to

---

FYI 13.1 RN SUCCESS TOOLS

To succeed as a nurse, you must have the tools needed to do the following:
- Become a registered nurse who will advance yourself as well as the profession
- Be accountable to yourself and the profession within the nursing role
- Maintain self-esteem and motivation as a means to becoming an expert nurse

---

recognize your role in the continuation of knowledge and skill acquisition. We investigate the Quality and Safety Education for Nurses (QSEN) standards and what they mean for you and then move on to personal and professional accountability in relation to nurse practice acts, professional practice standards, and standards of care; recruiting help; and assessing outcomes through quality of care issues. These topics are explored in relationship to the RN's role in maintaining educational competency. This chapter also helps you understand where you will be (educationally and experientially) upon graduation, how to continue acquiring knowledge and experience to advance in nursing, ways to maintain accountability for professional and personal development, and how to maintain personal motivation and self-esteem (FYI 13.1).

CLASSIFICATION OF NURSING SKILL LEVEL

Benner (1984) suggests that the graduate nurse enter the workforce as an advanced beginner. Del Bueno (2000) believes that the expectation for the novice RN is safe practice within set performance standards. While acquiring experience and skills, as well as continuing with learning, the nurse will advance in a predictable pattern toward becoming an expert nurse (Benner, 1984; Benner et al., 1996; Del Bueno, 2000). Specific characteristics distinguish the novice, competent, proficient, and expert nurses, and each type of nurse makes decisions and gives care in specific ways.

A **novice nurse** is a beginner with only basic skills and little experience. Generally, a novice is rule-driven, is a concrete thinker, and believes and trusts whoever has authority or whatever direction is perceived to have come from someone in authority. Novice nurses have inflexible thinking, and rules learned are applied in a generic, one-size-fits-all fashion. Basically, they do exactly as they are told. As an LPN/LVN, it is unlikely you will enter registered nursing as a novice. Your previous knowledge and experience have prepared you beyond this level. This is an example of how transitions can be highly variable and somewhat unpredictable. While you may be an expert in the LPN/LVN role, it is likely you will enter into the fullness of registered nursing at the advanced beginner or competent level. The **advanced beginner** has gained experience in the field and demonstrates a solid performance. The experience gained allows for understanding to begin forming meanings and principles that may guide later practice. A **competent nurse** has more experience (usually 2 or 3 years in the new role) and has developed safe organizational skills to get through the day's tasks efficiently. Flexibility within the nursing role is difficult to manage at this point, and when deviations from the schedule occur, the nurse generally has a feeling of unease. However, movement toward abstract, analytical thinking improves efficiency.

A **proficient nurse** has much experience and a beginning ability to recognize patterns and think both holistically and critically, basing many decisions on experience. The proficient nurse is able to adapt to change and might have garnered the admiration and respect of peers. An **expert nurse** has had a great deal of experience and is flexible and adaptable, responding to change with ease. The expert nurse is a skilled critical thinker and demonstrates an intuitive understanding of clinical conditions, making performance within the role exceptional.

Performance evaluations are designed to distinguish the RN's performance as being at the novice/safe level, the competent level, or an expert level (Del Bueno, 2000). The RN gains expertise and improved critical thinking through experience and knowledge acquisition. Additionally, while gaining experience, the RN begins to think more broadly and deeply. As you gain experience in the RN role, you will be comfortable investigating the human experiences of the patient, which enables you to make more accurate clinical judgments. As an expert you will recognize minute changes in patient conditions that will assist in planning and managing precisely individualized care, ultimately improving patient outcomes (Benner et al., 1996). A minimum expectation is that you will strive for excellence and maintain and improve skills and knowledge through continuing professional education. Adherence to educational and professional standards contributes to excellent role performance.

EDUCATIONAL AND PROFESSIONAL STANDARDS

It is likely that in your practice as an LPN/LVN you have encountered changes within the health care system in response to the 1999 Institute of Medicine (IOM) publication *To Err Is Human.* In this publication the IOM identified that more people die in hospitals every year from preventable errors than from motor vehicle accidents, breast cancer, and AIDS combined! The IOM identified the areas with the highest ratio of errors to be in ICUs, ORs, and EDs. Since then, major health care quality organizations have stepped up to address this astounding issue. The Agency for Healthcare Research and Quality (AHRQ) called for the creation of a **culture of safety,** or a commitment on both individual and organizational levels to accept accountability to attain excellence in performance by directing resources toward the problems. The National Quality Forum (NQF) created and has since expanded and revised a list of *never events* that are categorized into six areas: surgical events, product or device events, patient protection events, care management events, environmental events, and criminal events (AHRQ, 2012). Consider this list for a moment. Who is most likely to be able to make a difference in any of these areas, if not the RN? As an RN, you will be front and center in the battle to protect your patients while in your care.

Quality and Safety Education for Nurses

It is precisely for these reasons that the Robert Wood Johnson Foundation (RWJF) funded the Quality and Safety Education for Nurses (QSEN, 2014) project. The goal of QSEN is to ensure that all nurses develop the knowledge, skills, and attitudes (KSAs) to be pivotal in the quest for continuous quality and safety improvement.

BOX 13.1 COMPETENCIES FOR KNOWLEDGE, SKILLS, AND ATTITUDES FOR PRELICENSURE PROGRAMS

- **Patient-Centered Care:** Recognize the patient or designee as the source of control and full partner in providing compassionate and coordinated care based on respect for patient's preferences, values, and needs.
- **Teamwork and Collaboration:** Function effectively within nursing and inter-professional teams, fostering open communication, mutual respect, and shared decision making to achieve quality patient care.
- **Evidence-Based Practice (EBP):** Integrate best current evidence with clinical exper-tise and patient/family preferences and values for delivery of optimal health care.
- **Quality Improvement (QI):** Use data to monitor the outcomes of care processes and use improvement methods to design and test changes to continuously improve the quality and safety of health care systems.
- **Safety:** Minimize risk of harm to patients and providers through both system effectiveness and individual performance.
- **Informatics:** Use information and technology to communicate, manage knowledge, mitigate error, and support decision making.

The KSAs for prelicensure programs in nursing (the kind of program you are attending) are categorized into six primary competencies: patient-centered care, teamwork and collaboration, evidence-based practice, quality improvement, safety, and informatics. The competencies you will attain in each of these areas are explic-itly defined in Box 13.1. Please visit http://qsen.org/competencies/pre-licensure-ksas/ and carefully read the KSAs for examples of knowledge, skills, and attitudes that are necessary to achieve each of the competencies. Once there you can download a .pdf version of the page to keep handy for your reference. For those who go on to advanced degrees in nursing, there are graduate level competencies and KSAs as well (qsen.org, 2014). As you go through your prelicensure nursing program, you will find that the culture of quality and safety is infused into every act and thought of the registered professional nurse in providing care; however, it is more than being attentive to your specific care but awareness of how your care is connected to the rest of the experience a patient receives.

Dolansky and Moore (2013) state that in addition to "vigilant individual care," "vigilant systems care" is necessary (para 7). Nurses must be taught **systems think-ing** and practice it routinely in planning, implementing, and evaluating patient care. Systems thinking means that you recognize how each individual act is interconnected with all the other care processes provided by all of the other health care providers in the care of the patient, family, group, community, or population. The outcomes of engaging in systems thinking include decreasing errors, increasing the accuracy of delegation and priority setting, improving problem solving and successful decision making, improving interactions with both the patient and other health care providers involved in the patient's care, and increasing participation in quality improvement initiatives for individual practice, the organization, and the profession. Keep systems thinking in mind as you complete Exercise 13.1 and consider your role in attaining the QSEN competencies.

? EXERCISE 13.1

Write at least one example of how you will work toward attainment of each of the six QSEN competencies. If you believe you already engage in activities related to one or more of these competencies in your current role, explain how you believe that activity will change as you take on the role of the RN.
1. Patient-centered care:_____
2. Teamwork and collaboration: _____
3. Evidence-based practice: _____
4. Quality improvement: _____
5. Safety: _____
6. Informatics: _____

Professional Accountability

Accountability is being answerable for the actions or interventions one performs as a nurse. Accountability also means taking responsibility for your professional growth. Although individuals are ultimately accountable to themselves, the RN is particularly accountable to the patient, society, and profession.

The nurse has been given professional capacity through licensure and by the job description. Standards of practice and standards of care are set by the profession as the benchmarks for judging nursing care. Individual state boards of nursing define the scope of practice and licensure requirements for RNs and LPN/LVNs, or the **standards of practice.** Each state establishes a nurse practice act, which sets legal boundaries for nursing. Boards of nursing have jurisdiction over RN and LPN/LVN licenses and decide on legal action to be taken against them. State and national nursing organizations and specialty organizations establish policies and provide position statements defining **standards of care** for nurses, in general and in specialty areas. Held to high standards of practice and care, the RN must know and understand both the state practice acts and the position statements on practice standards. To this end, there is clearly personal accountability required within the RN role.

Personal Accountability

The individual RN should maintain a current level of expertise. nurse practice acts mandate specific individual RN responsibilities related to continued education and competency updates. State boards of nursing may maintain specific requirements of continuing educational units. Professional standards of care as defined by peers through professional organizations, such as the National League for Nursing and the American Nurses Association (ANA), outline expected levels of expertise and experience for clinical areas.

In some states, failing to maintain currency through continuing education may result in the inability to renew the RN license. Although it benefits an institution for staff LPN/LVNs and RNs to have current experience and expertise, your place of employment will not necessarily meet all of your continuing education needs. Unit-specific orientation with formal courses may be provided by the institution, and additional unit-specific updates are often provided regarding procedural or equipment changes or treatment plans. The scope of RN practice is much broader than these courses, however, and the RN must seek other means to remain current.

⚑ FYI 13.2   ACCOUNTABILITY IN REGISTERED NURSING

1. The RN is accountable to self, patients, and the profession of nursing.
2. Practice standards, policies, and state nurse practice acts define limits as well as the scope of the RN's role.
3. Patients deserve quality, caring, compassionate nursing.
4. An RN who strives for excellence will gain greater trust from patients.

The new graduate must make an honest assessment of weaknesses and strengths related to the chosen work area. Write out your personal and professional goals, as well as steps toward accomplishment of those goals, and place them where you will see them daily. The new RN needs to schedule monthly evaluations with the supervisor to determine how well the goals are being met. The RN who uses this or a similarly proactive approach to development is assuming both professional and personal accountability. See FYI 13.2 for highlights of accountability in registered nursing.

Professional Practice Standards and Standards of Care

The ANA has established a policy statement regarding the need for the RN to use the nursing process when developing plans of care. The assumption is that the RN works in collaboration with the physician and other health care professionals to establish plans of care. As an independent care practitioner, the RN must use knowledge, skills, and experience to make decisions. The autonomy of RNs is thus a practice standard.

Professional nursing organizations such as the ANA, NLN, and Critical Care Nurses Association (and other specialty organizations) set policies and practice standards. The ANA Code of Ethics defines the fundamental ethical standard under which the nurse will practice. In ethical and professional actions, the RN is expected to act fairly, judicially, and professionally. The RN's judgment must be based on continuous acquisition of knowledge. The code also requires the RN to provide quality care in a collaborative effort with other health care team members to meet the needs of the patient. (See Chapter 12 for more on ethics in your practice.)

As an RN you are responsible for meeting the needs of the patient. Your decisions will be judged against the practice standard and may have legal and ethical implications. Practice standards determine ideals, identifying what the prudent RN should do within the role. Your decisions will be judged against those made by other RNs in a similar situation. Just as RNs are judged against their peers, patients and families also evaluate the quality of care given. Answer the questions related to quality and priority of care in Exercise 13.2.

Accountability is a practice standard, and clinical judgment should demonstrate that you are willing to be accountable. If inadequate or inaccurate data are being gathered, then the quality of care suffers, and patient length of stay and health costs increase. In the scenario in Exercise 13.2, clinical judgment regarding the level of

---

? EXERCISE 13.2

In a one-on-one clinical session, an instructor questions an LPN/LVN transition student with regard to the priority of care. The student is unsure why the patient is still on a monitored floor and is sent to investigate. On return, the student explains that just 2 days ago, the patient had pulmonary edema from fluid volume overload, and, with the change in medications the patient received, the physicians required that the patient be closely monitored to ensure that the pulmonary edema did not recur. The instructor then asks what the patient's intake and output have been for the last 24 hours and what the patient's weight has been. The student reports that the patient has not been saving the urine for the nurses to measure and the weight check was not done this morning.

1. Identify the outcome priority.
2. What areas of accountability are in question in this situation?
3. Identify the standard of practice and determine whether it has been breached.
4. How does the outcome of this situation affect cost?
5. What are your responsibilities as an RN?

---

care will be faulty if the standards are not followed. Additionally, how will quality of care be addressed if the RN is negligent in adhering to basic practice standards and agency policy? The RN is in an ideal position to increase quality of care and reduce costs if acting responsibly and accepting accountability for establishing and maintaining the plan of care. This includes the need to adhere to the policies of the unit and agency to ensure that all data are available to make decisions regarding the plan of care.

The need to be accountable for every action may seem overwhelming to the beginning RN. As an RN, you will need to make independent decisions regarding the plan of care and implementing interventions. This freedom can be a powerful tool if acted on judiciously, but accountability cannot happen in a vacuum. RNs must collaborate with all members of the health care team and elicit their expertise and cooperation. Nurses are frequently the team leaders when decisions affecting patient care are addressed, and likewise, it is often the RN who assumes the risks while managing patient care.

MANAGING CARE ABERRANCES

A health team member may defer or avoid asking for assistance from a supervisor to resolve a problem or to report an error for fear it will hurt his or her professional reputation. One may feel that going to the supervisor will set up a confrontational situation where the only resolution to the problem or mistake will be disciplinary action. The nurse may feel powerless to request help.

The RN must act judiciously and prudently in the delivery of care. By not going to the supervisor when a mistake is made and failing to demonstrate accountability for contributing to the mistake, the RN risks not only harm to the patient but also potential legal and ethical consequences. The RN needs to take a proactive approach with administration so that issues of accountability will not be so difficult to resolve.

Occurrence Reports

Reconsider the statistic that preventable errors are attributable to more deaths in hospitals than motor vehicle accidents, AIDS, and breast cancer combined (IOM, 1999). In an earlier chapter you read the staggering statistic that as many as 400,000 preventable deaths occur each year in our hospitals across the nation. That is just astounding! It is OUR job as the RN to do everything possible to decrease the number of errors in whatever way available to us. The RN directly involved in an error or who discovers an error completes the **occurrence report** to document errors in omission or commission and to document measures taken to safeguard the patient. According to Nurses Service Organization, a major supplier of nursing malpractice insurance, the purposes of the occurrence report are to: "jog your memory," "trigger a rapid response," and "facilitate decisions about restitution" (nso.com, n.d., para 1-4). It is important when completing an occurrence report that you include just the facts, with no opinion or emotion. The occurrence report, which is mandated by health care facilities of all types, provides critical data that inform decisions related to practice in everything from medications and processes to a procedure and equipment. This surveillance and monitoring of data and trends are a part of quality assurance and risk management practice standards. Risk managers can identify areas of weakness through patterns seen in these occurrence reports, and a plan to decrease errors can then be designed. It is our responsibility to know and comply with all risk management policies and procedures in the facilities in which we work (Martin, 2006).

However, some nurses are reluctant to complete the occurrence reports as they perceive the reports as punitive and that they will result in disciplinary action, or they think that the reports will be placed in the employee's permanent file, which is not the case. Some nurses think the reports "fall on deaf ears," and so they believe that it is not worth the effort to complete the form. Some are even afraid that if they complete the report that they will be named in any possible legal action that may result. All of these concerns, though they may seem real to the nurse, are no excuse for failing to complete and submit the reports in any situation that warrants it to be done. It is part of our covenant with the public when we become professional nurses (Martin, 2006).

Root-Cause Analysis

Root-cause analysis of an occurrence identifies the underlying causes. Root-cause analysis is designed to seek errors of process, rather than lay blame on individuals or groups. Most errors result from one or more breaks in a chain of events.

One example would be where a nurse gives the wrong medication to a patient. In a root-cause analysis, a committee is formed, which would include in this case a facilitator (usually the risk manager or performance improvement director), the nurse or nurses involved, a pharmacist, the physician, and the team leader or supervisor. The purpose of the committee is to reconstruct the events leading up to the error. By looking at the process, the committee may discover that the physician's order was unclear, that two drugs with similar names were placed next to each other in the medication-dispensing unit, or that the unit of measure for the drug was unclear. Even though the process of dispensing medications is typically safeguarded with redundant checks and balances, nurses are the last check against a medication error.

Acute health care hospitals that use the root-cause analysis process gener-ally identify solutions more accurately than hospitals that do not. These solutions include further individual or staff education, correction of a policy or procedure, or, if needed, discipline. By not making negative consequences, such as discipline, the main focus of correcting systemic or procedural problems, greater reporting of errors or problems will hopefully occur. Whether it is an individual, communica-tion, system, or procedural problem, occurrence reporting provides a way to track and identify problem areas, which can ensure better outcomes when put through the analysis process.

The nurse must view an occurrence report as a positive step toward improving care. Quality care will not happen without evaluation. The report can identify staffing inadequacies or disparities as well as educational or training needs. Positive change cannot happen without understanding the need for change. A dialogue between staff nurses and unit management should be initiated to ensure that occurrence reports are used in a positive way. Unless gross negligence, assault, or battery or another felony has occurred, the occurrence report should not be used in a punitive way. Individual problems can be handled with greater supervision, education, training, and a specific plan that will help the individual achieve a higher level of function. Unit-specific problems may require education, increased staff support, or a greater supervisory role. All care providers, both licensed and unlicensed personnel, must be held accountable for their actions, and occurrence reporting is a means to establish accountability.

Involving Management in Decision Making

Accountability also extends to times when the nurse must involve supervisors, department managers, or the nursing or hospital administrators in the decision-making process. The RN must recognize those times when management is needed to facilitate care or to assist in operational decisions affecting care given on a unit. For example, the staff RN is often reluctant to call unit managers, house supervisors, or administration when bed availability issues arise. This includes times when you are required to find beds in another unit or even in another facility for transfers. Although these tasks may be within the RN's collaborative role, you will need to know when this task should be delegated to those who do not have direct patient care duties, such as the unit or house supervisor or the bed-utilization nurse. If the problem will take more than a phone call to resolve, it would be taking time and energy away from patient care, and you will have to be judicious with your priorities in such cases.

PATIENT AND FAMILY COMPLAINTS

Patient and family complaints are another area in which the RN may not have the experience, time, and information to intervene appropriately. As an LPN/LVN, on the other hand, you may be no stranger to these challenging situations. You will need to determine when you can handle a problem personally or if you need to refer it to another appropriate resource. Resolved or not, the outcome will depend on how well the patient or family perceives that needs are being met. As an RN you will need to understand the experiences, responsibilities, and accountabilities of different health care team members when it comes to accessing them. Be prepared to resolve certain patient problems through a phone call to the unit manager or house supervisor. Pastoral care services or social services may be able to assist with other issues.

Chain of Command

The RN may be reluctant to use the **chain of command** when a need arises to correct a problem that threatens patient care. Each health care system has an established chain of command, including individuals with defined management responsibilities, from the board of directors to the health care administrator or chief operating officer, through the various levels of management, down to the nursing staff. The nurse resolves problems by beginning with the immediate supervisor and, if necessary, working up the chain of command to higher levels of authority. If the RN knows how to use the chain of command effectively, most problems can be resolved without a compromise to patient care. For nurses, the final step most often occurs at the director of nursing level, but the process could continue to the board of directors, if necessary.

Difficulties with communication between a physician and a nurse may lead to conflicts that compromise the standard of care. The RN must remember that not going up the chain of command in an attempt to resolve the conflict makes him or her accountable if patient care continues to be compromised. You are the advocate in these situations. It is better to raise the questions and point out the issues than to remain silent. Accountability requires us to be the advocates.

Failing to gain cooperation from the other health care team members may make the RN's load much heavier than necessary. Input from the supervisory level can often facilitate accomplishing actions in a more timely fashion. Consistently using the appropriate chain of command reinforces the team effort to uphold the standard of patient care. The RN is accountable for the care given, and the care must be given in a judicious manner.

Quality of Care Measurement

Quality of care measurement tools gauge patient satisfaction, cost of care, and effectiveness of care. The RN, as the coordinator of care, is directly accountable for these issues. Generally, quality of care is measured through patient satisfaction surveys, chart reviews, and core measures and quality indicator studies that look at specific aspects of care and the performance of the facility in specific areas. Patient satisfaction has a direct influence on the revenue that the hospital receives because patient satisfaction drives the patient's decision to use the health care facility again. Therefore, the RN must pay attention to quality care ratings given to health care facilities, as well as to units within these facilities.

More importantly, when an individual patient is unhappy and behaving in a negative manner, the RN must investigate this behavior and determine its source. Often it is related to pain, angst, sorrow, or anxiety. Once the source of the behavior is identified, the RN must attempt to resolve the problem with good communication and management techniques. Not surprisingly, patients are more satisfied with care that includes listening, empathy, and understanding than when the nurse has a detached, all-business, or seemingly uncaring manner. We are accountable to ensure that our patients and their families are satisfied with the care they receive.

KEY POINTS

After completion of this chapter, you have learned:

- As a student, you are being prepared to become an RN. Accountability, quality care, and personal satisfaction are important concepts to keep in mind.
- The graduate nurse enters the workforce as an advanced beginner. Moving toward proficiency, the new RN acquires experience, continues learning, and gains skills and with further progress advances to become an expert nurse.
- QSEN competencies help to prepare the nurse to provide high-quality care.
- It is your responsibility to ensure that you attain and maintain competency and to continually strive toward excellence in patient care.
- The RN is also accountable to the patient to provide the best care possible that is safe and effective in moving the patient to a prior or higher level of function.
- The RN must also be accountable to the nursing profession because the profession sets practice standards that, with standards of care, provide benchmarks for judging nursing care.
- A standard of practice is that RNs maintain a level of expertise for their area.
- Additionally, the RN needs to recognize situations that call for assistance from managers or supervisors.

▌ CRITICAL THINKING QUESTIONS

The answers to each of the following questions should use the elements of critical thinking: purpose, questions at issue, available information, basic concepts, assumptions, inferences and interpretations, implications and consequences, and point of view.

1. Identify five things about the role of the RN you believe to be important. Rank them from most important to least important to you. Get together with one other student in your class, and from your two lists, come up with three facts that you both agree are most important. Then identify two other students who do not have the same facts, and repeat, agreeing on just three facts that the four of you believe to be most important. For each fact, answer the following questions:
   a. How would you go about supporting your assumption that these items are highly important to the role of the RN?
   b. What information would you need to prove or disprove your claim?
   c. What are the possible outcomes of not holding these to be true?
2. You are the RN in charge. An LPN/LVN has just reported that she has just hung the O-negative blood on Mr. Smith. The blood had been ordered, but you were unaware that the type and cross-match had been completed and the blood was ready.

a. What are the standards of practice for the incident, and what action must you, as RN, take?

b. Write out the incident report as it should be documented, as well as the nurse's notes.

3. Your patient is to receive a bolus of 4 mg of morphine sulfate IVP and has a standing PRN order for 2 to 4 mg IVP q1h. The unit-dose syringe is 10 mg per 1 mL. After giving the 4-mg bolus, you decide that, rather than waste the rest of the medication, you will place the medication in the patient's drawer to give later. A team member RN later reports giving your patient 4 mg of the morphine from the drawer stash and wasting the rest of the medication. He wants you to cosign the pharmacy sheet to account for the waste.

a. What are the professional and legal issues?

b. What assumption can you make, and how would you go about collecting information to support the assumptions?

4. In order to improve your systems thinking ability, think of a care process that you routinely engage in with your patients. Now in a flowchart, write out every step involved in that care process including all of the people involved in this process. Think deeply and comprehensively and add as many levels in the flowchart as you can. How many levels or steps surround your specific care? What would happen if one small step included an error or miscalculation of some sort? Who else would be affected and why?

5. Think of a problem that you encountered or know of in caring for a patient. Conduct a root-cause analysis, moving beyond individual blame and look for understanding how a system may have contributed to the problem. Perhaps consider a medication error for this scenario.

WEB RESOURCES

http://ahrq.gov/
http://qsen.org/
http://systems-thinking.org/rca/rootca.htm
www.nso.org

REFERENCES

Agency for Healthcare Research and Quality [AHRQ]. (2012). *Never events*. Retrieved from http://psnet.ahrq.gov/primer.aspx?primerID=3.

Benner, P. (1984). *From novice to expert: excellence and power in clinical nursing practice.* Menlo Park, CA: Addison-Wesley.

Benner, P., Tanner, C. A., & Chesla, C. A. (1996). *Expertise in nursing practice: caring, clinical judgment, and ethics.* New York, NY: Springer.

Del Bueno, D. J. (2000). *A model for competence and success. Presentation given at Northeast Baptist Hospital.* San Antonio: TX. March 2000.

Dolansky, M. A., & Moore, S. M. (2013). Quality and safety education for nurses (QSEN): the key is systems thinking. *The Online Journal of Issues in Nursing, 18*(3). Retrieved from http://www.nursingworld.org/Quality-and-Safety-Education-for-Nurses.html.

Institute of Medicine. (1999). *To err is human: shaping the future of healthcare.* Retrieved from http://nap.edu/books/0309068371/html/.

Martin, R. H. (2006). *Incident reports.* Retrieved from nursing.advancedweb.com.

Nurses Service Organization. (n.d.). *Why incident reports are a must.* Retrieved from http://www.nso.com/risk-education/individuals/articles/Pages/Why-Incident-Reports-Are-A-Must.aspx.

Quality and Safety Education for Nurses [QSEN]. (2014). *Pre-licensure KSAs.* Retrieved from http://qsen.org/competencies/pre-licensure-ksas/.

UNIT 4

The RN as Manager of Care

CHAPTER

14

Leading, Delegating, and Collaborating

⊝volve WEBSITE

Additional resources are available online at:
http://evolve.elsevier.com/Claywell/transitions

OBJECTIVES

After completing this chapter, the student will be prepared to:

1. Define leadership.
2. Describe the leadership role in nursing.
3. Compare leadership styles.
4. Analyze his or her own leadership style.
5. Delegate according to professional principles.
6. Collaborate as a part of the health care team.
7. Describe the accountability embedded in leadership.
8. Describe the role of advocate.
9. Analyze strategies for conflict management.

KEY TERMS

accountability	decision making	quantum leadership
advocacy	democratic leadership	sacrifice resolution
autocratic leadership	Emotional Intelligence	servant leadership
caring	interpersonal conflict	transactional
collaboration	laissez-faire leadership	leadership
competition resolution	leadership	transformational
conflict	manage	leadership
culture	problem solving	win-win resolution

OVERVIEW

Part of the professional nursing role is to serve as a leader. However, leadership development takes time to cultivate specific knowledge, skills, and abilities. As an LPN/LVN you may have served in numerous management/coordinator capacities. Being a manager of care *is* a major role of the RN, who is expected to become primarily responsible for managing the plan of care for several patients. As a registered professional nurse, you will be not only a well-organized coordinator but also a knowledgeable collaborator and skilled delegator within a team delivering safe, effective care. Ultimately, the nursing profession needs leadership to grow, develop, and sustain excellence among its members. It is important to recognize that not all leaders are managers and not all managers are leaders. Leadership in nursing is required at all levels in the organization, including at the point of care. This chapter presents leadership characteristics and styles as well as other components of your new role, such as task delegation, collaboration, accountability, advocacy, and conflict management.

LEADERS, MANAGERS, AND FOLLOWERS

Leaders, managers, and followers are complementary to one another, and professional RNs will experience each role (Yoder-Wise, 2015). The term **leadership** has many definitions. Older definitions focused on behaviors and traits, while contemporary definitions focus on leadership as a process of influencing and interacting with others (Marquis & Huston, 2015). Leaders influence patients, families, and others toward a vision or a goal. They empower those working with them, communicate a sense of direction, and demonstrate self-confidence. Characteristics of a leader include competence, trustworthiness, self-assuredness, decision-making ability, and the skills to prioritize (Yoder-Wise, 2015). Tasks of leadership include envisioning goals, affirming values, motivating others, managing, achieving workable unity, developing trust, explaining, serving as a symbol, representing the group, and renewing the self (Gardner, 1990, as cited in Yoder-Wise, 2015). Registered nurses can develop leadership skills by volunteering for leadership roles in the workplace and involvement with professional organizations (Kerfoot, 1999, as cited in Yoder-Wise, 2015). Staff nurses should share their ideas for future improvements by volunteering for committees and other opportunities to lead (Yoder-Wise, 2015).

Management provides the structure and direction necessary to accomplish goals and outcomes that are known and where there is a system in place to achieve the outcomes (Marquis & Huston, 2015). The term *manager* should not be thought of as meaning only those in top positions of authority, because any staff member who bears responsibility for the work of others or who must ensure the completion of an organizational process may be considered a manager. Managers guide the processes necessary to accomplish tasks necessary to achieve organizational outcomes (Yoder-Wise, 2015).

Followership is not a passive process but rather actively uses personal behaviors that contribute to the health care team's goals. The follower demonstrates collaboration, influence, and action with the leader or manager in order to accomplish goals and outcomes. Followers should be willing to question, debate, compromise, collaborate, act on, and be accountable for those actions (Yoder-Wise, 2015). Accomplishing organizational goals and outcomes is not only dependent on the skills of the leader and manager but is equally dependent on the skills of the follower.

LEADERSHIP CHARACTERISTICS

Implementation of the plan of care for several patients takes organization and **leadership**—the ability to influence outcomes through positive interactions with team members. A strong leader recognizes the strengths and weaknesses within the team and manages them to effect a positive outcome from a plan of care. Morrison, Jones, and Fuller (1997) contend that an important aspect of leadership is empowerment of all the team members to do the jobs of which they are most capable.

Defining the Leadership Role

Basic to the leadership role is the ability to know the defined roles of each team member, as well as his or her strengths and weakness. A strong leader delegates assignments, tasks, and duties to the best individuals for the particular jobs. A strong leader empowers the team members through delegation of tasks within their capacity and by the trust placed in them to complete these tasks. Morrison and colleagues conclude that job satisfaction increases when there is empowerment. Laschinger and colleagues (1999) suggest that a leader's empowerment behavior predicts a lower level of job tension and more effective work.

To **manage** is directing or supervising others as a means to control a situation (Marquis & Huston, 2015). Managing patient care means overseeing the plan of care and directing others to implement the plan toward achievement of the desired outcomes. A manager has leadership qualities, acts as an advisor, and influences the beliefs of others. With the RN as a patient care manager, the leadership role is both an expectation as well as an earned role. It is an assumption that a strong leader has expertise in the practice area or clinical specialty. A strong leader knows about the patients and is able to anticipate their needs. Within this role, the RN is confident, in control of the day, and willing to help when needed.

The RN leader is decisive, practices sound judgment, and is able to articulate fluently. Perra (1999) associates a sound leader with self-knowledge, respect, trust, integrity, vision, participation, learning, communication, and catalyzing change. Respect and trust are mutual and inclusive between the leader and team members. Respect comes to the leader with integrity, who reliably does the right thing by all and for the profession. Leadership fosters participation from others in the critical thinking process as sources of information, expertise, and specific knowledge. The leader with integrity advocates diversity of opinion and beliefs within the team and is thus open to critiques of actions and decisions. The strong leader is a critical and rational thinker. Such an RN leader is better equipped to influence the other health care team members and gain their cooperation and respect.

Leadership Styles

Leadership styles emerge as ways to relate to others and influence the outcomes of situations. Each style has distinct qualities that define it and make it suitable for meeting a particular situation's team objectives. The three main styles are demo-cratic, autocratic, and laissez-faire leadership. You need to know when to use which leadership type, based on your assessment of the situation:

- The **democratic** leader bases decisions on *consensus,* or mutual agreement, within the group. This leader delegates duties according to the strengths within the team. With each team member solicited for input, however, outcomes are slow in coming.
- Authoritarian and **autocratic** leaders use power to influence others and affect outcomes. If the autocratic leader just assumes power without earning the subor-dinates' respect, though, that power can foster resentment. Authoritarian power exerted in an acute crisis situation, however, can effectively influence outcomes.
- A **laissez-faire,** or nondirective, leader deliberately intervenes as little as possible. When team members are independently motivated but cohesive, much can be accomplished over a period of time. Chaos can occur, however, if individual needs and agendas interfere with the overall goals of the group.

Additionally, a group may have more than one leader, requiring either a co-lead-ership approach or a rotating leadership approach. The dynamics of the group as well as the individual leaders generally dictate the success of such a group.

Leadership Approaches

Leadership has also been described in relation to one of three popular approaches: transactional, transformational, and servant leadership. Each influences change through empowerment of the nurse and team members (Morrison et al., 1997; Trofino, 1995).

The RN's style of leadership should reflect the personalities of the group members as well as respond to the situation. Individual personalities affect the group interac-tion. A strong leader understands such dynamics and capitalizes on them. An example might be when the RN is determining patient assignments. Knowing the personalities of the group, the RN makes assignments so that each member will use his or her best attributes and best work together with the others. For example, an RN team leader could assign an LPN/LVN who does not need much direction to be supervised by an RN who is known to expect independence from the LPN/LVNs. In another example, the RN team leader may make patient assignments based on the critical nature of the situation, delegating critical patient care to the most experienced RN.

Generally, the RN incorporates one or more styles of leadership to meet the needs of the patient. Judicious leadership takes open communication between the group members. Clear goals and objectives must be a part of the plan of care, and each member of the team must understand his or her role in meeting the goals. When a team works together for a common goal, communicating positive patient outcomes and patient satisfaction to the team members can give a sense of pride and accom-plishment (Morrison et al., 1997).

Transactional Leadership

In **transactional leadership,** the traditional boss makes decisions without staff input. This type of leadership motivates followers in three ways: offering rewards, moni-toring work performance and correcting the staff member immediately, or waiting until a problem occurs and dealing with it later (Dunham-Taylor, 2000, as cited in Yoder-Wise, 2015). This type of leadership relies on power and authority to reward or punish performance and is usually found in stable work environments (Yoder-Wise, 2015).

Transformational Leadership

Transformational leadership, in contrast, seeks and welcomes input from staff to set goals and make decisions and brings out the best in people (Yoder-Wise, 2015). The transformational leader identifies common values, is committed, is visionary, examines outcomes, and empowers others. This type of leader is charismatic, inspirational, motivational, intellectually stimulating, and treats others as unique individuals (individualized consideration) (Marquis & Huston, 2015). Research conducted by McGuire and Kennerly (2006) found that followers have a higher sense of organizational commitment when working with the transformational leader. The transformational leader motivates followers to reach their fullest potential (Northouse, 2004). The transformational leader influences change through empowering the followers to do the work of change. Within a group process, this leadership style supports the competencies of the individual members, allowing them to take responsibility and authority for their decisions. This leadership style fosters support for creativity, uniqueness in problem solving, and an individual spirit of freedom. Team members feel empowered to do their work and often perform at a higher level than expected. Fundamental trust is established between leader and follower, and the task of the team is fulfilled with a high degree of patient satisfaction.

Servant Leadership

Servant leadership emphasizes service to others, including employees, customers, and the community as a first priority (Marquis & Huston, 2015). Servant leaders focus on the needs of others, empathize with them, and are attentive to the concerns of followers (Northouse, 2004). The term *servant leadership* originated with Robert Greenleaf in 1979, but the concept goes back thousands of years in religious and humanistic teachings. The characteristics central to service learning are listening, empathy, healing, persuasion, awareness, foresight, conceptualization, commitment to the growth of people, stewardship, and building community (Marquis & Huston, 2015). Servant leadership is taught in colleges and universities and is practiced in many settings, as more emphasis is placed on the ability of leaders, managers, and followers to positively interact with others.

Quantum Leadership

According to Curtain (2013) both the traditional, hierarchical perspective of leadership and the new, dynamic quantum approach are important in the life of an organization. **Quantum leadership** seems most effective in times of chaos and change. It is during these times when leaders who have the following characteristics arise and excel:

- A strong "moral purpose to make a positive difference" (para. 6) for others
- The ability to establish and promote nurturing relationships
- Who approach decision making through empowered followers

Porter-O'Gradey and Mallach (2015), internationally renowned experts in nursing and health care leadership, explain how chaos theory, complexity theory, and quantum theory come together to help health care leaders of today deal with the reality of health care in a time of harsh limitation of resources in the face of the social, political, and economic drivers toward transformation. Ultimately they reveal that in order to understand complexity, first we must recognize that everything and everyone are connected in some way. We may not actually be able to concretely see the connections, but they are there nonetheless, and great leaders are able both to live in the actual moment reality and to perceive the potential reality and act upon and plan for what might be coming. If nurses focus only on what they are specifically doing at any moment in time and pay no attention to the team or the greater system at work, they miss the opportunity to anticipate when and where change is needed for improved outcomes at every level. In practicing quantum leadership, nurses must recognize and adhere to Porter-O'Grady and Mallach's (2015) ten leadership principles (Box 14.1).

BOX 14.1

- Principle 1: "Wholes are not just the sum of their parts" (p. 55) but rather how the parts function interdependently.
- Principle 2: "All health care is local" (p. 59). Everything we do is directed to improve the actual point of care that is carried out individually but affected by every part of the system.
- Principle 3: "Value is now the centerpiece of service delivery" (p. 62). All effort is directed at adding value within the components of the systems but within context of the whole.
- Principle 4: "Simple systems aggregate to complex systems" (p. 65). All parts of a system are little systems in themselves and must be developed and managed with the larger system in focus.
- Principle 5: "Diversity is essential to life" (p. 67). The wisdom that is the collective of various perspectives is necessary for organizations to be able to adapt and thrive.
- Principle 6: "Error is essential to success" (p. 69). Error is the catalyst for learning, growth, and change when viewed as opportunities for improvement.
- Principle 7: "Systems thrive when all of their functions intersect and interact" (p. 71). Nurses as leaders influence the point at which the greatest interactions take place at the point of care.
- Principle 8: "Equilibrium and disequilibrium are in constant tension" (p. 75). It is at the edge of stability and chaos where change can be made, and nurse leaders reside at the intersection where decisions about care are made.
- Principle 9: "Change is generated from the center outward" (p. 79). Nurses are at the center with the patient, and all improvements must come from this perspective.
- Principle 10: "Revolution results from the aggregation of local changes" (p. 82). Nurses are positioned as leaders to serve as change agents that lead to transformation of care.

LEADING AND EMOTIONAL INTELLIGENCE

Leading occurs within and outside of the work setting. The way we lead has an impact on followers, whether they are people in the community, family, or friends. The leader's skill in dealing with people, motivating, giving feedback, and developing trust is crucial to success, because others in the workplace are affected by the leader's behaviors and will have a tremendous impact on the team. Daniel Goleman's concept of **Emotional Intelligence** (EI) has gained popularity since his 1995 book *Emotional Intelligence,* in which he states that there are four major domains of EI: self-awareness, self-management, social awareness, and relationship management (Porter-O'Grady, 2003).

Organizations, including health care organizations, are fighting and struggling to survive, and yet they often miss the impact of positive and empathetic leadership on the workplace (Porter-O'Grady, 2003). Empathy, caring, and the importance of developing the therapeutic relationship are familiar concepts to nurses, and these same concepts are found in EI. EI refers to recognizing and regulating emotions in ourselves and others. Because nurses must have good rapport with patients as well as the ability to understand patient needs, nurses can easily become emotionally drained, and the nurse must be able to recognize and manage his or her emotions.

While caring, empathy, and the development of the therapeutic relationship are nothing new to nursing, the concept is new within the context of leadership. Looking within ourselves helps us to interact positively with others. Given the complexity of the nursing profession, EI becomes increasingly important, especially given the high-stress environment of nursing. Nurse leaders are in an ideal position to demonstrate and apply the concepts of EI in health care. Applying the concepts of EI, leaders can improve staff relationships and patient outcomes, motivate others, resolve conflict, and create a healthy work environment. EI is a win-win situation for patients, staff nurses, nurse leaders, and health care organizations.

ETHICS AND CULTURE: CENTRAL TO LEADERSHIP

Ethics and Leadership

Leadership has a moral, or ethical, dimension. As you will learn, ethics examines whether an action is right or wrong. Whether leaders ethically base their decision making on possible consequences or on whether an action is right or wrong no matter what the cost may be, they must be able to accurately assess a situation (Johnson, 2005). Leaders can face many ethical challenges. For instance, the leader may need to decide if staff have a right to know that a patient is HIV-positive or has a contagious disease. Northouse (2004) names five principles of ethical leadership: serving others, showing justice, respecting others, honesty, and building community.

Leaders have the ethical responsibility to treat followers with dignity and respect and to be sensitive to their interests, needs, and concerns. Because of the influence that the leader has on followers, as well as the need to accomplish mutual goals and establish organizational values, ethics is central to effective leadership (Northouse, 2004). Advocacy roles and accountability to the profession increase the likelihood that nurse managers, leaders, and followers will be faced with an ethical issue

(Yoder-Wise, 2015). The complex interactions in organizations, generational differences, cultural differences, and differences in values and beliefs require that the professional RN understand the role of ethics in health care.

Culture and Leadership

Cultural competence extends not only to the recipients of health care but also to the workplace. The professional RN must understand how **culture** influences working relationships. Some examples of cultural diversity include values, beliefs, customs, practices, race, nationality, religious affiliation, language, physical size, gender, sexual orientation, age, and disability (Campinha-Bacote, 2003). One of the most difficult cultural differences to overcome in the workplace is generational. Nurses are likely to work with individuals from four generations: the Veteran generation, the Baby Boom generation, Generation X, and the Millennial generation.

See Chapter 9 for a detailed discussion of the impact of generational differences in communication. Generational differences may make some parts of the leadership role, such as delegation, more challenging.

DELEGATION

Delegation is the process of assigning tasks or duties to an entrusted individual. Marquis and Huston (2015) define *delegation* as "getting work done through others or as directing the performance of one or more people to accomplish organizational goals" (p. 330). Appropriate delegation requires the RN to base judgments on who is most qualified for the job. An RN does not inherently know, but must learn, the job descriptions or the state board limitations on the LPN/LVN or the state regulations of unlicensed personnel. The LPN/LVN or health care aide is then an assumed representative of the RN, acting under the authority of the RN. The LPN/LVN or health care aide is expected to report to the RN the results of the intervention as well as the patient's response.

As an RN, your supervisory and accountability responsibilities will increase. In your work as an LPN/LVN, you have undoubtedly delegated tasks to nursing assistants or unlicensed assistive personnel (UAP). In your new role as an RN, you will be required to delegate to LPN/LVNs as well.

Principles of Delegation

Chapter 9 of this text provides additional information regarding delegation where communication with co-workers is concerned. The NCSBN, in 2015 created the National Guidelines for Nursing Delgation, found here, https://www.ncsbn.org/NCSBN_Delegat ion_Guidelines.pdf. These guidelines identify the difference between and an assignment and delegation and also the associated "responsibilities of the employer, nurse leader, delegating nurse, and delegatee..." (p. 5). See Fig. 14.1. Below are the responsibilities of the licensed nurse regarding delagating nursing activities:

- The licensed nurse must determine when and what to delegate based on the practice setting, the patients' needs and condition, the state/jurisdiction's provisions for delegation, and the employer policies and procedures regarding delegating a specific responsibility (NCSBN, 2016, p. 10).

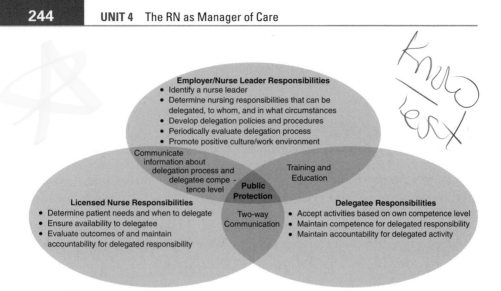

FIG. 14.1 From National Council of State Boards of Nursing (2016): National guidelines for nursing delegation. Journal of Nursing Regulation 7(1), 5-14.

- The licensed nurse must communicate with the delegatee who will be assisting in providing patient care (NCBSN, 2016, p. 10).
- The licensed nurse must be available to the delegatee for guidance and questions, including assisting with the delegated responsibility, if necessary, or performing it him/herself if the patient's condition or other circumstances warrant doing so, (NCSBN, 2016, p. 10).
- The licensed nurse must follow up with the delegatee and the patient after the delegated responsibility has been completed (NCSBN, 2016, p. 11).
- The licensed nurse must provide feedback information about the delegation process and any issues regarding delegatee competence level to the nurse leader (NCSBN, 2016, p. 11).

Employer/Nurse Leader Responsibilities regarding delegation include:
- The employer must identify a nurse leader responsible for oversight of delegated responsibilities for the facility (NCSBN, 2016, p. 9).
- The designated nurse leader responsible for delegation, ideally with a committee (consisting of other nurse leaders) formed for the purposes of addressing delegation, must determine which nursing responsibilities may be delegated, to whom, and under what circumstances (NCSBN, 2016, p. 9).
- Policies and procedures for delegation must be developed (NCSBN, 2016, p. 9).
- The employer/nurse leader must communicate information about delegation to the licensed nurses and UAP and educate them about what responsibilities can be delegated (NCSBN, 2016, p. 9).
- All delegatees must demonstrate knowledge and competency on how to perform a delegated responsibility (NCSBN, 2016, p. 9).
- The nurse leader responsible for delegation, along with other nurse leaders and administrators within the facility, must periodically evaluate the delegation process (NCSBN, 2016, p. 10).
- The employer/nurse leader must promote a positive culture and work environment for delegation (NCSBN, 2016, p. 10).

Delegatee responsibilities regarding delegation include:

- The delegatee must accept only the delegated responsibilities that he or she is appropriately trained and educated to perform and feels comfortable doing given the specific circumstances in the health care setting and patient's condition (NCSBN, 2016, p. 11).
- The delegatee must maintain competency for the delegated responsibility (NCSBN, 2016, p. 11).
- The delegatee must communicate with the licensed nurse in charge of the patient (NCSBN, 2016, p. 11).
- Once the delegatee verifies acceptance of the delegated responsibility, the delegatee is accountable for carrying out the delegated responsibility correctly and completing timely and accurate documentation per facility policy (NCSBN, 2016, p. 11).

When delegating tasks, interventions, and duties to other team members, the RN must always maintain patient safety. The RN must therefore understand the *scopes of practice* of the LPN/LVNs, health care aides, therapists, and other providers on the health care team, in addition to their knowledge and skill levels.

The RN must respect each team member and be respected by them for delegation to be effective. The RN will build trust and be appreciated because of consistent, appropriate delegation; encouragement; and compassionate understanding of each team member. Take, for example, the RN who appears to consistently make patient assignments to minimize his or her own workload. When others are working hard to get through the day, this RN does not offer support or assistance but rather is seen to be spending time doing comparatively very little. In contrast, consider the RN who both delegates difficult assignments to appropriate individuals and has an equally difficult assignment or is available to assist the other team members. This RN will be a highly regarded team leader, gain more cooperation from the others, and experience greater patient satisfaction and positive patient outcomes.

Issues Related to Delegation

Delegating fairly does not mean delegating equally. The leader bases assignments on individual capability, which means the experienced RN's assignment may be challenging and the inexperienced RN's relatively less challenging. Every member of the team should understand the role, capacity, and responsibility of every other member. As the experience level of the team members equalizes, so too will the assignments. The lead RN may have difficulty communicating apparent assignment disparities to all the team members involved. If the RN shows understanding of this while helping the others recognize the differences between them, this may facilitate cooperation. However, the RN must be alert to a potential for conflict and use the skills presented in the following section to head off or resolve conflict.

The three elements of nursing that may not be delegated are the initial and subsequent nursing assessments that require professional judgment; the determination of nursing diagnoses, goals, plans of care, and progress; and interventions that require the application of professional knowledge and skills. Even if organizational protocols permit staff to perform a task for the RN, that employee must be competent to perform the task (Yoder-Wise, 2015; ANA & NCSBN, 2006). This requires that the RN be diligent in assessing performance and be able to identify learning needs, as well as provide the education necessary for the UAP to perform safely. Yoder-Wise (2015) states that delegation is a matter of trust and that providing deadlines and avoiding the tendency to over supervise will reduce the likelihood that the delegatee loses confidence or becomes frustrated.

Subordinates may resist delegation for a number of reasons, such as being overwhelmed, a lack of self-confidence, resistance to authority, or overdelegation of routine tasks (Marquis & Huston, 2015). Dealing with this type of problem requires that the RN first assess the reason for the resistance or refusal to perform a specific task and then take appropriate action to remedy the situation. For example, the UAP may lack the knowledge and skills to perform a task or may have a physical or psychological condition that makes it difficult to perform a task. The UAP may be bored, anxious, or upset, and the RN must investigate. Most state boards of nursing provide a decision-making tree for the appropriate delegation of tasks, and you are encouraged to make yourself familiar with it. Figure 9-1 in Chapter 9 is the diagram created by the ANA and NCSBN in their Joint Statement on Delegation to help you make appropriate delegation decisions. Consult your state board of nursing for the Decision Tree that governs your practice specifically. *Remember that if the patient has not been assessed by an RN, delegation should not occur* (Yoder-Wise, 2015). If you find it difficult to delegate to others, you must ask yourself why and then work hard to overcome those barriers. Collaboration is inherent in delegation, and both concepts and practices must be integrated to achieve successful outcomes.

COLLABORATING IN PROVIDING CARE

Collaboration

Collaboration is a partnership arrangement between two or more individuals where there is mutual agreement to work together. Each partner brings to the group unique talents and skills, which will be used to create the best possible outcome or to meet specific goals. The RN, recognizing that the health care team is made up of unique individuals, takes into account the many resources available, such as these specific skills and knowledge, when designing the plan of care.

Collaborative health care provides better patient outcomes, but in order for a team to collaborate successfully, several conditions must be present. The health care team must agree on the plan of care and the prioritization of the components of the plan. There must be excellent communication among the team members regarding all aspects of care, changes in condition, and updates to the plan of care. There must be mutual recognition and respect for all of the varying knowledge, experiences, skills, and abilities within the health care team. In addition to delegation, other concepts related to the collaborator of care role are accountability, advocacy, and respect for self and for other health care workers.

Accountability

The RN is accountable for patient outcomes as they apply to the plans of care for the patients. When delegating responsibilities to the team members or collaborating with other departments to extend care, the RN must evaluate the effectiveness of the plan of care. **Accountability** means the RN must ensure that the medical and nursing plan of care are implemented, evaluated, and possibly modified so that the patient outcomes are the best they possibly can be.

For example, based on what you have just learned about delegation, consider that the RN is accountable for delegating appropriately. If the RN knowingly delegates an assignment beyond someone's qualifications or scope of practice, then the RN assumes responsibility for any negative consequences. For example, an RN gives a medication to a health care aide with instructions to make sure the patient takes it. The health care aide, not instructed in the Five Rights, fails to identify the patient correctly, which results in giving the medication to the wrong patient, who is harmed as a result. The coordinating RN has clearly failed to follow standards of practice as well as policies and the Nurse Practice Act. The RN should be reprimanded and risks sanctions from the board of nursing.

Many situations regarding delegation and accountability are not completely clear, yet the RN must be aware of conditions, however subtle, that will place patients at risk. For example, the RN delegates a patient's dressing change to an LPN/LVN who has learned sterile technique and can do dressing changes. The patient develops a wound infection, however. If the RN had not adequately assessed the wound, only relying on the LPN/LVN's assessment, and knew the patient was at risk for developing an infection, then the RN failed to render safe care, neglecting a fundamental duty to the patient.

Job descriptions, policies, procedures, and licensure dictate the roles and responsibilities of each member of the team. The RN is not accountable for the LPN/LVN or health care aide who willfully neglects a patient or steps over the bounds of legal limitations. Whoever is acting in a reckless or neglectful manner is responsible. For example, the LPN/LVN who makes a medication error is responsible for the error, unless the error was made in collaboration with the RN. In any case, the RN would be accountable for taking steps to minimize the effects of the negligence, document the incident, and appropriately communicate the incident per hospital policy and procedure as well as board of nursing guidelines.

Professional Advocacy

A central role in nursing is **advocacy.** Yoder-Wise (2015, p. 241) describes an advocate as one who:
- Defends or promotes the rights of others
- Changes systems to meet the needs of others
- Empowers and promotes self-determination in others
- Promotes autonomy of diverse cultures and social groups
- Ensures respect, equality, and dignity for others
- Cares for the humanness of all

Advocacy occurs when one individual promotes someone else or someone else's idea. As a patient advocate, the RN promotes the patient's decisions in a nonjudgmental manner. By being involved in the plan of care, the patient is informed and can express feelings and preferences. Additionally, the RN should know what the physician tells the patient with regard to the condition and treatment plan. If possible, the RN should make rounds with the physician to be available to take orders and understand the medical plan of care. If the RN is not able to make rounds with the physician, then the RN must assess the patient's level of understanding the physician. Clarification of the medical plan of care can then be given if necessary. The RN can help write down questions for the patient to refer to when the physician comes by again. If the patient is unable to articulate his or her own needs, then the RN reports the wishes or questions to the physician.

The RN is responsible for assessing the patient's understanding of the plan of care and ensuring that the patient has all the information needed to make informed decisions. An informed patient is empowered to make choices that best meet his or her needs. The RN must be certain that the patient understands the implications of every decision. Furthermore, the RN is in a better position to advocate for the patient who understands the plan of care.

The RN must be a caring individual to be a patient advocate. **Caring** implies that the RN has a commitment to preserving the patient's humanity, personal worth, and dignity. The patient's humanity is the part that makes him or her unique. It is a mixture of culture, beliefs, spirituality, thoughts, and feelings. The patient who has an acute, chronic, or terminal illness is facing many challenges. The RN demonstrates a caring nature through actions and words that encourages the patient toward holistic wellness. This means that the RN takes an interest in the patient's concerns, establishes dialogue for understanding, and develops a plan of care to meet these needs. Caring means the RN accepts responsibility for providing the best possible care.

These same principles of advocacy apply to leaders, managers, and followers, who must create a safe environment where employees feel valued and appreciated and where concerns, needs, and dilemmas can be openly discussed. Even though a nurse may be seen as a troublemaker, it does not excuse inaction (Marquis & Huston, 2015). The ANA *Code of Ethics for Nurses* (2015) states that acquiescing to and accepting unsafe or inappropriate practices, even if the individual does not participate in the specific practice, are the same as condoning unsafe practices.

Nurses must speak up concerning unsafe conditions because patient safety is paramount. Professional advocacy also includes advocating for the public and the nursing profession through involvement with professional organizations and becoming active in legal issues concerning health care policy. More information related to advocacy, policy statements, and political issues can be found on the ANA website.

Finally, advocacy extends to the self. Understaffing and mandatory overtime, for instance, may not only lead to compromised patient safety, increased errors, and patient harm, but it is also likely to result in physical and emotional burnout for the nurse.

Collaborating and Advocating Through the Medical Plan of Care

Part of the RN role of advocating for the patient is directing the medical plan of care, but the physician is the manager of the medical plan of care. Medical management of patient care is influenced by an increasing amount of state and federal regulations that restrict payments and limit the number of reimbursable hospital days. For example, physicians must manage care within diagnosis related group (DRG) designations that set the amount of payment for each medical diagnosis and procedure.

The physician, as the medical manager of care, trusts that the plan is implemented in an efficient and effective manner. The RN must anticipate the medical direction, understand the orders written, and foresee how they will affect the patient and patient care. Understanding how a patient responds to the illness as well as to the treatment plan is essential to designing an individualized plan of care. It will also ensure that diagnostic procedures, medications, and treatments ordered by the physician are carried out efficiently and safely. The RN is acting as a patient advocate when making sure that the physician's orders are carried out in a timely fashion. The RN must not cause a delay in diagnosis or treatment based on an incorrect schedule. Equally important is to ensure that the patient's response to one treatment or diagnostic test will not interfere with recovery. Recognizing the adverse effects that may occur at certain times, the RN can take measures to minimize or eliminate them.

More than one physician may be managing different medical problems for one patient. The RN must understand each of these roles and be able to communicate information to whichever physician has a need for it, averting time delays and minimizing physician frustration. Delays in care could place the patient in a compromised position, extend patient care days, and potentially cause harm.

When making a phone call to a physician about a change in patient status, the RN needs to anticipate all the data and information the physician will require to make a decision regarding the medical plan of care. Organizing the data and reporting them in a coherent manner are key to establishing a professional relationship with the physician, not to mention speeding the healing process and positively affecting patient outcomes.

All aspects of patient care require the RN to know how to communicate key information. In collaborative practice the RN is aware of the requirements of each department. Being well organized is important when requesting information, ordering treatments, and communicating with various health care agencies (Exercise 14.1).

The RN must understand the complexities of patient care management in order to advocate for the patient. The RN, either directly or by delegation, must communicate with the physician regarding changes in patient status and priority of care. To advocate in this way, the RN helps the patient receive the best care at the appropriate level and for the least cost. Effective communication includes knowing who is in control of patient discharge or transfer. Generally, the admitting physician is the doctor of record and the one to write discharge orders or to be consulted for transfers. If the patient's problems are related to or compromise the system being managed by the specialist, then this physician will determine the need and write the orders for the change in patient care.

In execution of physician orders, the RN must take into account policies and procedures as well as standing or unit-specific orders. A physician may order medications or treatments that are experimental or not FDA approved for the specific medical disorder of the patient. The RN must be aware of when medications or treatments are

---

? EXERCISE 14.1

A patient with end-stage renal disease is being admitted for complications from an imbalance in fluid and electrolytes. The outcome priority is _____, which includes correcting the fluid overload and electrolyte disturbances. The admitting physician, the patient's nephrologist, has called in an endocrinologist to manage the patient's type 2 diabetes and an internal medicine physician to rule out a potential stress-related peptic ulcer. The following are the admission orders:

- Chem. 12 and ABGs to be drawn now
- Flat plate abdomen and chest x-ray
- Blood cultures
- NG to intermittent suction

The patient has 200 mL of dark red secretions, testing positive for blood, from the NG tube within the first hour. The patient complains of thirst, and the glucometer reading is 260.

1. When the results come back, who will need to have the information?
2. What other questions need to be answered before calling one or both of the physicians?

---

being used for anything other than the labeled, intended use. Being a patient advocate means the RN must protect the patient's right to be fully informed. Experimental treatments must have a protocol, and the patient must give informed consent before being included in the treatment plan.

The RN promotes each member of the health care team through understanding and respecting his or her role and seeking his or her expertise. This widens the RN's pool of resources. The RN can call upon a respiratory therapist with questions regarding the patient's breathing problems and then include the recommended interventions in the plan of care. Working in collaboration with the medical lab, the RN will coordinate the timing of blood draws based on medication, electrolytes, or IV solution.

DECISION MAKING AND PROBLEM SOLVING

Decision making and problem solving are closely related and use a similar process to arrive at a decision. **Problem solving** involves making a decision that is focused on trying to solve an immediate problem. **Decision making** is a purposeful and goal-directed process aimed at identifying and selecting options as part of problem solving, planned change, or improvement. Yoder-Wise (2015) identifies a step-by-step decision-making process: defining objectives, identifying options, identifying the advantages and disadvantages of each option, selecting an option, implementing the option, and evaluating the result.

Decision making can be complicated by ethical and legal issues because values have a tremendous impact on decision making. There are many different decision-making and problem-solving models. Using a model increases the probability that a sound decision will be made (Marquis & Huston, 2015). Poorly identified objectives are likely to lead to poor-quality decisions (Yoder-Wise, 2015). Decision making is influenced by personal values, life experiences, individual preferences, and individual ways of thinking and decision making (Marquis & Huston, 2015). Yoder-Wise (2015) suggests the following steps for effective decision making and problem solving:

- Gather data from many sources.
- Learn different approaches to problem situations.
- Observe positive role models in action.
- Talk to a colleague or superior who is an effective problem solver and decision maker.
- Perform research to increase your knowledge base.
- Take risks using new approaches to problem solving.

CONFLICT MANAGEMENT

Conflict is an opposition of feelings, beliefs, desires, or goals. Conflict is generally considered to be a negative occurrence or state, but in reality it is neutral because either positive or negative outcomes can result. Conflict can be intrapersonal, within one individual; interpersonal, between two or more individuals; intragroup, within one group; or intergroup, between two or more groups (Marquis & Huston, 2015; Smith, 1992; Sullivan & Decker, 1988). The individual and group responses to conflict may create problems within the workplace. A conflict has a preceding causative event that sets up a perceived or felt antagonism. Conflict within the health care workplace becomes a source of discord when a disruption occurs in patient care activities. Examples of possible causative events are staffing mixes, ethical decisions, and punitive measures. Perceived differences in care management, patient load responsibility, and personality differences can also be sources of conflict between the RN coordinator of patient care and others on the care team. Lack of mutual respect between the RN and the others may result from unresolved conflict.

Interpersonal conflict, or conflict between two or more people, may need a more immediate approach to resolution because it may result in compromised patient care. The first steps are for the RN to recognize that those involved each have points of view worth considering, think through each point of view in a logical manner, and ask the parties to assist in helping to clarify the issues. An assertive, logical, and reasoned approach is necessary for assessing the situation. The RN must not act with emotion but always stay focused on the facts of the issue or, more important, on the potential consequences for patient safety if resolution were not to occur. The RN must also articulate his or her own point of view as team leader in an equally clear and rational manner.

The RN may need to be autocratic if the situation is critical and the behavior of one of the parties is impeding timely resolution of a patient problem. In a less critical situation, the RN may have more time for a more collaborative approach. A win-win situation can occur if the RN is willing to work toward common goals and objectives rather than just putting forth his or her own agenda. Exercise 14.2 illustrates an interpersonal conflict situation between an RN and an aide.

Any discussion regarding conflict should be done in an area that gives as much privacy as possible, especially away from patient care areas where patients or families may overhear the discussion. The key focus must be on patient care and patient safety. Both parties must be willing to talk calmly and rationally. If the other party is angry and out of control, then you must stop the discussion. You can then explain

? EXERCISE 14.2

A new RN on a busy medical–surgical unit is attempting to direct a patient care aide who is being argumentative and disruptive with regard to her patient care assignment. The health care aide has refused to assist a patient with ambulating, complaining that RNs have learned to ambulate patients, and he should do it, not her. The RN needs the aide to complete vital signs on a new surgical patient each hour over the next 3 hours, as well as ambulate a patient who is 2 days postoperation. The following conversation takes place between the RN and the health care aide in the break room:

RN: "You have stated that you refuse to ambulate the patient in room 769. Help me understand your reason for refusal."

Health care aide: "You're new to this floor. What gives you the authority to tell me what I'm supposed to do? You've been taught how to walk a patient. I think you should walk him."

RN: "How is my role different from that of the other RNs?"

Health care aide: "You need to know your place on this floor. I have more experience than you. I know my job, and I do it well. You don't need to tell me what to do."

1. What is the health care aide's main issue?
2. What is the best way for the RN to proceed with resolving this conflict?
3. What is the priority of care that the RN should remember in dealing with this conflict?

✦ FYI 14.1   STEPS TO COLLABORATIVE CONFLICT RESOLUTION

1. Open a dialogue that brings forth and is respectful of each individual's point of view.
2. Determine a group or shared goal.
3. Identify the expertise and contribution of each individual as the group agrees on the shared goal.
4. Review the goal and move to honestly accept or reject it (acceptance requires the consensus of the group).
5. Design a plan to meet the new goal, using the expertise of the group to design interventions to meet the goal.
6. Determine the roles of the members in carrying out the interventions. A role must be within the capacity of the member and mutually accepted as fairly defined.
7. Set an evaluation point and include all individuals in the evaluation process. Maintain respect for everyone's input or contribution, and focus on interventions and actions rather than personalities, feelings, or prejudices.

that you will take up the discussion at a later time. If and when you cannot resolve a conflict, you must know when to stop and recruit a manager to assist.

Conflict management is a challenging skill that the RN must master in order to lead a team in the role of manager of care (FYI 14.1). You can learn and practice basic principles of conflict management, such as sacrifice resolution, competition resolution, and win-win resolution.

Sacrifice Resolution

When two people compromise to resolve conflict, they both give up their positions. Neither gets exactly what he or she wants, but both are able to live with the decision. Conversely, in **sacrifice resolution** one may strongly want to avoid or end the conflict and will therefore accommodate the other by essentially sacrificing his or her position, thus allowing the other to have his or her way. The one who continually sacrifices in order to accommodate others may build up resentment that could eventually surface inappropriately.

Competition Resolution

Competition resolution is another form of conflict resolution in which one or both of the parties work competitively, instead of cooperatively, toward resolution. The problem with resolving conflicts in this manner is that one side wins and the other loses. The obvious result is resentment or jealousy on the part of the individual who lost. An example of this type of conflict resolution is when a unit manager posts a memo regarding holiday or vacation schedule requests. If clear rules are not in place that direct a fair distribution of days off among the staff members, certain individuals may view this as an opportunity to "win" their preferred days off at the expense of others. A policy of "first come, first served" would be unfair in this situation. In that case, staff members working the shift when the schedule comes out would be in a better position to request days off before others who are not there. This practice of competitive conflict resolution pits staff members against one another and creates resentment toward the manager, as well as toward the individuals who take advantage of it.

Win-Win Resolution

Setting up a **win-win resolution** requires a collaborative method of conflict resolution (Marquis & Houston, 2015). The two opposing parties come together to decide on mutual goals, design interventions to meet these goals, and work together to evaluate the outcomes. Because the parties agree on how to deal with the situation, all parties involved have a sense of ownership and will generally work together to achieve the best outcome for all. Engaging in collaborative steps to resolve conflict may assist the RN in managing conflicts that threaten to derail the team and ultimately impede patient care. If the example in the previous section were handled with win-win resolution, the manager might post the memo with a deadline for sign-up and then hold a staff meeting to discuss it.

KEY POINTS

After completion of this chapter, you have learned:
- Being a manager of care is a crucial role for the RN. The patient and the entire health care team have come to rely on the RN for direction and management of minute-to-minute patient care.
- The manager of care role requires the RN to be a leader with knowledge of the health care team's strengths and weaknesses. The strong leader uses this knowledge

to empower the health care team to meet the complex and unique needs of each patient. There are different styles and approaches to leadership.

- Leaders must adhere to ethics and take into consideration cultural differences.
- Emotional Intelligence is a strong leadership quality.
- Delegation is a critical nursing role with principles for its application to practice.
- Collaboration with other health care professionals in carrying out the plan of care is essential, and the nurse is ultimately responsible for coordinating all aspects of patient care within and between the various disciplines.
- Conflict is inevitable for the manager of care, but the RN can use certain tools to find the optimal resolution.

CRITICAL THINKING QUESTIONS

1. As an RN on a medical–surgical unit, you have a care team that includes two LPN/LVNs and a patient care aide. One of the LPN/LVNs is a 12-year veteran with IV certification and training to do unit-specific IV pushes. The second LPN/ LVN has just 2 months of experience, is not IV certified, and has been known to need assistance with complex dressing changes as well as with organizing her day. The patient care aide has 10 years of experience and has had advanced aid training, including urinary catheter insertion, simple enemas, and advanced skin care. Assignments and duties for the day include an I&O catheter, an antibiotic IV push, a complex dressing change, a prep for a barium enema, small and large bowel tests, a surgical skin prep, and a patient who will need close supervision due to confusion.
   a. What are the safest and most effective patient assignments for each of the team members?
   b. Describe the way you would delegate care for a new admission to each of the health care workers.
2. An RN must decide not only when to call a physician but what information the physician will need to know. A patient with a history of chronic airway insufficiency has been given a diuretic for fluid retention and slight pulmonary edema. A serum potassium level of 3.2 came back after the diuretic was given.
   a. What assessment must be done before notifying the physician?
   b. What information must be included when the physician is called regarding the potassium level?
3. Patient assignments have been made when you overhear an RN state, "I can't believe it! The third day in a row I got this assignment. What does she think she is doing? I get all of the hard assignments, and that Jenny gets all of the easy assignments. Just 2 months out of nursing school, and she gets preferential treatment."
   a. How would you respond to this apparent conflict?
   b. What may be the basis for the apparent discrepancy in assignments?
   c. What information do you need to resolve this conflict?

CASE STUDY 1

Sam is a new nurse working the day shift on a busy medical–surgical unit. He asks his aide to walk the patient in Room 244 while he admits another patient. The patient in Room 244 is postangioplasty, and it would be the first time he has ambulated since the procedure. Sam tells his aide to walk the patient only to the nurse's station and back. He also says that if the patient's heart rate rises more than 20 beats/min above the resting rate, the aide should stop, have the patient sit, and inform Sam immediately.

A. Did Sam appropriately delegate in this scenario? If not, which of the rights of delegation was not followed? Why?

B. The aide misunderstands Sam's instructions and instead ambulates the patient in Room 234, who is 3 days post-hysterectomy and has been walking in the halls for 2 days. Where did the breakdown in communication occur?

C. Who would be accountable for the outcomes if the patient in Room 234 had fallen and broken a hip during ambulation? Would it be Sam, who directed the aide to ambulate the patient in Room 244, or the aide, who actually ambulated the patient in Room 234?

CASE STUDY 2

Kim is a student nurse in her final medical–surgical rotation. Her patient has a new left forearm arteriovenous graft for dialysis. As part of her clinical assignment, Kim must select a task that could be delegated regarding the care of her patient. The instructor also requires Kim to include how she would communicate, supervise, and provide feedback to a nursing assistant. Kim describes how she could delegate taking the vital signs to the nursing assistant. She states that she would ask if the assistant had ever taken vital signs before, ask her to demonstrate the task, clearly state how often the vital signs needed to be completed as well as parameters for the vital signs, and provide feedback on the performance.

The instructor says that she is pleased with Kim's thoroughness and allows her to delegate the vital signs to the nursing assistant, Juanita, who accepts the task. After 3 hours, Kim notes the patient's graft arm has decreased pulses and is cool to the touch. She asks Juanita if she noted the same findings. The assistant responds, "I thought it was strange that you asked me to check her blood pressure on her left arm, but I figured you knew what you were doing and had checked it with your instructor."

A. What went wrong in this scenario?

B. How were the five rights applied to this scenario?

C. Who retains accountability for the outcome? Why?

CASE STUDY 3

John is a new nurse, still in orientation with a preceptor, on the intermediate care unit. These patients are currently on the unit:

- 230—A 48-year-old admitted yesterday evening with an acute myocardial infarction; waiting for an angiogram
- 231—A 72-year-old patient with chronic congestive heart failure; taking multiple medications for blood pressure
- 232—A 51-year-old patient who had a coronary artery bypass graft 3 days ago; waiting for discharge

Continued

CASE STUDY 3—cont'd

- 233—A 54-year-old patient in the ED with a medical diagnosis of uncontrolled atrial fibrillation; waiting for admitting orders

John is caring for the patients under the supervision of Dana, his preceptor, who is also the day shift charge nurse. He has completed the first assessment and is looking at the medications for his patients. He notes multiple medications ordered for bed 231, new medications ordered for bed 230, and medication teaching needed for bed 232. As he makes the notations to himself, Dana gives him the abnormal lab values for the patients, with instructions to notify the attending physicians. She also reminds him of the admit waiting in ED. The nursing assistant points out that the patient in 232 is very impatient; he is waiting for his diet and medication instructions so that he can be discharged. At this point, John becomes frustrated trying to juggle all the demands on his time.

A. Identify the resources available to John regarding available personnel to whom he might delegate tasks.
B. Of those individuals identified as resources, which tasks could be delegated to each person?
C. Write at least one appropriate outcome for each patient and identify the right person to assist John in achieving the outcomes. Describe how John would evaluate the outcome.
D. Which of the patients can John delegate assessment to a licensed practical nurse?
E. When in doubt about delegating to other health care professionals, where would you find information about which actions you can delegate and to whom?
F. Construct a case scenario that demonstrates how John would correctly implement the five rights of delegation based on one of the answers listed.

CASE STUDY 4

You are the nurse caring for a postoperative appendectomy patient who had surgery 6 hours ago. The following tasks need completing:
- Assess the patient's ability to drink clear liquids.
- Determine the amount eaten.
- Document the patient's tolerance of clear liquids.
- Assess the patient's tolerance for sitting at the side of the bed.
- Assess the patient's tolerance for ambulating.
- Document the patient's tolerance for activity.
- Assess the patient's pain level.
- Provide education about activity levels.
  A. Which of the tasks can be delegated, and to whom can they be delegated?
  B. If the patient were 2 days postoperative, would this change how you delegate?
  C. To whom could the tasks be delegated if your co-workers included the following: licensed practical nurse, medication aide, and nursing assistant?
  D. Select one of the tasks and describe how you would delegate to an appropriate person by using the five rights. Specify how you would meet each of the rights.
  E. Select one of the tasks and develop an outcome. How would you evaluate the ability of the patient to achieve the outcome if the task was delegated to the appropriate person?

WEB RESOURCES

NCSBN: Delegation https://www.ncsbn.org/1625.htm
NCSBM and ANA Joint Statement on Delegation https://www.ncsbn.org/Delegation
_joint_statement_NCSBN-ANA.pdf
http://ncbi.nlm.nih.gov/pubmed/16787469
http://managementhelp.org/intrpsnl/basics.htm
http://foundationcoalition.org/publications/brochures/conflict.pdf

REFERENCES

American Nurses Association (ANA). (2015). *Guide to the code of ethics for nurses: inter-pretation and application.* Silver Spring, MD: Author.

American Nurses Association (ANA) & the National Council of State Boards of Nursing (NCSBN). (2006). *Joint statement on delegation.* Retrieved from https://ncsbn.org/Joint_statement.pdf.

Campinha-Bacote, J. C. (2003). Many faces: addressing diversity in health care. *Online Journal of Issues in Nursing, 8*(1). Retrieved from http://nursingworld.org.

Curtain, L. (2013). Quantum leadership: upside down. *American Nurse Today, 8*(3). Retrieved from https://www.americannursetoday.com/quantum-leadership-upside-down/.

Johnson, C. (2005). *Meeting the ethical challenges of leadership: casting light or shadow* (2nd ed.). Thousand Oaks, CA: Sage Publications.

Laschinger, H. K., Wong, C., McMahon, L., & Kaufmann, C. (1999). Leadership behavior impact on staff nurse empowerment, job tension, and work effectiveness. *Journal of Nursing Administration, 29*(5), 28–39.

Marquis, B. L., & Huston, C. J. (2015). *Leadership roles and management functions in nursing: theory and application* (8th ed.). Philadelphia, PA: Lippincott.

McGuire, E., & Kennerly, S. M. (2006). Nurse managers as transformational and transactional leaders. *Nurse Economics, 24*(4), 179–185.

Morrison, R. S., Jones, L., & Fuller, B. (1997). The relation between leadership style and empowerment on job satisfaction of nurses. *Journal of Nursing Administration, 27*(5), 27–34.

National Council of State Boards of Nursing (NCSBN), (2016). National guidelines for nursing delegation. Journal of Nursing Regulation, 7(6), 5–14. Retrieved from https://www.ncsbn.org/NCSBN_Delegation_Guidelines.pdf.

Northouse, P. G. (2004). *Leadership theory and practice.* Thousand Oaks, CA: Sage Publications.

Perra, B. M. (1999). The leader in you. *Nursing Management, 30*(1), 35–39.

Porter-O'Grady, T. (2003). A different age for leadership, part 1. *Journal of Nursing Administration, 33*(2), 105–110. Retrieved from Academic Research Premier.

Porter-O'Grady, T., & Mallach, K. (2015). *Quantum leadership: building better partnerships for sustainable health* (4th ed.). Burlington, MA: Jones & Bartlett Learning.

Smith, S. (1992). *Communications in nursing: communicating assertively and responsibly in nursing: a guidebook.* St. Louis, MO: Mosby.

Sullivan, E. J., & Decker, P. J. (1988). *Effective management in nursing* (2nd ed.). Menlo Park, CA: Addison-Wesley.

Trofino, J. (1995). Transformational leadership in health care. *Nursing Management, 26*(8), 42–47.

Yoder-Wise, P. (2015). *Leading and managing in nursing* (6th ed.). St. Louis, MO: Elsevier.

CHAPTER

15

Promoting Healthful Living in the Primary Care Setting

*e*volve WEBSITE

Additional resources are available online at:
http://evolve.elsevier.com/Claywell/transitions

OBJECTIVES

After completing this chapter, the student will be prepared to:
1. Define the health-illness continuum.
2. Describe the theoretical basis of self-care.
3. Analyze the RN's role in health promotion.
4. Explain environmental influences on health promotion.

KEY TERMS

community health promotion	health promotion matrix	self-care deficit
developmental need	*Healthy People 2020*	self-care requisite
health-deviation need	physical environment	self-health promotion
health-illness continuum	primary health care	universal need
	self-care ability	

OVERVIEW

Primary health care establishes an environment conducive to a healthy lifestyle. Interventions that promote a healthy lifestyle include health screening, immunization, teaching, and role modeling (of a healthy lifestyle). To develop individualized plans of care based on health promotion, you must have an understanding of environmental factors that influence health promotion within society and with your individual patients.

This chapter addresses primary health care within a theoretical framework. Included are basic tools that will assist you in understanding your role in health

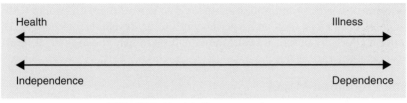

FIG. 15.1 Health-illness continuum.

promotion and a discussion of the relationship between your own health and the ability to affect your patients' self-health behaviors.

THEORETICAL FRAMEWORK

Every person moves along a **health-illness continuum,** between states of illness and wellness, throughout life, as well as between independence of and dependence on health care services (Fig. 15.1). During times of illness, a person seeks assistance from health care services. The initial level of need can be minimal to nearly complete dependence, but the patient will gain the knowledge and skills necessary to regain independence. **Primary health care** promotes independence and involves many interventions, with the goal of maintaining independent, healthy individuals in a community.

Self-Care

Orem (2001) believes that every individual has some **self-care ability,** which is the day-to-day personal care needed to function and develop. This ability is affected by several things, including but not limited to the individual's age, developmental stage, health, and environmental factors.

Orem states that the goal for all adults is to have the power and capability to care for themselves. Adults seek assistance when they have a **self-care deficit,** having needs that go beyond their resources to manage. They seek nursing care because of the specific knowledge nurses have and because of their ability to act in association with other health care professionals to assist the patient in regaining self-care ability. Health promotion deals with "what is known about (1) human structure and functioning and (2) specific diseases or interferences with the normal human condition" (p. 130). Orem assumes that the responsibility of primary health promotion is with the individual adult. Within the realm of health promotion, someone may seek a higher level of function or development, thus seeking out nurses who have special knowledge of ways to achieve this goal. Nurses are involved in health promotion when the following take place:

1. People are under the direct care of a nurse.
2. The nurse is engaging in practices that prevent or interrupt the disease process in the environment of the patient.
3. The nurse is guiding people toward health prevention methods.
4. The nurse is incorporating factual information about the patient into the plan of care.
5. The nurse is aware that the adult or responsible adult will be the primary person to carry out the plan of care.

In terms of health promotion, the nurse's role is working with people with generally good health but who are experiencing life or development changes. Health promotion efforts by nurses are educational efforts to help the individual remain an independent self-care agent.

Health Promotion Model

Pender and colleagues (2011) present a revised health promotion model that makes specific assertions with regard to health promotion. Key to the model is characteristics and experiences as influenced by the individual's perceptions, as well as the interpersonal and situational influences on health. Pender and colleagues (2011) do not state that a clear association exists between any one influence and the healthy behavior outcomes, including individual commitment to health-promoting behaviors. An example is the differences in two individuals' responses to a broken leg. One sees an opportunity to take time off from work, is challenged to figure out how to complete activities of daily living (ADLs), and is looking forward to catching up on reading. The other finds the experience to be limiting, gets angry when not able to do something easily or when needing help with ADLs, and gets bored not being able to go to work. The first person is easygoing, takes day-to-day challenges in stride, and has no problem seeking assistance when situations warrant. The second finds working pleasurable at the expense of recreation and has trouble delegating or seeking consultation from fellow workers or friends. Pender and colleagues (2011) infer that every factor has some degree of influence on healthy behaviors, and consideration of these will need to take place for the nurse to know how to assist these patients.

The nurse should engage in health protective behaviors as well as health promotion behaviors. Health protective behaviors take a person away from a dangerous situation or from a dangerous habit. Deciding not to smoke, not going near a burning building, and not crossing the street except at designated crosswalks all protect one's health. Health promotion behaviors move an individual to a higher level of health, greater vigor, or energy to do more than he or she is currently capable of doing.

HEALTH PROMOTION PRINCIPLES

Gorin and Arnold (1998) envision a **health promotion matrix** as a clinical tool for the RN. This model recognizes that the individual is surrounded and influenced by patient systems of family, group, and community. These systems can have a positive, supportive influence or a negative influence on the patient's health promotion. These systems formulate the patient's image and image processing of his or her health, health behaviors, and ability to seek help for them. Thus, a family of smokers and perhaps several peer smokers may influence an individual who is a smoker. Their perceptions or images of their health behavior and willingness to stop smoking may be strongly influenced by the systems. If family members do not support the cessation efforts of the individual, the attempt to successfully quit smoking will be compromised. Your role as an RN in this situation may be to gather other support systems, such as smoking cessation support groups, in order to optimize the individual's chances of cessation success.

Orem (2001) considers self-care as meeting one's own basic needs, including the self-care requisites of universal, developmental, and health-deviation needs. A **universal need** is an essential requirement for everyone: food, shelter, air, water, and other basic needs. A **developmental need,** such as trust, love, and belonging, changes as a person moves through each life-cycle period. A **health-deviation need** is based on an individual's genetic or constitutional deviations from normal.

Orem recognizes that to meet self-care requisites, a person must have knowledge of the self-care requisite need. A **self-care requisite** could be a universal need, an essential that everyone must have to sustain and nurture life. Such needs are basic to human life (food, water, rest, and so on) in addition to specific cultural, social, environmental, and enrichment requirements that the individual deems necessary for growth and development. Individuals also need a supportive environment, and they must be willing to engage in internal and external orientation activities that promote health. Thus, an individual may engage in a weight reduction program in which he or she may meet once a week with others to be supported in his or her effort (external orientation). This individual may also engage in reading self-help books to discover ways to rid himself or herself of negative feelings that promote the unhealthy eating habits (internal orientation). A person must also be willing and able to access available resources to meet the self-care requisite needs (FYI 15.1).

The importance of external and internal influences on a person's health promotion is evident, and we must assess these influences to begin the health promotion plan of care. A holistic assessment process takes into consideration all factors that assist in or inhibit meeting goals.

Health Promotion Plan of Care

A health promotion plan of care includes education and self-actualization exercises to help the individual seek a higher level of health. For example, someone may need to gain an understanding of why he or she is overweight before getting involved in a weight reduction program. The plan of care should allow the person time to come to terms with the basis of the weight problem. The comprehensive health care plan reflects all health concerns, rather than focusing on just weight reduction, so the RN in this case needs to assess for such weight-related problems as hypertension, hyperlipidemia, and diabetes as well. A holistic plan of care takes into account the total person and how all of his or her characteristics influence outcomes.

The priority of care for health promotion is to help a patient regain control over his or her health. The priority nursing diagnoses include *Health-seeking behaviors* or *Knowledge deficit.* Outcome criteria and the measurement of outcomes focus on the progress toward the primary goal of a higher level of health. The patient will need to be included in planning the care as a means to empowerment and compliance.

The RN's Role in Health Promotion

Besides designing individual plans of care, the RN can also be proactive in health promotion on a local or regional political level. One way to become politically involved is to provide expert testimony to governing bodies in an attempt to promote a more positive health environment. For example, a nurse can testify on the effects

FYI 15.1 SELF-CARE REQUISITES

To meet self-care requisites, the RN does the following:
- Identifies potential and actual social support systems
- Understands the patient's point of view
- Considers the developmental task
- Understands the patient's self-care abilities

Assessment

Assess individual or group:
1. Level of wellness
   a. What are the individual or group self-care abilities?
   b. What factors are interfering in the maintenance of a wellness state (e.g., smoking, high cholesterol level, poor sleep habits, stress)?
2. Readiness to change to a higher state of health
   a. What is the motivation to change?
   b. What will actually or potentially interfere with change?
   c. Is the environment suitable for learning?
3. Understanding self-care needs
   a. What cultural, spiritual, and social needs exist?
   b. What language and educational needs exist?
   c. What limitations of sight, hearing, or speech exist?
   d. What self-care limitations exist?
4. Understanding self-care knowledge
   a. What information does the individual or group have?
   b. What myths, assumptions, or inferences exist?
   c. What questions are being presented?
   d. What concerns are being voiced?

Outcome Identification

Voiced satisfaction of level of understanding, compliance with wellness plan of care, specific measurable criteria related to individualized plan of care (e.g., weight loss, cholesterol levels lowered, blood pressure under control)

Planning

Decide whether the following exist:
1. A knowledge deficit related to at-risk behaviors, noncompliance with healthy lifestyle
2. Health-seeking behavior related to new diagnosis/treatment and/or voicing of concerns with current treatment plan, voiced need to change life to a healthy lifestyle

Implementation

Support of self-care ability:
1. Provide education at an individual level of understanding, using a preferred learning style.
2. Assist the individual or group in setting a schedule or plan with clear, measurable goals.
3. Reinforce progress.
4. Help patient cope with disappointments or setbacks; be available for venting of frustrations.
5. Use support groups or individual counseling as a means to share difficulties and progress.
6. Provide information on classes or other avenues (e.g., the Internet) for further education.
7. Individualize tools for reminders if there is a need for scheduled events (e.g., handmade calendars, refrigerator magnet reminders, 7-day pill dispensers); be creative and incorporate the individual's suggestions.

Evaluation

Evaluate effectiveness:
1. Stick to set time frames for evaluating progress.
2. Use outcome criteria as a basis for evaluation.
3. Assess patient satisfaction for progress toward a higher level of wellness.

of environmental pollution on the health of a community or lobby through letters to representatives, advocating changes in legislation with regard to pollution. On a local level, the RN can offer services to church groups, parent-teacher associations, or neighborhood organizations as educators or by assisting with public awareness of problems identified within the community. As RNs, we recognize the importance of research as a way to identify cause-and-effect situations and support or provide interventions to make a change. If we actively engage in health promotion, we will be of value to the communities in which we live.

ENVIRONMENTAL INFLUENCES ON HEALTH PROMOTION

Everyone exists within an environment—the surroundings or conditions that exert an influence on, and affect the health of, a person. One's environment is made up of physical, cultural, spiritual, social, economic, and developmental components (FYI 15.2). The environment can be supportive of a healthy lifestyle, or it can be a source of stress. The RN must recognize the influence of the environment on people's health care abilities.

Physical

The **physical environment** is composed of tangible factors where the individual lives, from housing, furniture, and food to pollution, air, temperature, and bacteria. Physical factors have concrete characteristics that can be seen, felt, tasted, touched, or measured in some way.

The degree to which the physical environment influences the individual can generally be detected through direct measurement. For example, air pollution has been studied in relation to many respiratory conditions. Many research studies show that individuals with asthma have more acute attacks when higher pollen counts or high smog numbers are present. Community public health departments often lead such studies and will make recommendations or issue public announcements warning of the increased risks during periods of air-quality problems. Another example, with perhaps longer-term consequences, is the relationship between high levels of lead in public housing and the number of health problems suffered by children living in this environment.

Health promotion related to the physical environment begins with assessment of the characteristics of the environment that have been implicated as causing health

---

FYI 15.2 ENVIRONMENTS THAT INFLUENCE HEALTH PROMOTION

- Cultural
- Developmental
- Economic
- Physical
- Social
- Spiritual or religious

variations for the individual or the community. A plan of care is developed to minimize the negative influence of the physical environment (Exercise 15.1). Interventions focus on either avoidance of the environmental factors or modifying lifestyles to minimize their effects.

Patient satisfaction with modifications in lifestyle will be an important component in evaluating any plan of care that attempts to change behavior to minimize environmental influence. For example, an individual with great affection for pets may also be allergic to them. The obvious solution, avoiding pets, may not be an acceptable intervention. A creative approach will be needed to minimize the person's response to the allergens while including the pets in the life plan. The pet owner may still have an acceptable level of allergic response, which will be part of the individual's definition of health. The RN must accept such patient decisions, while promoting a healthier lifestyle.

Cultural, Spiritual, and Social

The cultural, spiritual, and social components of the environment play a major role in how an individual views health and illness. One's personal beliefs are generally formed as he or she grows up. As part of the community, the RN is in a position to understand how these individual beliefs can influence the general health of the community, as well as the health of the individual. By being able to evaluate these environmental influences, the nurse can begin to formulate a list of potential health risks and actual problems.

Cultural influences on health are most obviously observed in the form of dietary habits. For example, as a whole, Americans consume a higher degree of fat and empty calories in their diet than do other cultures. As a result, a large percentage of the United States' population develops negative health consequences, such as peripheral vascular disease, coronary artery disease, hypertension, obesity, and diabetes. Culture may have a more subtle influence on the way individuals seek health care. In some cultures, people are not encouraged to seek help. The RN should recognize cultural influences that will bias the health-seeking behaviors of individuals because this information will help define the needs of each person within a community.

Spiritual or religious support for health promotion may come from a person's perception of help from a higher power (Gorin & Arnold, 1998). Spiritual wellness comes from a person's connection to others and to the universe. Spiritual wellness involves developing an inner connection and harmony between yourself and the

---

💡 EXERCISE 15.1

An individual is diagnosed with asthmatic allergies, and cedar pollen has been identified as one of the allergic triggers for asthma events. In planning interventions, the nurse should know that airborne allergens are difficult to avoid.
1. How could the plan incorporate measures to minimize exposure to cedar pollen?
2. What interventions would not only minimize the effects of the allergens but also support the patient's need to remain independent?

wonder, majesty, and mystery of the universe. This may manifest itself in practices dictated by a religious body's beliefs that are geared to promote physical as well as spiritual health, such as prayer for health and rituals believed to be health promoting and life affirming. Activities that promote finding purpose and meaning in life help to promote spiritual wellness. Additionally, many spiritual practices, such as therapeutic touch, prayer, and spiritualism, are engaged in to regain health or restore spiritual well-being. Cues that a person is in need of spiritual care include emotional turmoil, anxiety, or fear. These may exhibit differently among different cultures, and thus it is important for the RN to actively assess for the need for spiritual intervention. Simply asking the patient about his or her need is a direct approach that may yield important information. The RN has the opportunity to encourage or support spiritual activities that promote an individual's health (Exercise 15.2).

Social support can come from immediate family members, friends, employers and co-workers, neighbors, the community (e.g., community centers), and state and national agencies (e.g., Red Cross, United Way, Social Security Administration, and U.S. Department of Health and Human Services). People who are gainfully employed and normally able to provide for their own basic needs may still require access to social support to help them cope with life stresses. People who are not as fortunate may access local or federal agencies for support for basic needs as well as for coping with life stresses. Everyone defines the support that he or she needs.

Systems of support are frameworks developed by the individual to assist in networking within the community. The two basic systems of support are closed and open systems. Someone with a closed system seeks support within the immediate or defined family. Someone with an open system looks beyond the family for sources of support. Most people move along the continuum from a closed to an open system as needs dictate. Healthy individuals generally have a balance of internal and external support systems.

Economic

The economic environment may influence health-seeking behavior. Low-income families generally access the health care system for preventive care less frequently than families with moderate to upper levels of income. Additionally, it is more likely that women and children of low socioeconomic status will not be insured (Drevdahl, 1999; Johnson, 2001; Polivka et al., 2000; Swider, 2002).

Many health promotion options are available for low-income families and individuals. Public health and private, nonprofit organizations provide many low-cost or essentially free services. Well-baby and women's health clinics are public, subsidized

---

? EXERCISE 15.2

Religion plays an important role in health-seeking behaviors and in health promotion. For example, your patient's religious beliefs forbid the use of vaccines.
1. What would a health promotion plan of care look like?
2. Without trying to change the individual's beliefs, how would you as RN in the educator role encourage a healthier lifestyle?

health promotion sites for low-income individuals. Private practice wellness clinics and "fast-track" clinics are now emerging as replacements for, or alternatives to, public health programs. The incentive of these emerging clinics is to provide medical assistance directly to infants, children, and families, and they establish a system of care that minimizes the need to use emergency departments for minor or nonemergent health concerns.

The economic health of a community affects the primary health care offering. If the economy is not strong, an agency that could otherwise support the community will not have the resources to meet preventive health needs. For example, smoking cessation classes and well-baby clinics that focus on illness prevention will be sacrificed for the community's more universal infrastructure needs, such as roads and sanitation.

Establishing continuity of care in populations that traditionally place a burden on community resources provides the community with a cost benefit. However, barriers may still exist that prevent access to these health promotion sites. Transportation to and from the clinics can be cost-prohibitive to people unable to afford their own transportation and without access to public transportation.

Perception of potential or actual economic consequences to one's wellness state can influence health-seeking behavior. If the cost of improving health or maintaining a current level of health is perceived as being greater than the individual can manage, then the healthy behaviors may be ignored. For example, even if an individual understands that he or she needs to take antilipid medication prescribed by the physician, without insurance or financial resources, it is unlikely that he or she will continue the medication or even fill the prescription in the first place. Low-income families may not have enough money to afford even reduced copayments for preventive medications, much less maintain a supply of healthy foods.

Church and other nonprofit organizations may become invaluable partners for an RN formulating a plan of care. Matching the resources of community organizations with people in need is part of coordinating a far-reaching health plan. An RN can thus be a catalyst for change in the overall health of the neighborhood, town, state, and nation.

DEVELOPMENTAL

Age-related and developmental factors also affect health-seeking behaviors. Developmental theorists attempt to define the process of physical and psychosocial growth as being predictable and orderly (Taylor et al., 2015). Development has many influences, including heredity, temperament, and emotion, as well as the physical, psychological, and social environments. Eric Erikson is probably the most influential developmental theorist relative to nursing. His theory bases psychosocial development on the process of socialization, or how people interact with and react to the world. Erikson recognized the influences of social interactions, the environment, and biology on the eight stages of life. Each person moves from or stays at a developmental level as a result of resolution of conflicts there (Potter et al., 2017; Taylor et al., 2015). FYI 15.3 lists Erikson's eight stages of development.

🔨 FYI 15.3 **ERIKSON'S EIGHT STAGES OF DEVELOPMENT**	
STAGE	**ASSOCIATED TASK**
Infancy	Trust versus mistrust
Toddler	Autonomy versus shame and doubt
Early childhood	Initiative versus guilt
Middle childhood	Industry versus inferiority
Adolescence	Identity versus role confusion
Adulthood	Intimacy versus isolation
Middle age	Generativity versus stagnation
Old age	Integrity versus despair

Fundamental concepts of developmental theory include adaptive potential; that adaptive abilities derive in part from cultural, hereditary, and environmental influences; and that each person strives for self-actualization within his or her world (Potter et al., 2017). *Self-actualization* is an individual's understanding of his or her abilities and roles within a culture, community, society, or world.

These developmental concepts describe positive or negative influences on health-seeking behaviors or compliance with a health promotion plan of care. For example, a 40-year-old man may be working to provide for a growing family and plan for a future retirement. Health promotion may be on his mind, but he may be caught up in self-imposed time constraints that may make it difficult for him to maintain a healthy lifestyle and may not perceive that he has the time or energy to take up the task of self-health promotion. The RN must understand this individual's developmental tasks and view before developing a trusting relationship. Trust is needed to develop a collaborative plan that takes into consideration the individual's need to maintain current life goals as much as possible.

Development progresses in an orderly fashion throughout the life span. Each individual progresses at his or her own rate, which means that some people's developmental levels may not correlate with age expectations. For example, a 50-year-old man who engages in drag racing on public streets or in unsafe sexual practices is modeling the high-risk behavior more typical of the developmental stage of early adulthood or late adolescence. The RN, in collaborating with this person on a health promotion plan of care, may come to realize that what this man considers important may actually interfere with his ability to understand the relationship of health promotion and decreasing high-risk behavior. The health promotion plan of care needs to include an exploration of why he continues to engage in high-risk behavior before interventions can be implemented to assist in changing the behavior.

Many factors influence the developmental age of the individual and can influence the response to health-seeking behaviors. Individuals under stress tend to rely on successful adaptive measures learned in the past, behaviors that may be health-promoting or in fact detracting from health. For example, a woman who quit smoking 5 years ago is now facing the possibility of a divorce. This life change has great significance and a high degree of stress. Remembering the times when she would smoke to calm herself when she was feeling anxious, the woman decides to start smoking again. A health promotion plan of care must focus on redirecting the unhealthy attempt to cope with healthier alternatives, such as support groups, counseling, or other positive-diversion activities.

Nursing diagnoses for developmental plans of care include *Health-seeking behaviors; High risk for ineffective coping, individual/family;* and *Knowledge deficit.* The priority of care is to maintain an environment that is optimal for growth and development. Outcome criteria are individualized but should include indicators that developmental milestones are being met and that the person is maintaining a healthy lifestyle and is satisfied with the progress being made. The RN who is willing to collaborate with the individual can design a strong health promotion plan of care.

PRIMARY HEALTH CARE SYSTEMS

While health promotion is a portion of the nurse's role, many other organizations and individuals provide primary health care. The family nurse practitioner and the family practice physician are primary health care providers. Patients seek them out and trust that their counsel will help keep them well. The primary services they provide include physicals, immunizations, screening for potential health problems, and monitoring health and well-being. The RN can refer to the family practice physician or the nurse practitioner as part of the health promotion plan of care.

Public health is another area with a focus on health promotion. Generally, public health promotion centers on a framework of public policies that dictate the economic and bureaucratic structure of the agencies. From the World Health Organization to the state and local health departments, the main focus is setting standards for health, implementing interventions to meet the standards, and monitoring the outcomes in an effort to improve the general health of the community. Constraints and benefits are often linked to an agency's ability to maintain the intended level of health promotion. On a national level, legislative regulations, budgetary concerns, and patients' rights can dictate the effectiveness of the programs. Federal and state regulations focus on actions that minimize potentially widespread health problems. Programs of vaccination, preschool health screening, reporting of specific diseases, and gathering of health statistics minimize the influence of potential or actual health concerns.

GLOBAL HEALTH PROMOTION

Gorin and Arnold (1998) present health promotion as a multidimensional effort by numerous agencies and individuals at the global, national, and local levels. Health promotion has both individual and social contexts. It includes both diverse and complementary approaches to effecting positive health behaviors. Health promotion can directly eliminate hazards or threats to health, as in the efforts of the Environmental Protection Agency, or be indirect, such as educational programs that present lifestyle changes and inoculation programs that hope to decrease the incidence of disease. Nurses work with government, private, nonprofit, and community agencies in the delivery of health promotion services.

Healthy People 2020 is an example of a national effort to improve the lives and health of all Americans. For 30 years, the government has encouraged informed decisions about healthful living through collaboration across all communities of interest. The topical objectives for *Healthy People 2020* are:

Access to Health Services
Adolescent Health
Arthritis, Osteoporosis, and Chronic Back Conditions
Blood Disorders and Blood Safety
Cancer
Chronic Kidney Disease
Dementias, including Alzheimer's Disease
Diabetes
Disability and Health
Early and Middle Childhood
Educational and Community-Based Programs
Environmental Health
Family Planning
Food Safety
Genomics
Global Health
Health Communication and Health Information Technology
Healthcare-Associated Infections
Health-Related Quality of Life and Well-Being
Hearing and Other Sensory or Communication Disorders
Heart Disease and Stroke
HIV
Immunization and Infectious Diseases
Injury and Violence Prevention
Lesbian, Gay, Bisexual, and Transgender Health
Maternal, Infant, and Child Health
Medical Product Safety
Mental Health and Mental Disorders
Nutrition and Weight Status
Occupational Safety and Health
Older Adults
Oral Health
Physical Activity
Preparedness
Public Health Infrastructure
Respiratory Diseases
Sexually Transmitted Diseases
Sleep Health
Social Determinants of Health

Substance Abuse
Tobacco Use
Vision

It is expected that through the help of governmental partners and their resources, states, cities, communities, and individual people will be able to achieve the objectives in each of the topic categories by 2020 (U.S. Department of Health and Human Services, 2013). You can find more details on each objective at healthypeople.gov. As you look over the list, consider which topical areas are of interest to you, both personally and professionally. As an RN, you have a responsibility to promote these healthy objectives for both you and your patients.

COMMUNITY HEALTH PROMOTION

An evolving role of the RN is that of Public Health Nurse who engages in **community health promotion** and primary prevention in partnership with both communities and populations. Community health promotion includes assessing, addressing, and advocating for the health and social problems, particularly of vulnerable groups. Solutions are often drawn from engaging with, gathering, and aligning available resources and agencies (Kulbok et al., 2012). The Centers for Disease Control and Prevention (CDC, 2014) has an entire website devoted to their Division of Community Health (DCH): Making Healthy Living Easier that can be accessed at http://www.cdc.gov/nccdphp/dch/programs/index.htm. Nurses can access multiple resources and even funding in support of community health promotion initiatives at this site.

SELF-HEALTH PROMOTION

As an LPN/LVN, maintaining a healthy lifestyle is important. Remaining healthy will optimize your transition through school to become an RN. A healthy lifestyle also bolsters self-confidence, which is even more important as you assume the responsibilities of an RN. Furthermore, to promote healthy lifestyles in your patients, you first must model a healthy lifestyle. As an RN, you need to practice what you preach. It would be difficult to help a patient stop smoking if you smoke. Modeling a healthy lifestyle empowers others to emulate the good habits, especially if we share our stories along the way. **Self-health promotion** also lends credibility to your role as patient advocate.

KEY POINTS

After completion of this chapter, you have learned:
- On an individual patient basis, the RN recognizes that many extenuating environmental circumstances can interfere with a healthy lifestyle and with health promotion efforts.
- Innumerable global and local factors affect the health of the individual as well as that of the collective population.
- The RN is in a position to take a lead in health promotion through role-modeling a healthy lifestyle.

- In collaboration with other health care team members, the RN can design a plan of care with consideration of the needs and influences of the individual, family, and community.
- The goal of health promotion efforts is a higher level of function and development to allow the patient independence and empowerment to make healthy life choices.
- *Healthy People 2020* is the national effort to help people live longer, healthier lives, and RNs are in the perfect position to effect change to that end.

CRITICAL THINKING QUESTIONS

1. Working at a health fair, you screen a participant who presents with a blood pressure reading of 190/110 mm Hg. She tells you she has a history of hypertension, but she does not like to take pills. "My mother kept us well without medications, and when she died, she was on at least 10 different medications. I just don't trust a system that hands out pills for every little thing."
   a. What questions would you ask this person?
   b. What is the definitive care priority that is related to the health promotion or prevention need?
2. A minister at your church approaches you to give a talk at a Tuesday Family Night gathering. You would like to do a health promotion talk but are unsure of the best topic.
   a. What assessment questions would you formulate to identify an important health promotion need?
   b. What potential health concern would a person who was raised within a Catholic, Jewish, Protestant, American Indian, Mexican American, or other subculture have?
   c. What would be the health promotion care priority for this cultural health concern?
3. The physician has ordered a weight reduction diet for an overweight individual with high cholesterol. The physician does not want the patient to have more than 20% fat in his diet.
   a. Of an 1800-calorie diet, how many calories should be fat?
   b. What would a typical day's balanced menu look like when the approximate weight or portion size of each of the items has been taken into account?
4. Considering the list of topical objectives for *Healthy People 2020,* which areas are of interest to you personally and professionally? How do you see your role as an RN expanding to meet the *Healthy People 2020* primary health care needs?

WEB RESOURCES

Healthy People 2020, http://healthypeople.gov/2020/default.aspx
CDC Division of Community Health (DCH): Making Healthy Living Easier http://www.cdc.gov/nccdphp/dch/programs/index.htm
World Health Organization, http://who.int/topics/health_promotion/en
Office of Disease Prevention and Health Promotion, http://odphp.osophs.dhhs.gov
American Journal of Health Promotion, http://healthpromotionjournal.com

REFERENCES

Drevdahl, D. (1999). Meanings of community in a community health center. *Public Health Nursing, 16*(6), 417–425.

Gorin, S. S., & Arnold, J. (1998). *Health promotion handbook.* St. Louis, MO: Mosby.

Johnson, M. O. (2001). Meeting health care needs of a vulnerable population: perceived barriers. *Journal of Community Health Nursing, 18*(1), 35–52.

Kulbok, P. A., Thatcher, E., Park, E., & Meszaros, P. S. (May 31, 2012). Evolving Public Health, Nursing Roles: focus on community participatory health promotion and prevention. *OJIN: The Online Journal of Issues in Nursing, 17*(2). http://dx.doi.org/10.3912/OJIN. Vol17No02Man01. Manuscript 1.

Kulbok, P. A., Thatcher, E., Park, E., & Meszaros, P. S. (May 31, 2012). Evolving Public Health Nursing Roles: Focus on Community Participatory Health Promotion and Prevention. *OJIN: The Online Journal of Issues in Nursing, 17*(2). Manuscript 1.

Orem, D. E. (2001). *Nursing concepts of practice* (6th ed.). St. Louis, MO: Mosby.

Pender, N. J., Murdaugh, C. L., & Parsons, M. A. (2011). *Health promotion in nursing practice* (6th ed.). Upper Saddle River, NJ: Pearson.

Polivka, B. J., Nickel, J. T., Salsberry, P. J., Kuthy, R., Shapiro, N., & Slack, C. (2000). Hospital and emergency department use by young low-income children. *Nursing Research, 49*(5), 253–261.

Potter, P., Perry, A., Stockert, P. A., & Hall, A. M. (2017). *Fundamentals of nursing* (9th ed.). St. Louis, MO: Mosby.

Swider, S. M. (2002). Outcome effectiveness of community health workers: an integrative literature review. *Public Health Nursing, 19*(1), 11–20.

Taylor, C., Lillis, C., Lynn, P., & LeMone, P. (2015). *Fundamentals of nursing: the art and science of nursing* (8th ed.). Philadelphia, PA: Lippincott.

U. S. Department of Health and Human Services (USDHHS). (2013). *Healthy People 2020.* Retrieved from http://healthypeople.gov/2020/about/default.aspx.

chapter 16

Managing Care in Secondary and Tertiary Health Care

⊖volve WEBSITE

Additional resources are available online at:
http://evolve.elsevier.com/Claywell/transitions

OBJECTIVES

After completing this chapter, the student will be prepared to:
1. Discuss the theoretical framework for managing in secondary care.
2. Identify outcome priorities for secondary care.
3. Analyze factors influencing patient outcomes.
4. Define the purposes of tertiary care.

KEY TERMS

clinical pathway	manager of care	social support
consequence	secondary (acute) health	spiritual distress
cultural strain	care	tertiary care
dependent-care agency	self-care agency	

OVERVIEW

A person enters the acute health care setting when he or she is without sufficient resources for self-care and in need of the specialized skills of the nurse to meet the dependent care needs brought on by the illness. To varying degrees, the individual who enters the acute care setting enters into a collaborative relationship with the health care team. The realm of the RN, nursing, is managing care related to the patient's response to the acute illness state, the pharmacological interventions, and the surgical and medical plan of care. The RN becomes responsible, as the **manager of care,** to plan, implement, and evaluate the plan of care. This chapter assists you in gaining the tools necessary to be a strong manager of care within complex acute and extended-care settings.

273

THEORETICAL FRAMEWORK

In the previous chapter, you learned that Orem (2001) believes that individuals have self-care and **dependent-care abilities (or agencies)** that work together to meet regulatory functioning and developmental needs. At various times in life, a person will have either a self-care or dependent-care demand that exceeds his or her **self-care agency.** When this happens, the person is said to have a self-care or dependent-care deficit. When this deficit is such that the person needs health care professionals with specialized training, the person enters the health care setting and engages in a collaborative relationship with the RN and other health care team members.

Nurses have had specialized training to recognize the physiological, spiritual, social, emotional, and intellectual responses to illness states. Additionally, we understand that every medical, surgical, or nursing intervention has a **consequence,** which may be regarded as an outcome or a side effect. A consequence is any significant response to or effect of an intervention. An *outcome* is an expected consequence of an intervention and can be measured. An unexpected consequence is considered a *side effect* or adverse effect of an intervention.

Orem (2001) believes that the overall goal of nursing is to reestablish the health care agencies of the patient. The role of the acute care nurse has ended when the balance shifts away from the acute, dependent-care needs of the patient. The **dependent-care agency** returns to the patient or can be met by someone with other specific training to meet his or her short-term or extended needs beyond the acute care setting. The health care requirements within the **secondary (acute) health care** system are as follows (p. 131):

1. Prevention of complicating disease and adverse effects of specific disease and prolonged disability through early diagnosis and treatment (secondary treatment) and
2. Rehabilitation in the event of disfigurement and disability (tertiary level of prevention) are specified in relation to what is known about the nature and effects of specific diseases, valid methods of regulating disease, and the human potential for living with and overcoming the disabling effects of disease.

Acute health care requirements vary with the progress of the disease either toward a cure or through complications that can occur. The RN uses information from many different sources to identify potential and actual problems with the patient's progress. The overall focus is to prevent complications while promoting a higher level of health (FYI 16.1).

The priority of care is unique and dynamic, or constantly changing, for each patient in the acute care setting. Patients are entering and leaving the acute care

---

✎ FYI 16.1   SECONDARY CARE OUTCOME PRIORITIES

The outcome priorities for a patient entering the acute (secondary) health care setting are as follows:
- Ensuring more independence in self-care ability
- Avoiding complications as the patient progresses through the illness state

setting more dependent than in years past. The hospital setting is reserved for only the most acutely ill patients. Nurses are being increasingly challenged to understand and restore each individual's self-care abilities. The primary role of the RN is to recognize when the patient's needs change, either to a more independent or more dependent state. To best meet the needs of the patient and still use health care resources efficiently, the RN must continually evaluate each patient against outcome criteria and determine the extent of the patient's dependent-care needs. When the priority of care warrants, the RN should advocate for a change in the level of health care.

MANAGER OF CARE

The RN manages the nursing and collaborative plan of care for the patient. The LPN/LVN works as a team member to carry out tasks, including assessment of the patient's response to the illness and the medical plan of care. These responses are communicated to the RN, who is then responsible for collaboratively planning and modifying care to best meet the patient's needs. Since registered nurses are required to understand the pathophysiology and effects of disease, you will recognize such changes in the patient's condition as well as changes resulting from medication and other therapies used to treat the disease. You will manage the minute-to-minute and day-to-day changes that occur within multiple realms.

The manager of care must deal with unique problems that the acute care setting brings. These problems are associated with the technical and institutional influences on the patient as well as the issues associated with the individual's environmental, spiritual, cultural, developmental, and social needs and influences (FYI 16.2).

Environmental Influences

Prior experience with the acute health care setting may affect a given patient in either a positive or a negative way. A patient who is familiar with the hospital routine and with a need for the equipment may respond better than the patient who is unfamiliar with the experience. Negative previous experiences, however, can make the patient more anxious. The RN must include interventions to orient the patient to the physical environment of the acute care setting and implement continuous assessment of the patient's response to the environment.

Much within the environment of the acute care setting has the potential to extend the patient's length of stay by introducing unexpected complications. Moving the

---

✎ FYI 16.2 FACTORS INFLUENCING PATIENT OUTCOMES

- Cultural values and beliefs
- Developmental processes
- Environment, both internal and external
- Social roles and supports
- Spiritual values and beliefs

patient through the acute care setting effectively and safely requires the RN to pay attention as the patient responds to the environment as well as to anticipate the potential effects the environment, including staffing issues, may have. A common nursing diagnosis is "risk for infection," and nosocomial, or hospital-acquired, infections are just one of the problems that competent nursing management can prevent. The charge nurse can manage this environmental concern by basing bed assignments on the diagnoses of the patients and then subsequently basing caregiver assignment on qualifications. For a patient likely to require more advanced intervention, the RN or LPN/LVN with the most experience will be assigned whenever possible. However, newer nurses may be assigned more challenging patients when a more experienced nurse is available to assist.

Read the scenario in Exercise 16.1 and answer the questions concerning the environmental influences on a patient.

Spiritual Needs and Influences

Patients facing stressful health care–related events may also experience **spiritual distress.** Illness states can place a patient in a position that forces consideration of the fragile nature of life. Resulting from a potential life-or-death experience or a life-changing event, such as becoming paralyzed; losing a limb, sight, or hearing; or learning to live with a debilitating illness, spiritual distress may take on many manifestations. Much as in the grief process, the patient may display anger, blame, bargaining, or denial or may overtly cling to a spiritual guide. As RN, you assess for spiritual distress and implement interventions that will help the patient cope, such as facilitating the patient's spiritual connection either through a referral or just by respecting personal wishes. Often the patient will require a spiritual guide by his or her side.

Additionally, religious beliefs may affect the patient's willingness to participate in the medical plan of care. For example, some religions forbid their participants from receiving blood or blood products. The plan of care must be respectful of the patient's beliefs while still providing the optimal environment for recovery.

According to Gorin and Arnold (1998), the effect spirituality has on health and well-being has not been formally studied extensively. However, an apparent link exists between the individual's ability to cope with adverse situations and his or her spiritual

---

? EXERCISE 16.1

A patient is admitted to an intensive care unit with a peripheral and central line, with a chest tube, and on a five-lead cardiac monitor. The family is asking about the alarms that are sounding from the monitor and from the IV pumps. The patient is quiet but appears anxious.

1. What questions would you ask to assess the environmental influence on the patient's recovery?
2. What outcomes would you have for the nursing diagnosis *Coping, ineffective individual and family, related to inexperience/knowledge deficit of the intensive care environment, as evidenced by anxious look, frequent questions regarding equipment and alarms*?

strength. Gorin and Arnold note that spirituality can even become stronger in times of adversity. According to Hart (2008), using prayer in healing dates back millennia to ancient times when physicians and other healers used prayer as a means of gaining humility in the face of caring for those who were ill. In many cultures, such as Native Americans, spirituality is tied directly to health, and it is crucial that as the manager of care, you actively assess the spiritual dimension needs in your patients and their families and then act upon meeting those needs. Spirituality promotes effective coping in patients, families, and caregivers, and in attending to this need, overall health may be improved for the entire patient-family-caregiver system (Torosian & Verschka, 2005). In the acute care setting, we can easily overlook a person's spiritual needs when physical needs are clearly evident. Be certain to attend to your patients in a holistic manner.

Cultural Needs and Influences

Culture affects how people respond to situations as a result of patterns acquired over time through social and religious structures as well as through their intellect and artistic expression (Giger & Davidhizar, 2002). The Giger and Davidhizar Model of Transcultural Nursing can help you to fully address the cultural needs of your patients. Each of the following six areas requires assessment to create a culturally sensitive healing experience for your patient and the associated family group. The associated questions may help you to manage the required assessment:

Communication: What is the primary language? Are titles used? Is silence expected? Is nonverbal communication used? Is touch part of communication?

Time orientation: Is time relative to the situation, or is it strictly by the clock? Is time carefully guarded, and are schedules followed?

Spatial orientation: Is there personal space? What happens if it is invaded? What is a comfortable distance for strangers, caregivers, and family?

Social organization: Who is in the social circle? Is the person married? Have children? Does the person believe in one God, many, or none? What are the person's roles within their social circumstances? How do political or other views factor into his or her sense of being?

Environmental control: Where does one's power reside—inside or from outside? What is the person's concept of health and his or her ability to maintain it? Who normally treats illness? What beliefs exist that external forces can heal or cause illness?

Biological variation considerations: What genetic predispositions exist? Are there illnesses in the family? What are the specific unique characteristics of the body? What composes the normal daily diet?

Carefully attending to the assessment of the phenomena within this model will help to identify holistic, culturally sensitive care priorities. The acute care setting may place an individual in a position that involves conflict with his or her cultural makeup. This **cultural strain** is the tension or pressure experienced by someone who has beliefs tested or when the actions of others are contrary to the beliefs, placing him or her in a position that potentially compromises these beliefs and thus hinders the healing process as a result.

Cultural strain may be manifested in the patient's responses to the surroundings or to the plan of care. For example, consider one culture-derived concept mentioned in the preceding model: that of personal space, the distance surrounding a person considered to be part of his or her identity. Personal space is generally thought to be between 1 and 3 feet around a person, depending on the cultural upbringing and personal interpretation. A breach of that space by objects or another person may cause discomfort and stress.

Within the acute care setting, the patient's personal space is often breached by the RN and other health care workers. Direct touching required during physical examinations may be the first experience the patient has with giving up personal space. Recognizing that the patient may have this concern requires the nurse to be respectful and seek permission to "invade the personal space," with adequate explanation of the need.

Respecting the patient's personal space also occurs during the interview stage. Some cultures require eye contact, but others may be offended by what they consider to be the presumptive nature of eye contact. Body language sometimes reveals patient discomfort with the interview process. Paying attention to the patient's comfort level during history-taking will encourage the establishment of trust.

One patient may have grown up with family members with extensive hospitalization or illness, whereas another may have had minimal or no experience with the health care system. Additionally, since ideas about health and other values, including responses to the illness state, are largely formed within a particular culture, one patient may hide his or her emotions, and another may wear emotions on his or her sleeve. However, they may equally be in despair. Cultural beliefs and subsequent behavior must be respected by the health care team to optimize a positive environment for healing. The RN who fails to respond to patients with equal respect can create mistrust of the plan of care as well as of the health care system.

Developmental Needs and Influences

While moving through life, everyone experiences developmental milestones. An acute or chronic illness state may pose a threat to the patient's developmental tasks. Many factors, such as stress from the illness state, uncertainty over long-term effects on self-care abilities, and perception of the plan of care, can pose a threat to the developmental tasks of the patient. "Role strain" is an appropriate nursing diagnosis when exploring a patient's concern over future or current developmental weaknesses. Outcome criteria focus on the return of the patient to as high a level of function as possible.

Social Needs and Influences

Humans, for the most part, are social beings. The acute care facility is a stressor to both patient and family. It can isolate the patient from the **social support** systems that he or she has in place. The needs of the family may not appear to be a priority for the nurse in planning the patient's care, but they must be considered for the patient to receive ample social support. The rest of the family is facing some of the same stresses as the hospitalized family member. They may need assistance coping with hospitalization of the patient or with the prospect of a poor prognosis (Appleyard et al., 2000; De Jong & Beatty, 2000; Gavaghan & Carroll, 2002; Kosco & Warren, 2000; Mendonca & Warren, 1998; Tin, French, & Leung, 1999).

The family of a patient facing acute illness needs open, honest information about their hospitalized family member. The nurse should anticipate providing updates and other information without the family's having to solicit it, easing some of their concerns.

Family members need to be with the patient as much as possible. Allowing access is an essential component to the plan of care, especially at times when the patient's prognosis may be poor. It will help both the family and the patient cope.

Monitoring the patient's response to family visitations is an important consideration for the RN. Often the family visits can be stressful to the patient rather than a source of comfort. Ensure that the patient's needs are held as the top priority. You may need to restrict visits on behalf of the patient.

Social support for the patient may come from others who are not legal relatives. Since people live and work within a community, friendships and companionship outside of family may become as important to someone as family. Many nontraditional definitions of "family" exist, which may include many combinations of significant individuals. Such nontraditional family relationships may present legal and ethical consequences within the acute care setting. For example, questions of confidentiality and privacy may need to be answered before planning care that includes keeping such people informed about the patient's progress.

The RN must recognize strain within the patient's social support system. *Ineffective individual or family coping, high risk for, related to multiple stress situations of hospitalization* would be a potential nursing diagnosis for patients experiencing decreased or ineffectual social support.

RESOURCE MANAGER

As a manager of care within the acute care setting, you will be responsible for recognizing that limited funds are available to provide acute health care. Within the limits set by administration, staffing mixes, and restrictions on equipment and supplies, the RN must provide the patient with consistently safe and effective care, including managing resources. Each day a patient is in the hospital, valuable human, equipment, and supply resources are being used. The RN must then continue to evaluate the priority of care for each patient to advocate safe and efficient transitions to a less acute level of care.

Clinical Pathways

A **clinical pathway** is a standardized care map that defines nursing care, outcome criteria, and evaluation time frames for specific disorders. Clinical pathways are designed to manage the resources of the health care agency, as well as enable consistent, safe care for patients. A clinical pathway defines the standard assessment data and frequency of the collection of the data needed for a specific illness or surgical procedure. These data include medical diagnostic tests, laboratory results, and vital signs, as well as fluid intake and output, for example. The pathway time frame also includes assessment points with defined outcome criteria. The responsibility of the RN is to evaluate the effectiveness of the plan of care and the patient's progress toward discharge.

Managing patient care requires the RN to ensure that the standard laboratory results, interventions, medications, and assessment data flow as outlined in the pathway. An RN learns to recognize and understand deviations from normal and is in a position, through collaboration with the physician and other health care team members, to adjust the plan of care to fit the individual needs of the patient. Strict adherence to evaluation points and efficient adjustments to the plan of care through collaboration will minimize the possibility of large deviations from the clinical pathway, which would increase the cost of care.

Discharge Planning

Patients moving through the acute care setting will eventually be discharged. The medical plan of care will have progressed to a point that the level of nursing care will have changed. The nursing plan of care will also change to a point that will require the RN to plan for discharge. In some facilities, discharge planning is a collaboration with the health care team and generally begins soon after admission. Patient outcome criteria are defined by the physician as well as the RN and are the source of evaluation of the patient's progress. If clinical pathways are used, then discharge dates may be identified as well.

Discharge planning requires assessing the patient plan of care to determine whether the outcome criteria are met. If a need exists for continuation of the plan of care, then the RN must evaluate whether the patient and family can continue with the necessary interventions or whether they need assistance. If the patient and the family are able to continue the plan of care, discharge teaching with regard to the continued care is needed. Discharge teaching will require the RN to assess the level of the patient's understanding with regard to his or her illness state and treatment regimen.

After discharge from an acute care facility, the patient may still need some level of nursing care or other specialized care beyond the patient's self-care ability, despite his or her having regained some independence. The physician will provide discharge orders that include the level of care needed. Occupational and physical therapy are continued for many patients discharged from acute care settings. Evaluation may reveal that a patient needs extended care.

TERTIARY CARE REFERRALS

The purposes of **tertiary care** are to provide health restoration and maintenance and to continue with health promotion (FYI 16.3). Health promotion and restoration assist the patient in achieving a higher level of functioning. For the patient with a progressive or terminal disorder, health maintenance focuses on at least sustaining the current level of functioning, slowing or preventing the effects of the disease. The goal of health maintenance is the establishment or continuation of dignity and respect during a condition of infirmity. Recognizing that the patient will require some level of dependent care, it becomes crucial to help the patient retain as much control and independence as possible.

A patient to be discharged to an extended-care facility is generally evaluated by a caseworker, who is usually a social worker or an RN with special training to evaluate the needs and the extent of care requirements of the patient. The discharge RN notifies

> **⚖ FYI 16.3   TERTIARY HEALTH CARE**
>
> - Tertiary health care involves health promotion and health maintenance.
> - The outcome priority of tertiary health care is to ensure that the patient regains or attains as much independence as possible.

the caseworker and reports the patient's history of the present acute illness state along with the progress to date. The caseworker, having knowledge of the services within different facilities, makes recommendations and assists in making arrangements for transfer to the facility chosen. The caseworker considers the economic needs of the patient and assists family in managing insurance or other forms of payment for care.

The RN may need to make a referral to hospice care when a patient has approximately 6 months or less to live. Hospice care helps the patient and family cope with the end-of-life experience. The priority of care is the patient's peaceful and dignified death after living life, even its very end, to the fullest. The hospice nurse assesses the continued needs of the patient and works with a physician to provide comfort measures for the patients. Pain and nutrition are important components in managing a patient at the end of life.

A patient who leaves the hospital with a chronic illness state will perhaps go home under the care of the family. Chronic care of a patient can take a toll on other family members. Respite care, services provided by persons trained in the care of people with special needs, can be given within the home or through adult day care centers. It is intended to offer the patient's family members time off from their dependent-care duties.

Home health care provides assistance to a patient and family for a short period of time after discharge to home from the acute care setting. Home health care agencies provide a variety of care, depending on patient needs, such as physical therapy, respiratory therapy, or occupational therapy. Home health care is capable of providing health promotion, health restoration, and health maintenance care. The needs of the patient are generally assessed with an intake interview and assessment by an RN case manager. The level of care and the treatment plan are then determined accordingly.

KEY POINTS

After completion of this chapter, you have learned:
- Secondary, or acute, health care uses the principles of health restoration and health maintenance.
- A person seeks secondary care when in need of specialized, around-the-clock nursing care, having an imbalance between health care abilities and dependent-care needs.
- The RN is trained to take care of the patient's holistic needs on a minute-to-minute basis.
- The continued-care needs of the patient are met within the varied realm of the tertiary health care system.
- In many cases, tertiary care is carried out either in long-term facilities or in the home with the assistance of both family and health care personnel. Both secondary and tertiary care needs are considered upon admission to a health care setting.

▌ CRITICAL THINKING QUESTIONS

1. A 74-year-old patient is admitted to an intensive care bed with a medical diagnosis of exacerbation of congestive heart failure and pulmonary edema. The patient has the following assessment data available: pulse 120–130 beats/min (A-Fib); respiration 26 breaths/min, labored, with crackles to the bases and coarse rhonchi throughout; oxygen per nasal cannula at 4 L, pulse oximetry 96%; 2+ pitting dependent edema bilateral lower extremities and to the coccyx area.
   a. What further questions need to be asked?
   b. What is the definitive care priority?
   c. What patient problems are identified, and what are the outcome criteria?
   d. Identify the developmental stage of the patient and the possible influence the disease response will have on the patient's perception of the future.
2. You enter your patient's room to do a shift assessment. The patient's family is gathered around the bed being led in prayer by a *curandera* (faith healer). The room is decorated with candles and religious paraphernalia. The ritual has a supernatural feel, and the patient is being offered a potent herbal tea mix.
   a. What questions do you need to ask?
   b. What interventions, if any, are necessary?
   c. To what extent would you report or chart the findings?
3. A patient is to receive an IVPB of 20 mEq K^+ in a bolus for a K^+ level of 3.0. On hand you have an IVPB of 20 mEq K^+ in 100 mL of 0.9% NS. The K^+ should be run no faster than 10 mEq/hr.
   a. At what setting would you place the pump to comply with the recommended IV rate?
   b. The patient complains that the IV is burning, and on assessment the IV site is red and slightly raised. What is your next step?
   c. The lab has been notified to draw a K^+ level 1 hour after the finish of the IVPB. You have already put in the order for the lab to draw 3 hours after the initial start. What action would be correct at this point?

WEB RESOURCES

Agency for Healthcare Research and Quality: http://ahrq.gov/qual/kt/
Open Clinical: Clinical Pathways: http://openclinical.org/clinicalpathways.html
European [clinical] Pathway Association: http://e-p-a.org/000000979b08f9803/index.html
The Cochrane Collaboration: http://cochrane.org/

REFERENCES

Appleyard, M. E., Gavaghan, S. R., Gonzalez, C., Ananian, L., & Tyrell, R. (2000). Nurse-coached interventions for the families of patients in critical care units. *Critical Care Nurse, 20*(3), 40–48.
De Jong, M. J., & Beatty, D. S. (2000). Family perceptions of support interventions in the intensive care unit. *Dimensions in Critical Care Nursing, 19*(5), 40–47.
Gavaghan, S. R., & Carroll, D. L. (2002). Families of critically ill patients and the effects of nursing intervention. *Dimensions in Critical Care Nursing, 21*(2), 64–71.

Giger, J. N., & Davidhizar, R. E. (2002). The Giger and Davidhizar transcultural assessment model. *Journal of Transcultural Nursing, 13*, 185–188.

Gorin, S. S., & Arnold, J. (1998). *Health promotion handbook.* St. Louis, MO: Mosby.

Hart, J. (2008). Spirituality and healing. Retrieved from http://thirdage.com/spirituality/spirituality-and-healing.

Kosco, M., & Warren, N. A. (2000). Critical care nurses' perceptions of family needs as met. *Critical Care Nursing Quarterly, 23*(2), 60–72.

Mendonca, D., & Warren, N. (1998). Perceived and unmet needs of critical care family members. *Critical Care Nursing Quarterly, 21*(1), 58–67.

Orem, D. E. (2001). *Nursing concepts of practice* (6th ed.). St. Louis, MO: Mosby.

Tin, M. K., French, P., & Leung, K. K. (1999). The needs of the family of critically ill neurosurgical patients: a comparison of nurses' and family members' perceptions. *Journal of Neuroscience Nursing, 31*(6), 348–356.

Torosian, M. H., & Verschka, R. B. (2005). Spirituality and healing. *Seminars in Oncology, 32*(2), 232–236.

UNIT 5

Putting It All Together

CHAPTER

17

Reflecting on Your Transition

⊖volve WEBSITE

Additional resources are available online at:
http://evolve.elsevier.com/Claywell/transitions

OBJECTIVES

After completing this chapter, the student will be prepared to:
1. Apply the nursing process to transitioning from LPN/LVN to RN.

KEY TERMS

critical reflection

┃OVERVIEW

Change takes effort. You have decided to make a major change in your life and have put forth effort to get to where you are in the process of becoming an RN. Along the way you have been given the tools necessary to make the change. You have been asked to set forth a plan to assist you through your program of study.

This chapter uses the nursing process to assist you in reflecting on your journey thus far and to challenge you to develop a portfolio, a map to your future. You will reassess your strengths and weaknesses, make a diagnosis, plan goals, decide what tools you need to implement your plan, identify what might be stopping you from progressing or ways you are enduring, and evaluate your readiness to embark on the next leg of your journey. If you set a course for excellence and have a lamp to light your way, then the road to success will not seem so difficult to travel.

284

ASSESSMENT

Early in this text, you were asked to "sketch your experiential résumé." You were asked to look at this résumé and determine experiences with positive and negative influences on your learning. After defining yourself, you identified and prioritized short-term and long-term personal and professional goals and your personal-care priority. You finalized your plan with a timeline for meeting these goals.

In the journey you have taken to this point, you have had the opportunity to learn and use new tools and expand your horizon through a broader base of knowledge. Brown and Gillis (1999) report that reflective thinking is an effective method for students to develop professional and personal philosophies. Development of a professional philosophy is an important component for the transition of a student with no nursing background into the role of professional nurse. The LPN/LVN mobility student, also being in a role transition, would benefit from reflective thinking to develop a personal and professional philosophy as well. Brown and Gillis demonstrate the relationship between reflective thinking and critical thinking. Through their literature search, the authors show how reflection is a dynamic process of analysis that forces the student to examine prejudices, beliefs, feelings, thoughts, and experiences in light of new nursing knowledge. Consider the process of reflection as a proactive way to challenge former assumptions and inferences about the role of the RN.

CRITICAL REFLECTION

To begin **critical reflection,** you must ask yourself tough questions about your beliefs. What are the differences between your beliefs about the role of the RN from what you know of the role of the LPN/LVN? If you answer truthfully, you will be able to identify areas for needed role development. Del Bueno (2000) remarks that the beginning RN must meet a minimum set of competencies, such as listed below, to be safe in the new role:

1. Ability to recognize problems from presenting signs and symptoms
2. Awareness of the urgency of a situation and acting appropriately to the level of urgency
3. Capacity to design a plan of care that safely meets the needs of the patient
4. Understanding the nature of the plan of care in relation to the patient's medical and nursing problems

Additional competencies of the beginning RN include strong interpersonal skills (e.g., teamwork, team building, conflict resolution, and patient interactions) and a competent level of clinical skills (Del Bueno, 2000). The implications to you as a soon-to-be graduate are out in the "real world," without the safety net of school. You will be asked to apply the knowledge, skills, and values you have learned in order to be a safe and effective practitioner.

Within the academic setting, you will demonstrate sufficient knowledge and skill to manage several patients in a safe, holistic manner. The graduate RN leaves school with the knowledge and skills of a generalist within the nursing profession. However, the journey of learning and skill acquisition is far from over. Your

---

⁉ EXERCISE 17.1

A patient presents to you with the following signs and symptoms: blood pressure 148/60 mm Hg; pulse 140 beats/min; respirations 18 breaths/min and deep with a fruity odor; blood sugar 485; lethargic, with slurring speech; and flushed and warm.

Ask yourself these questions: Are you able to recognize patient problems from the presenting signs and symptoms? Do you understand the significance and urgency of the patient information? Can you design a plan of care that effectively manages the patient problems and will assist the patient toward health? Do you know the reasons behind your nursing plan and the medical plan of care and the relationship between the presenting patient signs and symptoms and problems?

When you are done with this brief evaluation, form a group in class where you can discuss your findings and defend yourself.

What assumptions that you made were not supported by the data presented?

Did you make any prejudicial assumptions?

How did these assumptions influence your plan of care?

---

professional development begins with a reflection on your past as a means to better understand the lessons you have learned. The philosophy of nursing you develop will serve as the basis for your future plan. Use Exercise 17.1 to begin the reflective process.

When you began your journey to becoming an RN, you may have wanted to know more about the nursing care you were giving, what the signs and symptoms meant, and how the plan of care would affect your patients' outcomes. This curiosity is as important now as it was then. Curiosity will lead you to continued education, which will improve your nursing care. Understanding the relationship of the disease process to the interventions provided by nursing and by other members of the health care team will help you to become a safe practitioner. The standard of practice for all nurses is to become an informed caregiver who is able to recognize significant changes in patient conditions, anticipate needs, and implement appropriate interventions.

In Exercise 17.2, and after reviewing the plan you developed early in this text, begin a retrospective assessment of where you are to date. You may be near graduation, or that exciting event may be further off, yet here you are now, one semester closer to graduation. Either way, hopefully your course of study and this textbook will have provided you with new insights.

From the problems you identified in Exercise 17.2, which ones are priorities to you? Did you choose improvements that will enhance your critical thinking abilities, broaden your knowledge base, and help with your skills? You need to recognize areas that pertain to your most immediate needs first, as well as ensure your ability to provide safe care. Remember that critical reflection is unbiased and does not let your ego interfere with the search for truth.

In planning care, pointing out and leveraging strengths are as important as identifying and correcting weaknesses. Capitalize on your strengths in your plan of action as tools to be built upon. In Exercise 17.3, read the scenario and answer the questions about your strengths and weaknesses.

ⓘ EXERCISE 17.2

STRENGTHS (GIFTS)	WEAKNESSES (BARRIERS)

How have your strengths and weaknesses changed since you listed them in Chapter 2?

Write a problem statement for each of your weaknesses.

WEAKNESS	PROBLEM STATEMENT

Which of these problems are priorities for you to resolve?

ⓘ EXERCISE 17.3

Hypothetically, consider that you have difficulty finding the correct way to interact with a patient or family member who is having trouble coping with hospitalization or illness. You may decide that this reflects a problem with your own ability to effectively use the catchphrases that are a part of therapeutic communication. You feel that your strength lies in recognizing that people need to have someone to talk with who is empathetic, but you feel awkward trying to be that someone.

1. How would you state the problems, and what would they be related to?
2. How would you go about using the strengths you identified to assist you with weaknesses you've identified?
3. Is there a catchphrase that you can believe in that will allow you to display empathy?
4. Is there a way for you to show empathy while also calling on another health care team member, such as the chaplain, to assist the patient in this time of need?
5. What steps would you take to improve your communication skills?

Your strengths will also assist you in your quest to become the best you can be. Clustering the strengths across from the weaknesses (see Exercise 17.2), can you identify how you will be able to draw from them to assist you in gaining experience and expertise? As an LPN/LVN, many treatment skills have become second nature to you. As a graduate from a mobility program, not needing to concentrate on practicing basic psychomotor skills, you will be more open to the evolving changes in the conditions that define the needs of your patients. Thus, your unique set of strengths will have enhanced a critical component of your ability to provide safe, effective care.

MAKING THE DIAGNOSIS

In clustering your strengths and weaknesses (see Exercise 17.2), you have a chance to identify diagnostic statements. These problem (or strength) areas will assist you in continued planning. If you have kept a journal, review it to see whether the problem areas that you have identified in Exercise 17.2 are part of your past problem list. If so, a revision of a preexisting plan of action may be all that is needed. A self-diagnosis should be specific to the problem, as should a plan to capitalize on and extend a strength. For example, if you have determined that you are not sure of all of the signs and symptoms to expect from a patient experiencing an exacerbation of a disorder, then your problem statement might be written like this: *Cognitive deficit, inability to identify pertinent data to make sound clinical judgment.* As in any diagnostic statement, you should identify what the problem is related to. A problem can be resolved only after you know the reasons behind it.

What could the problem's cause be for you? You might have worked too much at your job and not had enough time to study. You may have chosen to settle for a minimum grade point average or study only for a specific test rather than seeking deep understanding and true knowledge. Whatever the cause of the problem, you should be honest in conducting your critical reflection. Determining a problem's cause, or at least conditions that seem to lead to the problem, should assist you in developing a plan that focuses on your problem areas.

In Exercise 17.2, you created problem statements that apply to those areas of weakness. Prioritize the problems to develop a plan to work on the problems of greatest importance first. You may need to solicit the advice of a faculty member or your mentor in making decisions on how to prioritize.

PLANNING

Now is the time to formulate personal and professional goals that will assist you with the transition into your new role as a safe beginning RN. Use the weaknesses you identified in Exercise 17.2 as problem areas to establish goals and outcome criteria. As in Chapter 1, establish your short-term and long-term goals. Short-term goals may assist you in meeting the needs of your family, seeking a job, or getting oriented to a new town, as well as passing the NCLEX-RN examination. Long-term goals can assist you during the orientation period in establishing and maintaining your mentor relationship and planning your future education. Long-term goals will also assist you in your professional development, such as planning for certification in a specialty area, earning an advanced degree, or even becoming an advanced practice registered nurse (APRN). The destination is yours to determine.

Professional development is an expected part of the role of the RN, but being a professional is more than being licensed as an RN. Becoming a professional means establishing yourself as capable, competent, and safe. It also means that you act to advance the practice of nursing through your actions and your skills. Orem (2001) defines *profession* in nursing as "the basis for distinguishing nurses prepared for entry to the beginning professional level of nursing practice who move themselves to become advanced professional practitioners from nurses prepared in technical

---

? EXERCISE 17.4

	GOALS	OUTCOME CRITERIA
Personal		
Professional		

---

programs preparatory for nursing" (p. 465). The LPN/LVN is trained at the technical level, and the RN receives education at the beginning professional level. Orem's definition implies that your professional development includes an obligation to advance yourself within the practice of nursing and does not stop at the end of your formal educational process. To be a part of the nursing profession, you must set goals that advance your professional development, building up your knowledge, skill, and critical thinking abilities.

In Exercise 17.4, write your personal and professional goals and outcome criteria associated with those goals. Include a personal development plan that is in balance with your professional plan. You should reestablish personal relationships to help cope with the transition into your new role. You might have neglected those closest to you during your schooling. The stress and pressure to complete a program that is abbreviated may have left you little time to spend with family and friends. Once-important relaxation activities, such as exercise, hobbies, and entertainment, might have been set aside while you were concentrating on your RN education. Remember, your self-definition is more than as an RN because you may also be a mother or father, sister or brother, potter, sewer, triathlete, actor, or friend. All the aspects of who you are help make you a better RN.

IMPLEMENTATION

Now that you have set your goals, you can implement your plan of action. Interventions to achieve your goals will assist you in establishing discipline and dedication to your professional development. Reflect on the interventions that assisted you in achieving your goal to graduate from your nursing program. Add to those the interventions that assisted you in achieving your new goal derived from the tools you have learned.

Remember to set time aside each day as study time. As a new graduate, your studying will be focused on the common patient problems presented in your work environment. You should also focus on reviewing for the NCLEX-RN examination. Will you take a review course or buy review books? Will you do both? Will you form a study circle, or are you a solitary learner?

?	EXERCISE 17.5

TOOL	MAINTENANCE PLAN

Your interventions will be unique for you. However, certain common interventions can be helpful in your role transition. Because learning is better when it has direct application or when it will be used soon after it has taken place, one intervention is to request a patient assignment that complements your area of need. You will learn more about complications of hypertension, for example, if you take a patient with hypertension than if you just read about one. Another way to enhance your knowledge base is to ask your mentor or preceptor questions that help you understand how he or she arrived at a conclusion or decision.

It will be important for you to communicate with your nurse manager or director when your role changes from LPN/LVN to RN. It may be the case that your manager may expect more from you because you were previously a proficient LPN/LVN. However, take the opportunity to remind him or her that as you begin your new role as an RN, you are a novice and wish to be treated like any other new graduate RN. Studies have found that this understanding between manager and new graduate is crucial in supporting you in your period of transition from one role to another (Goodwin-Esola & Gallagher-Ford, 2009; Miller & Leadingham, 2010). Consider including in your routine after-graduation-study, working through patient care scenarios where you first consider what your previous LPN/LVN duties would have been and then envision how your role expands and changes within the scenario as an RN. This may help you more quickly assimilate to your new role (Goodwin-Esola & Gallagher-Ford, 2009).

Recognize that you will need to decide if you are more likely to socialize appropriately into your new role and feel supported if you move to a new division rather than staying on the same unit in which you functioned as a practical/vocational nurse. Perhaps establishing yourself as a new RN graduate in a new environment may allow a more comfortable transition into the RN role. Consider discussing this with a director or mentor.

Your New Tools

In approaching graduation, you bring with you many new tools related to knowledge, skills, and values. List these tools in Exercise 17.5. Cluster these tools into categories, such as those you may use daily, weekly, or occasionally. If you find a tool or skill that you might use infrequently, how will you maintain expertise with it? Competency requires that you maintain currency in all aspects of your job. All aspects of the RN's role must be carried out safely and with the utmost proficiency to ensure patient satisfaction and positive outcomes. For example, if you are called upon to start an intravenous line, your proficiency in doing so will decrease patient stress and minimize risks.

<table>
<tr><td colspan="2">**⟨?⟩ EXERCISE 17.6**</td></tr>
<tr><td>**BARRIERS**</td><td>**PLAN TO MEET AND BREAK BARRIERS**</td></tr>
</table>

BARRIERS	PLAN TO MEET AND BREAK BARRIERS

What's Stopping You?

You have demonstrated commitment in your journey through the educational process. You have learned much along the way and are now ready to begin your new role, but are you truly ready to take on your new role? Have you subconsciously or even consciously set up barriers that keep you from moving into your new role?

Change can provoke anxiety, especially at the initiation of a whole new direction in life. Within your nursing program, you have been guided and had a safety net. Now you are going to be making decisions on your own, with patients and a team depending on you. You will be required to manage care based on the soundness of your knowledge and skills. This alone could be a source of anxiety and could give you pause. Yet, keep in mind the "gifts" you have gained, the knowledge and the tools you have. This will assist you in gaining confidence. In Exercise 17.6, list the barriers you have identified that may be keeping you from doing your best. Next to each, state what you can do to break through the barrier.

Confidence will come with experience. You must overcome the urge to resist change and continue in the more comfortable role of the LPN/LVN. An RN who is not accepting the need to change is placing patients at risk. You have learned that the RN is an advocate for patients and, as an advocate, you must know how to make decisions that are sound and safe.

In your role as an LPN/LVN, you have had to rely on the RN to make patient care decisions. You may have known an RN who made poor decisions and many more who made correct decisions. As an LPN/LVN, you may even have believed that you could have solved a problem better than the RN. Now you have the power and the responsibility to make these decisions. What image do you want to project to the LPN/LVN who will be working with you?

EVALUATION

Until now, you have assessed your readiness, what you have learned, and how your philosophy has changed. Now it is up to you to evaluate the effectiveness of your efforts to become an RN. You have many ways in which to evaluate yourself. You can take an emotional inventory, asking during your orientation period whether you are ready to accept the emotional roller-coaster ride associated with the RN role. You may need to do a confidence inventory as well. How confident

? EXERCISE 17.7

On a piece of paper—heavy, colored construction paper if you choose—trace your right or left hand, and then cut around the tracing. Now decorate the cutout hand with encouraging words or phrases or bright and cheerful pictures. When you are satisfied with your creation, take the hand and mount it on the jamb of a door through which you will go at the beginning of every day and at the end of the day. Each time you pass the hand, give yourself a pat on the back and say to yourself, "I did a good job today" or "I am doing a good job and deserve to tell myself so." No matter how tough a day you've had, you should commend yourself and recognize the positive parts of your day. For each of the self-improvements you plan to make, find at least one strength or strategy that will get you there.

are you? You have acquired the tools necessary; now it is up to you to say, "I can do the job." Confidence will come with experience and with an established support system, such as a mentor, your family, or another significant person. Take a moment to complete Exercise 17.7, a tool that will help you make the transition to the RN role.

KEY POINTS

After completion of this chapter, you have learned:
- To evaluate your journey through the transition from LPN/LVN to RN. You were asked to reflect on your journey as a means to identify your philosophy of nursing as an RN.
- To apply the nursing process to your own transition into your new role.
- Socialization into your new role may require careful mentoring and an important conversation with your manager or director.
- As you journey through the rest of your RN career, your philosophy of nursing will likely evolve. Embrace the possibilities that a career in nursing, a life of nursing, has to offer, and do what you are called to do.

▌ CRITICAL THINKING QUESTIONS

1. Now you can develop your own critical thinking questions. Begin with a case scenario from your clinical experience. Consider the signs and symptoms and disease process. What assessments do you need to make? Develop a plan of care and make a prediction as to when your patient should reach the intended outcomes. Evaluate the effectiveness of the plan and explain the reasons for the outcomes that actually occurred. How is your role as an RN now different from what it was as an LPN/LVN in the same scenario?
2. Create a concept map, reflecting on your journey to this point considering what lies ahead. Run through the nursing process and create a diagram of your self-care plan.

CASE STUDY 1

Laurie is graduating from nursing school next month. As she prepares for graduation, she reflects on her experiences during nursing school. She remembers her fundamentals class; she was so nervous during her first nursing assessment that she fumbled with the blood pressure cuff and had it upside down. Smiling, she remembers how her patient patted her arm and told her she was doing fine. Laurie recalls holding a family member's hand while a patient passed away, feeling inadequate to handle the situation, but feeling powerful in that the family wanted her to stay with them. Then there was the pediatric rotation with that young boy who fell out of the tree and broke his arm. The babysitter heard him fall and called 911. During her assessment, Laurie found bruises all over his body and showed the nurse. She became sad as she recalled that when social services finished with the case, the babysitter was charged with abuse.

Laurie remembered how she ambulated dozens of patients miles and miles around the various nursing units. One patient asked questions about his newly diagnosed diabetes, and Laurie's mind froze. She felt embarrassed and humiliated that she couldn't respond to his inquiries quickly. Based on the interaction, Laurie created an educational plan for the patient, but when she arrived at the patient's room she found his wife and sister at the bedside. Again, she froze, but the family was kind and wanted to participate in the teaching. When she discussed the event during post conference, her classmates agreed with her teaching plan and discussed their fears about their own knowledge base of nursing. Her classmates supported her, validating her feelings and suggesting methods to overcome the fear associated with teaching. Finally, Laurie remembered her final medical–surgical rotations. She laughed as she recalled her horror over an assignment of three patients during the clinical rotation. With guidance from her clinical instructor, she managed and coordinated the care of the patients.

A. Describe how Laurie demonstrated evidence of the following roles of the traditional nurse.

WEB RESOURCES

Article: Teaching Critical Reflection, http://inspiredliving.com/business/reflection.htm

Article: Reflective thinking in clinical nursing education: a concept analysis, http://ncbi.nlm.nih.gov/pubmed/15712824

REFERENCES

Brown, S. C., & Gillis, M. A. (1999). Using reflective thinking to develop personal professional philosophies. *Journal of Nursing Education, 38*(4), 171–175.

Del Bueno, D. J. (2000). *A model for competence and success. Presentation at Northeast Baptist Hospital.* San Antonio: TX.

Goodwin-Esola, M., & Gallagher-Ford, L. (2009). Licensed practical nurse to registered nurse transition: developing a tailored orientation. *Journal for Nurses in Staff Development, 25*(5), E8–E12.

Miller, C. L., & Leadingham, C. (2010). A formalized mentoring program for LPN-to-RN students. *Teaching and Learning in Nursing, 5*, 149–153.

Orem, D. E. (2001). *Nursing: concepts of practice* (6th ed.). St. Louis, MO: Mosby.

CHAPTER 18

Passing the NCLEX-RN®

⊖volve WEBSITE

Additional resources are available online at:
http://evolve.elsevier.com/Claywell/transitions

OBJECTIVES

After completing this chapter, the student will be prepared to:
1. Discuss the development of the NCLEX-RN®.
2. Compare the differences between the NCLEX-RN® and the NCLEX-PN®.
3. Apply evidence-based strategies to achieve NCLEX-RN® success.

KEY TERMS

ANA	KATTS	test plan
CAT	NCSBN	the Five C's
estimated ability	question drill	

| OVERVIEW

As licensed practical or vocational nurses, you have already demonstrated your ability to take and pass a national licensing examination. Depending on how long it has been since you took and passed the examination, you may be surprised by how it has changed over the years. You may also be surprised to find that the Practical Nursing examination is actually quite different with regard to the levels and types of questions you will be asked. This chapter covers the development of the National Council Licensure Examination for Registered Nurses (NCLEX-RN®) examination and how it has changed over time. It will point out the differences between the Practical Nurse (PN) and Registered Nurse (RN) examinations. Finally, this chapter discusses the strategies you might use in order to improve your chances of success. The reason this chapter is important now, as you are just beginning your RN program, is that it is important to "begin with the end in mind" and to be able to envision what you will experience both along the way and at the end when the NCLEX-RN® is all that stands between you and this important professional move. This learning about the examination now is a proactive way to consciously prepare for it every day between now and then (stephencovey.com, n.d.).

EVOLUTION OF THE NCLEX-RN® EXAM

The American Nurses Association (**ANA**) began as and still is the organization representing and advocating for nurses. Its Council of State Boards of Nursing was responsible for the regulation and licensing of members of the profession. However, in 1978, the organization came to realize that carrying out both advocacy for and regulation of the profession may present a conflict of interest, and thus the National Council of State Boards of Nursing (**NCSBN**) was spun off as a separate organization with the charge to protect the public interest by ensuring that all nurses entering the profession have demonstrated knowledge and skills at a standard minimum level required for safe and effective practice as a newly licensed, entry-level nurse. The NCSBN continues to fulfill its charge to maintain the minimum standard for practice, continually evaluating and updating the examinations based on research regarding current nursing practice and the current practice environments (NCSBN).

From its inception until the mid-1990s, the NCLEX® examination was administered to large groups on a regional basis, in paper and pencil format. The testing center was often in a university and may have been far enough away to require a hotel stay overnight after a long drive. The test took up to 2 days to complete and was proctored closely by pacing officials. The waiting, both for test day to arrive and afterward for the results, could take weeks or months. The anxiety surrounding the situation could be dreadful. However, the testing experience began to change dramatically with the advent of Computer Adaptive Testing (CAT).

CAT

With **CAT,** students choose the times, dates, and testing centers that meet their needs. In 1994, the NCSBN instituted the use of CAT because it reliably estimates each test-taker's ability related to nursing knowledge and skills at the level of entry to the profession. In CAT, the student's answer to each question determines whether the next question will be easier or more difficult. Wrong answers prompt an easier question; correct answers prompt a more difficult next question. Every time you answer a question, the computer recalculates your **estimated ability** based on all of the questions answered to that point. The process continues with each question answered, until the computer has enough information to determine whether or not your ability meets the passing standard (NCSBN, 2016).

There are three means by which the computer can determine your pass or fail status. The first and most ordinarily applied rule is that the computer will continue to test you until it determines with 95% confidence that your ability either surpasses or does not meet the minimum passing standard. The second rule that may be applied is related to the length of the test. If by the 265th question, the computer has not been able to determine within 95% confidence that you have either surpassed or are clearly below the passing standard (in other words, you are right on the borderline), the computer will then estimate your ability. In this situation, meeting the standard is not considered passing; you must exceed the standard to pass. The third rule the computer uses to determine whether you have passed or failed the examination is the time limit. If you run out of time before you have completed at least 75 questions, the computer will determine that you have failed. If you have answered at least 75 questions, the computer will evaluate the last 60 ability calculations, and as long as each and every one exceeds the minimum passing standard, the computer will determine that you have passed. As you can see, this process is very complicated. Students may either pass or fail after answering 75 or up to 265 questions. Therefore, it is very difficult for the student to know the pass/fail status immediately following the test based only on the number of questions answered. Rigorous testing has concluded that the CAT is both reliable and valid, and the NCSBN continues to evaluate and make improvements over time (NCSBN, 2016).

In addition to consistently evaluating the testing process, the NCSBN also assesses and, from time to time, adjusts the minimum passing standard for the examinations. The passing standard was increased in 2010, in association with a change in the blueprint, or test plan, for the NCLEX-RN®. By the writing of this text, the last PN passing standard and test plan adjustments were implemented in 2011 (NCSBN, 2016). The current passing standard for the NCLEX-RN® remains unchanged and will remain so until at least March of 2019.

NCLEX TEST PLAN

The NCSBN engages in regular (every 3 years) practice analysis to determine the expectations of a newly licensed, entry-level nurse. Nursing care activities are analyzed in relation to the frequency of performance, impact on maintaining patient safety, and patient care settings where the activities are performed. As a result of these studies, officials can determine the foundational concepts, principles, and practices for which to assess in those seeking licensure. New items are continually tested and added to the exam, ensuring a reliably updated pool of questions. Items are written by experienced educators and practicing nurses who have been recruited and provided experiential opportunities in item writing and reviewing skills in order to maintain the rigorous standards adopted by the organization.

One such standard is the use of Bloom's taxonomy. The cognitive domain is used as a basis for writing and coding items for the examination. The NCLEX-RN® is composed mostly of items that are considered to assess knowledge, skills, and abilities at the application, analysis, synthesis, and evaluation levels within Bloom's taxonomy. The NCLEX-PN® has the majority of its items at levels up to and including analysis, with an emphasis on comprehension. In addition to the use of Bloom's taxonomy, the NCLEX exam uses Client Needs as its organizing framework, and all questions are organized into one of four primary patient needs categories.

The most recent revisions to the NCLEX-RN® **test plan** were effective as of April 2016; these revisions were a result of the 2014 analysis of 12,000 new RNs. Most items are at the application and higher levels. This test plan outlines four main categories of testing: Safe and Effective Care Environment, Health Promotion and Maintenance, Psychosocial Integrity, and Physiological Integrity. Safe, Effective Care Environment includes the subcategories of Management of Care and Safety and Infection Control; Physiological Integrity includes the subcategories of Basic Care and Comfort, Pharmacological and Parenteral Therapies, Reduction of Risk Potential, and Physiological Adaptation. Each category and subcategory have been assigned certain percentages of test questions that will be on the NCLEX-RN® examination. These categories and subcategories have been assigned the percentages (NCSBN, 2016) listed in Table 18.1.

Content that may be covered in each of the client needs categories is reflected in Box 18.1. It is imperative to familiarize yourself now with what will be on

TABLE 18.1 NCLEX-RN® TEST PLAN CATEGORIES

CLIENT NEEDS	PERCENTAGE OF ITEMS FROM EACH CATEGORY/SUBCATEGORY
Safe and Effective Care Environment	
Management of Care	17%–23%
Safety and Infection Control	9%–15%
Health Promotion and Maintenance	6%–12%
Psychosocial Integrity	6%–12%
Physiological Integrity	
Basic Care and Comfort	6%–12%
Pharmacological and Parenteral Therapies	12%–18%
Reduction of Risk Potential	9%–15%
Physiological Adaptation	11%–17%

From NCSBN, NCLEX-RN® Test Plan, 2016, p. 5.

BOX 18.1 CLIENT NEEDS CATEGORIES

Safe and Effective Care Environment
Management of Care
- Advance Directives
- Advocacy
- Assignment, Delegation, and Supervision
- Case Management
- Client Rights
- Collaboration with Interdisciplinary Team
- Concepts of Management

- Confidentiality/Information Security
- Continuity of Care
- Establishing Priorities
- Ethical Practice
- Informed Consent
- Information Technology
- Legal Rights and Responsibilities
- Performance Improvement (Quality Improvement)
- Referrals

Continued

BOX 18.1   CLIENT NEEDS CATEGORIES—cont'd

Safety and Infection Control
- Accident/Error/Injury Prevention
- Emergency Response Plan
- Ergonomic Principles
- Handling Hazardous and Infectious Materials
- Home Safety
- Reporting of Incident/Event/Irregular Occurrence/Variance
- Safe Use of Equipment
- Security Plan
- Standard Precautions/Transmission-Based Precautions/Surgical Asepsis
- Use of Restraints/Safety Devices

Health Promotion and Maintenance
- Aging Process
- Ante/Intra/Postpartum and Newborn Care
- Developmental Stages and Transitions
- Health Promotion/Disease Prevention
- Health Screening
- High-Risk Behaviors
- Lifestyle Choices
- Self-Care
- Techniques of Physical Assessment

Psychosocial Integrity
- Abuse/Neglect
- Behavioral Interventions
- Chemical and Other Dependencies
- Substance Use Disorder
- Coping Mechanisms
- Crisis Intervention
- Cultural Awareness/Cultural Influences on Health
- End-of-Life Care
- Family Dynamics
- Grief and Loss
- Mental Health Concepts
- Religious and Spiritual Influences on Health
- Sensory/Perceptual Alterations
- Stress Management
- Support Systems
- Therapeutic Communication
- Therapeutic Environment

Physiological Integrity
Basic Care and Comfort
- Assistive Devices
- Elimination
- Mobility/Immobility
- Nonpharmacological Comfort Interventions
- Nutrition and Oral Hydration
- Personal Hygiene
- Rest and Sleep

Pharmacological and Parenteral Therapies
- Adverse Effects/Contraindications/Side Effects/Interactions
- Blood and Blood Products
- Central Venous Access Devices
- Dosage Calculation
- Expected Actions/Outcomes
- Medication Administration
- Parenteral/Intravenous Therapies
- Pharmacological Pain Management
- Total Parenteral Nutrition

Reduction of Risk
- Changes/Abnormalities in Vital Signs
- Diagnostic Tests
- Laboratory Values
- Potential for Alterations in Body Systems
- Potential for Complications of Diagnostic Tests/Treatments/Procedures
- Potential for Complications from Surgical Procedures and Health Alterations
- System Specific Assessments
- Therapeutic Procedures

Physiological Adaptation
- Alterations in Body Systems
- Fluid and Electrolyte Imbalances
- Hemodynamics
- Illness Management
- Medical Emergencies
- Pathophysiology
- Unexpected Response to Therapies

From NCSBN, NCLEX-RN® Detailed Test Plan, 2016, pp. 6-8.

the test plan in order to optimize and focus your learning throughout the program. You are encouraged to access the latest detailed test plan online at http://www.ncsbn.org. To further improve your chances of success on your first attempt to pass the NCLEX-RN®, it will help you to understand and practice with the different types of items that will be included on the exam. The candidate version of the NCLEX-RN® test plan can be accessed at https://www.ncsbn.org/2016_RN_Test_Plan_Candidate.pdf.

NCLEX-RN® STYLE TEST ITEMS

Each candidate's examination is unique; however, it primarily consists of four-option multiple-choice questions, which include single- and multiple-response items (Fig. 18.1). The exam may also include fill-in-the-blank (Fig. 18.2); completing calculations; or using/analyzing exhibits, pictures, tables, or graphs. You may also be asked to click on a certain area on an image to indicate your answer; these are called "hot spot" items (Fig. 18.3). You may also be required to drag and drop items from one location to another on a screen indicating ordering or prioritizing (Fig. 18.4) (NCSBN, 2016).

It may be helpful to obtain an NCLEX-RN® review manual now to begin practicing with NCLEX-RN® style questions as you progress in your program; in addition, there are evidence-based strategies you can use that will help you improve your testing performance.

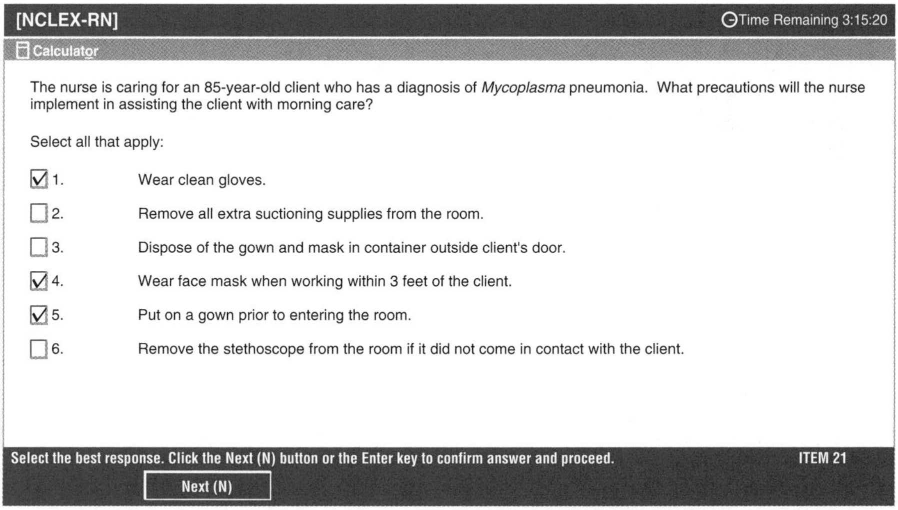

Answer: The answer is based on standard precautions, plus respiratory precautions for the pneumonia. Nothing should be removed from the room and the gown should be removed prior to leaving the room, not outside the room.

FIG. 18.1 Multiple response. (From Zerwekh, J & Garneau, A Z. (2018). *Nursing today: transitions and trends* (9th ed.). St. Louis: Elsevier.)

[NCLEX-RN]   ⏱Time Remaining 2:25:30

🖩 Calculator

A client is receiving IV antibiotic therapy. The order is for methicillin 750 mg IV. The nurse has a vial on hand that contains 1 g. The instructions for reconstitution say to add 1.5 mL sterile water. Reconstituted solution will contain 500 mg methicillin per milliliter. How much will the nurse give?

Answer: | 1.5 | mL

Enter the correct answer. Click the Next (N) button or the Enter key to confirm answer and proceed.   ITEM 20

Next (N)

Answer - 1.5 mL
Rationale: 500 mg: 1 mL :: 750 mg: x
Formula: 500 × X = 500X
1 × 750 = 750
X = 750/500 = 1.5
The dosage calculation cannot be made from the amount of solution added to the vial. The ratio of mg per mL after reconstitution is 500 mg per mL.

FIG. 18.2 Fill-in-the-blank. (From Zerwekh, J & Garneau, A Z. (2018). *Nursing today: transitions and trends* (9th ed.). St. Louis: Elsevier.)

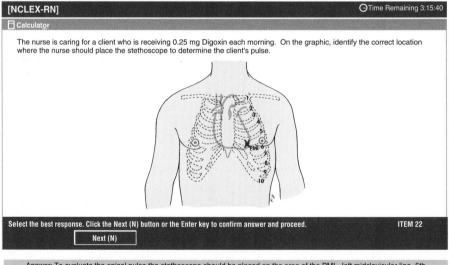

[NCLEX-RN]   ⊖Time Remaining 3:15:40

🖩 Calculator

The nurse is caring for a client who is receiving 0.25 mg Digoxin each morning. On the graphic, identify the correct location where the nurse should place the stethoscope to determine the client's pulse.

Select the best response. Click the Next (N) button or the Enter key to confirm answer and proceed.   ITEM 22

Next (N)

Answer: To evaluate the apical pulse the stethoscope should be placed on the area of the PMI - left midclavicular line, 5th intercostal space. To answer this question, you would simply click the area on the graphic. The correct location is noted in the figure.

FIG. 18.3 Hot spot. (From Zerwekh, J & Garneau, A Z. (2018). *Nursing today: transitions and trends* (9th ed.). St. Louis: Elsevier.)

```
[NCLEX-RN]                                                    ⊘Time Remaining 2:15:20
 ▯ Calculator
    The nurse is caring for a client with pneumonia.  He is dyspneic, his temperature is 102° orally, and he is complaining of
    chest pain. In what order would the nurse provide care for this client?

    Place all of the actions below in the order of priority for nursing care.  Use all of the options.

    Unordered options:                              Ordered Response:

    ⟮Encourage clear fluids            ⟯            ⟮Place in Semi-Fowler's position    ⟯
    ⟮Administer humidified oxygen      ⟯            ⟮Administer humidified oxygen       ⟯
    ⟮Place in Semi-Fowler's position   ⟯            ⟮                                   ⟯
    ⟮Administer antipyretic medication ⟯            ⟮                                   ⟯
    ⟮Instruct client regarding risk factors⟯        ⟮                                   ⟯



 Select the best response. Click the Next (N) button or the Enter key to confirm answer and proceed.        ITEM 23
            Next (N)
```

Need to know: Review each of the items in the list. Determine what is the most important action to take first, then second, etc. This question is asking you to provide care for a client who is experiencing difficulty breathing and has chest pain. The dyspnea and chest pain are most likely a result of the client's pneumonia. Position is the first thing that you can do that will benefit the client the most, then begin the oxygen, administer the antipyretic medication, encourage clear liquids, and teaching is last. Remember Maslow when setting priorities.

FIG. 18.4 Drag and drop (ordered response). (From Zerwekh, J & Garneau, A Z. (2018). *Nursing today: transitions and trends* (9th ed.). St. Louis: Elsevier.)

EVIDENCE-BASED STRATEGIES FOR TESTING SUCCESS

Think back to how you prepared for the NCLEX-PN® examination. Did you study notes and textbooks as you might have for tests in school? Did you attend a structured NCLEX-PN® review program or use NCLEX prep books? Perhaps you used a combination of these? When did you begin the process of review and preparation for the examination? Did you wait until after graduation, or did you begin while still in school? Often students wait until after graduation and then try to study notes and textbooks as they might for a content test in school. Preparation for passing the NCLEX-RN® should begin right now, at the beginning of your bridge program, and should include a range of testing strategies. The difference between school examinations and the RN licensure examination is that the RN exam tests critical and higher thinking skills, going beyond the recall and recognition of knowledge. Therefore, your preparation for passing the NCLEX-RN® should include not only a deep review of content-specific information but also practice with completing the multiple forms of test item types found on the NCLEX-RN®. There are both paid and free resources for NCLEX-RN® test preparation and both are recommended. Khan Academy has free practice questions and even videos for content review and can be accessed at https://www.khanacademy.org/test-prep/nclex-rn. Kaplan Nursing has paid NCLEX-RN® review courses and online practice tests as well as free practice questions and review available and can be accessed at https://www.kaptest.com/nursing/nclex-prep. There are numerous books with companion websites, and these are highly recommended. It is important to practice in the manner in which the test is given in order to prepare for the experience. In addition to practice, there are models and frameworks you can use to help you learn the best way to approach a test such as the NCLEX-RN®.

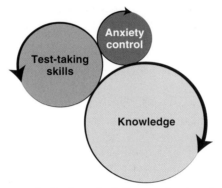

FIG. 18.5 KATTS framework. Each part of the mechanism is of equal importance; issues in one component will necessarily impact the others.

Your experience with the NCLEX-PN® should give you the advantage of having taken a similar test in the past.

KATTS FRAMEWORK

According to McDowell (2008), the factors that lead to passing the NCLEX-RN® exam can be categorized in two ways: academic and nonacademic. Academic factors are things such as cumulative grade point average, grades in science and nursing science classes, end-of-course standardized exams, and standardized, comprehensive end-of-program exams. Nonacademic factors include such things as test anxiety, self-esteem, fatigue, role strain, and responsibilities outside of being a student, such as work and family (McDowell, 2008; Thomas & Baker, 2011). The best review programs will incorporate materials and activities that address both academic and nonacademic factors.

The knowledge base, anxiety control, and test-taking strategy (**KATTS**) framework was developed in the 1990s as a test-taking theory to help students who were struggling with poor performance on tests. KATTS focuses on three primary components, each of equal importance: **k**nowledge base, **a**nxiety control, and **t**est-**t**aking **s**kills (McDowell, 2008). There are several activities that a student (with the help of a faculty advisor) can do to strengthen the knowledge components of the framework. Compile the results of any and all end-of-course and end-of-program standardized tests into a table, and compare with the current test plan for the NCLEX-RN®. Note any areas of deficit that are identified and formulate a study plan to address the gaps. Then, based on this study plan, seek test banks that allow selection of content areas of focus and practice specific content-area tests. Complete any NCLEX-RN® pretests that are available. Practicing taking the tests will also help to reduce the anxiety related to taking tests, but there are more specific strategies you can use to help actively control your anxiety level before and at test time (McDowell, 2008) (Fig. 18.5).

It's been said that attitude is everything, and having a positive attitude and believing that you will earn your RN designation by passing the NCLEX-RN® test are critical! Practicing self-care activities such as eating a balanced diet, getting adequate sleep, and exercising will help you maintain your feeling of well-being. Try to study both alone and with groups. The social nature of the group study may help to relieve tension, and the focused study will help you practice concentration. Complete a dry run through the pretesting activities that includes going to the testing center to familiarize yourself with its location, parking, and traffic. If a hotel stay is required near the testing center, be sure to arrive early the day before in order to allow time to relax and find the test location in relation to the hotel. At test time, use relaxation techniques such as meditation to find a sense of calm.

The well-practiced test-taker will have reduced anxiety when it comes time to take the test. Practicing with NCLEX-RN® style test questions is critical, but the KATTS framework suggests that multiple-question drill sets will improve your overall ability to take tests. A **question drill** means to complete at least 50 questions in 1 hour and then working up to 100 questions in 2 hours. The drill set includes checking your answers and then analyzing the results, looking for gaps in your knowledge and then adding the gap content to your personal study plan. Be certain that you understand the rationale for both the correct and incorrect answers. KATTS further guides students to complete 1 hour of focus content review for every 2 to 3 hours of question drill time. Ultimately, you should complete upward of 2500 NCLEX-RN®–style questions (McDowell, 2008) in preparation for taking the test. This process has to be started early and cannot wait until after graduation.

Another characteristic that can be practiced has to do with pacing during testing. Question drill can help in this area as well, in that the student can learn to be aware of his or her pace throughout the exam. In a study completed by Thomas and Baker (2011), it was found that while all study participants experienced a slowing of their pace as the test progressed, those who passed the test at 75 questions had a much quicker item response time than those who clearly did not pass at 75 questions. This finding is significant for you in that it emphasizes the need to practice being aware of time as you take tests in school and as you practice for the NCLEX-RN®.

THE FIVE C'S

Another model that can help you with the majority of the items on the NCLEX-RN® is called the **5 Cs** (Rollant, 2007) (Fig. 18.6). Each component of this model

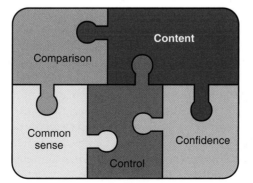

FIG. 18.6 The 5 Cs. Each component is important to creating a holistic approach to test success.

is interrelated with the others. That means the fluctuation of one component can affect all the others. The 5 C's are content, confidence, control, common sense, and comparison. The content component means that you must know the content; specific, focused study of the content is important. Confidence relates to your ability to say, "I know this and I can do this. I can figure it out." Control means being able to control the tension that will inevitably build as the test goes on. That is, toward the end of the test, even though you are tired, you are steady, not rushing, not giving up, but remaining positive. Common sense means to ask yourself what your intuition tells you might be the right answer. Finally, comparison means to narrow down the choices and then compare the last two possibilities before confirming your answer. This model is a practical guide for producing successful outcomes on tests throughout nursing school as well as on the NCLEX-RN®.

KEY POINTS

After completion of this chapter, you learned the following about the NCLEX-RN®:
- Originally it was the ANA that first advocated for and regulated/licensed nurses.
- In 1978, the NCSBN was formed out of the ANA as a separate organization to license nurses.
- The NCLEX examination was originally paper and pencil but in 1994 was changed to CAT.
- CAT is both a reliable and valid means of testing for entry-level nurse competency.
- CAT adjusts the level of difficulty of each question based on the accuracy of the previous answer.
- CAT calculates your estimated ability with each question answered.
- CAT uses a 95% confidence interval for determining the minimum passing standard for competency.
- The NCLEX-RN® test plan is updated every 3 years based on the findings of the RN Practice Analysis: Linking the NCLEX-RN® Examination to Practice. The NCLEX-RN® test items are written by expert educators and practicing nurses with additional training.
- The NCLEX-RN® test plan has four main content categories for testing: Safe and Effective Care Environment; Health Promotion and Maintenance; Psychosocial Integrity; and Physiological Integrity.
- The NCLEX-RN® may contain several forms of test items, including multiple choice, multiple response, fill-in-the-blank, calculations, and analysis of exhibits, pictures, graphs, or tables.
- It is best to begin to prepare for the NCLEX-RN® now, at the beginning of your program.
- Using the KATTS framework can help you prepare for and pass the NCLEX-RN® examination.
- You should engage in 2 to 3 hours of question drill for every one hour of focused content study.
- You should complete a minimum of 2500 NCLEX-RN®–style questions as part of your comprehensive preparation plan.

CRITICAL THINKING QUESTIONS

1. You are preparing for a final examination in a medical–surgical class. The test will consist of simple multiple-choice and multiple-select type questions. Explain how you might approach this exam using the 5 C's approach.
2. You have been cleared to take the NCLEX-RN® examination. How would you apply the KATTS framework in your preparation for the exam? Include at least three strategies in your response.

CASE STUDY

Carol just finished taking the NCLEX-RN® exam. One of the questions involved evaluating the outcomes from a nursing intervention. She recalled a similar experience from her position as a nursing assistant and how the nurse, who had six patients that day, performed the procedure in a way different from what Carol learned in school but with the same outcome. Carol answered the question based on this experience. The next question concerned delegating to a nursing assistant. Carol felt confident, knowing that she was an excellent nursing assistant and that her nurse delegated many tasks to her, especially complicated dressing changes and treatments. The subsequent question asked about the nursing care priority for a patient complaining of a new headache. Carol selected the response that involved completing a nursing intervention because she thought that turning off the lights would be more important than performing a nursing assessment.

A. Explain why Carol's dependence on her experiences from working as a nursing assistant might hinder her from responding appropriately to the first NCLEX question.
B. What error in judgment did Carol make in responding to the question concerning delegation?
C. How should Carol have responded to the question concerning the nursing priority for a patient with new onset of a headache?

WEB RESOURCES

National Council of State Boards of Nursing found at https://www.ncsbn.org/index.htm
NCSBN Learning Extension at http://learningext.com/
HESI/Saunders Online Review for the NCLEX-RN Examination at http://us.elsevier health.com/product.jsp?isbn=9781437706949
Test Prep Review at http://testprepreview.com/nclex_practice.htm
2016 NCLEX-RN test plan https://www.ncsbn.org/2016_RN_Test_Plan_Candidate.pdf
Khan Academy NCLEX-RN Practice https://www.khanacademy.org/test-prep/nclex-rn
Kaplan Nursing https://www.kaptest.com/nursing/nclex-prep

REFERENCES

McDowell, B. M. (2008). KATTS: a framework for maximizing NCLEX-RN performance. *Journal of Nursing Education, 47*(4), 183–186.

National Council of State Boards of Nursing [NCSBN]. (2016). *NCLEX-RN examination: Detailed test plan for the National Council Licensure Examination for Registered Nurses: Candidate Version.* Retrieved from https://www.ncsbn.org/2016_RN_Test_Plan_Candidate .pdf.

Rollant, P. D. (2007). How can I fail the NCLEX-RN with a 3.5 GPA? Approaches to help this high-risk group. In M. Oermann, & K. Heinrich (Eds.), *Annual review of nursing education volume 5, 2007: challenges and new directions in nursing education* (pp. 259–273). New York, NY: Springer Publishing.

Stephencovey.com. (n.d.) *Habit 2.* Retrieved from https://www.stephencovey.com/7habits/7h abits-habit2.php.

Thomas, M. H., & Baker, S. S. (2011). NCLEX-RN success: evidence-based strategies. *Nurse Educator, 36*(6), 246–249.

Basic Math Review: Preparing for Medication Calculations

⊖volve WEBSITE

Additional resources are available online at:
http://evolve.elsevier.com/Claywell/transitions

OVERVIEW

This appendix reintroduces some basic math functions encountered on a daily basis by most practicing nurses. Fractions, ratios, and proportions are examined and applied. Equivalent conversions among the metric, household, and apothecary systems of measurement are crucial concepts to practice. You will learn about the ratio and proportion method, the formula method, and the dimensional analysis (factor labeling) method of calculating medication dosages. Basic intravenous therapy calculations are also presented.

PREPARING FOR CALCULATIONS: BASIC MATH REVIEW

Fractions

A fraction is a common way of showing a number divided into equal portions. It is made up of two parts, the numerator and the denominator, separated by a line.

The **numerator** is the top number when a fraction's dividing line is horizontal, the left number when the line is a slash. It represents how many portions of the whole are represented. The **denominator,** the bottom or right number, gives the total number of equal portions. In other words, the denominator represents how many parts the whole has been divided into. Thinking of the denominator in this way helps you understand the fraction line's function. The fraction line indicates that the top number is divided by the bottom number.

Example: Fig. A.1 shows a whole circle and a circle divided into four sections. In the circle on the right, of ¾ the circle is shaded. The numerator, 3, represents 3 portions of the whole. The denominator, 4, indicates that the circle has 4 equal portions.

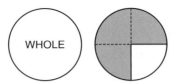

FIG. A.1 A circle as a whole (left) and a circle divided into four equal sections (right).

Reducing Fractions

You may recall the term *reduce* associated with fractions. **Reducing fractions** means finding the smallest numbers that can represent the numerator and denominator without changing the fraction's value. You must be able to divide the same number into both the numerator and the denominator.

Example	Reduce $^{12}\!/_{16}$
Steps	$^{12}\!/_{16}$ can be reduced by dividing both the numerator (12) and denominator (16) by 4
	$12 \div 4 = 3$, and $16 \div 4 = 4$
Solve	The answer is: $^{3}\!/_{4}$

Improper Fractions and Mixed Numbers

An **improper fraction** has a numerator greater than the denominator. When you reduce an improper fraction, the result will be either a whole number or a whole number plus a fraction, which is termed a *mixed fraction,* or *mixed number.*

You often have to change mixed numbers to improper fractions and improper fractions to mixed numbers when solving equations. To change an improper fraction to a mixed number, then vice versa, follow the steps in the following examples.

Example	Change the improper fraction $^{10}\!/_{3}$ to a mixed number
Steps	Divide the denominator into the numerator: $10 \div 3 = 3$, remainder 1
	The mixed number is the whole number, 3, plus the remainder, 1, over the denominator, 3
Solve	The answer is: $3\frac{1}{3}$

Example	Change the mixed number 3 into an improper fraction
Steps	Multiply the denominator by the whole number: $3 \times 3 = 9$
	Add the result to the numerator of the fraction: $9 + 1 = 10$
	Put this result over the denominator of the fraction, 3
Solve	The answer is: $^{10}\!/_{3}$

Lowest Common Denominator

Another function you must master to add and subtract fractions is finding the **lowest common denominator,** which is the lowest number into which all denominators in the problem can be evenly divided. Keep in mind that the lowest common denominator may be one of the denominators presented in the problem. Be careful not to overlook that. See the following examples.

Example	Find the lowest common denominator of ¾ and ⅔
Steps	Ask: Are either of these denominators evenly divisible by the other? No.
	To find the lowest number that is evenly divisible by both denominators, multiply the two denominators: 4 × 3 = 12
Solve	The answer is: 12
	The result of multiplying to find a common denominator can sometimes be reduced. For example, the lowest common denominator of ¼ and ⅙ is not 24; it is 12

Example	Change each fraction (¾ and ⅔) to a fraction of the same value with the lowest common denominator, 12
Steps	Divide the lowest common denominator, 12, by the denominator in the first fraction: 12 ÷ 4 = 3
	Multiply the result by the numerator of the fraction you are converting: 3 × 3 = 9
	Put this result over the lowest common denominator.
Solve	The answer is: 9/12, which is a fraction with equal value to the original fraction, ¾

Follow the same conversion procedure with the second fraction, ⅔. The resulting equivalent fraction with the lowest common denominator is 8/12.

Using a combination of the preceding methods, you are ready to apply such mathematic functions as adding, subtracting, multiplying, and dividing to fractions. Remember that to add and subtract fractions, you must find the lowest common denominator and convert all fractions within the equation to their equivalents.

Adding Fractions

To add fractions, whether simple (a fraction with no associated whole number) or mixed, first find the lowest common denominator and convert the fractions to equivalents. Add the numerators and put the result over that lowest common denominator. Always remember to reduce your answer fraction to its lowest terms.

Example	Solve: $\dfrac{1}{4} + \dfrac{2}{3}$
Steps	Multiply the denominators to find the lowest common denominator, which is 12
	Convert the two fractions so they have the same lowest common denominator:
	$\dfrac{1}{4} = \dfrac{3}{12}$ and $\dfrac{2}{3} = \dfrac{8}{12}$
Solve	Add these two fractions with the same denominator
	Therefore, $\dfrac{3}{12} + \dfrac{8}{12} = \dfrac{11}{12}$
	This answer is already in reduced form. It cannot be converted to an equivalent fraction with lower numbers

Subtracting Fractions

To subtract a fraction, you must also have the lowest common denominator for all the fractions in the equation. Subtract the second numerator from the first and place the result over the lowest common denominator. Then reduce, if applicable.

Example   Subtract $\frac{1}{3}$ from $1\frac{1}{2}$. That is, solve:

$$1\frac{1}{2} - \frac{1}{3}$$

Steps   Change the mixed number into an improper fraction:

$$1\frac{1}{2} = \frac{2}{3}$$

Apply the lowest common denominator, which is 6:

$$\frac{3}{2} = \frac{9}{6} \text{ and } \frac{1}{3} = \frac{2}{6}$$

Solve   Therefore,

$$\frac{9}{6} - \frac{2}{6} = \frac{7}{6}$$

If the final result is an improper fraction, such as this answer of 7/6, for clarity you may want to convert it back to a mixed number:

$$\frac{7}{6} = 1\frac{1}{6}$$

Note: Always use common sense by looking at your derived answer to determine whether it "seems" right. For instance, since we converted the final answer back to a mixed number, it is easy to see that the final answer, 1⅙, is slightly less than the initial larger figure, 1½. While this technique does not prove that your answer is correct, it can point out a glaring mistake.

Multiplying Fractions

When numbers are multiplied by each other, the answer is called the *product.* Multiplying fractions does not require conversion to the lowest common denominator. Follow the steps in the example.

Example   Solve $\frac{3}{4} \times \frac{1}{2}$

Steps   Multiply the numerators: $3 \times 1 = 3$
                   Multiply the denominators: $4 \times 2 = 8$
                   Place the product of the numerators over the product of the denominators

Solve   This answer is: ⅜. Reduce if needed, but ⅜ is already in its lowest terms

Canceling is a process that can make multiplying fractions easier. Canceling reduces each pair of opposite numerators and denominators to their lowest terms.

Example   Solve $\frac{3}{16} \times \frac{4}{6}$

You can multiply the numerators and then the denominators

$$\left(\frac{3}{16} \times \frac{4}{6} = \frac{12}{96} \right),$$

but this answer is awkward.
The following steps can be used instead.

Steps   Cancel the original fractions by reducing each pair of opposite numerators and denominators
                   For the first numerator and the second denominator, reduce each to the lowest common divisor (the lowest common divisor for 3 and 6 is 3)
                   For the second numerator and the first denominator, reduce each to the lowest common divisor (the lowest common divisor for 16 and 4 is 4)
                   The equation now looks like this: $\frac{1}{4} \times \frac{1}{2}$

Solve   The answer is: $\frac{1}{4} \times \frac{1}{2} = \frac{1}{8}$

Dividing Fractions

The trick to dividing fractions correctly is inverting the **divisor,** or the second fraction in the equation. The phrase to remember is "invert and multiply." Follow the steps in the example.

Example	Solve $\dfrac{3}{4} \div \dfrac{1}{2}$
Steps	Invert the divisor, so that $\dfrac{1}{2}$ is written as $\dfrac{2}{1}$
	Multiply the first fraction by the inverted divisor:
	$\dfrac{3}{4} \times \dfrac{2}{1}$
Solve	This answer is: $\dfrac{3}{4} \times \dfrac{2}{1} = \dfrac{6}{4}$
	Reduce: $\dfrac{6}{4} = \dfrac{3}{2} = 1\dfrac{1}{2}$

RATIO AND PROPORTION

A **ratio** is another way to represent a fraction. The ratio 1:10 is the same as $\frac{1}{10}$, which is the same as $1 \div 10$. This ratio is read, "1 to 10."

A **proportion** is an expression with two ratios separated by two colons, as with 3:6::4:8. The proportion is read, "3 is to 6 as 4 is to 8." In the preceding example, the 3 and the 8 are the *extremes,* and the 6 and the 4 are the *means.* This is important to know when you solve proportion problems.

A proportion problem is seen when one of the numbers (one of the means or one of the extremes) in the proportion is unknown, and it is represented by an x. Thus, we can solve for x. Follow the steps in the example to solve for x.

Example	Solve for x in the following proportion problem: 4:12::6:x
Steps	Multiply the means by each other: $12 \times 6 = 72$
	Multiply the extremes by each other: $4 \times x = 4x$
	Put the product with the x on the left and the other product on the right for the new equation, separated by an equals (=) sign: $4x = 72$.
	Divide both sides of the equation by the number associated with x, which is also called isolating the x
Solve	This answer is: $x = 18$
	Replace the x in the proportion with its derived value. The proportion is now: 4:12::6:18. This reads as, "4 is to 12 as 6 is to 18." Each side of the proportion is a ratio equivalent to 1/3.

Conversions of Units of Measurement

One of the most problematic areas for nursing students is converting amounts among the different systems of measurement that are widely used in health care. On any given day, the nurse may have to convert doses from metric and apothecary units to household units to help patients understand their medication doses. The nurse must also calculate amounts of medications to give when they are ordered according to a different measurement system from how they are supplied.

Metric System

The *metric system* is the system of measurement most commonly used in health care settings. Metric amounts are expressed with decimals rather than fractions. Orders of 10 are associated with prefixes appended to unit names. FYI A.1 provides a list of metric measures of weight, volume, and length.

You must memorize the information provided in FYI A.1. There is no alternative or shortcut. To calculate conversions, you can use the ratio and proportion method learned earlier. Later in this appendix, you will also find out how to simplify making conversions when calculating dosages by using dimensional analysis.

Example	Solve 2 g = _____ mg
Steps	Write the equivalent of grams to milligrams as a ratio:
	1 g:1000 mg
	Put the known from the equation in ratio to the unknown:
	2 g:x mg
	Write the two ratios as a proportion: 1 g:1000 mg::2 g:x mg
	Multiply extremes and means
Solve	The answer is: 1x = 2000 mg, or x = 2000 mg

Household Measurements

Household measurements are sometimes seen in acute care settings but are more frequently used in the home and home care settings. To communicate appropriate measurements to patients, who most likely use and understand household measurements, you must be able to convert metric to household and back. FYI A.2 provides a table of conversion of metric measures to household measures.

As with conversions between metrics, you must memorize the information contained in FYI A.2. You can use what you have learned about ratio and proportion to make the conversion in the example below.

Example	Solve 1½ tsp = _____ mL
Steps	Place what we know to be the equivalent for tsp and mL in the
	proportion:
	1 tsp:5 mL
	Combine the known and the unknown from the equation:
	1 tsp:5 mL::1½ tsp:x mL
	Multiply the extremes and the multiply the means: 1x = 5 × 1 1/2
	$$x = \frac{5}{1} \times \frac{3}{2} = \frac{15}{2} = 7\frac{1}{2} \text{ or } 7.5 \text{ mL}$$
Solve	The answer is: 7.5 mL

✏ FYI A.1   METRIC MEASURES OF WEIGHT, VOLUME, AND LENGTH

Weight
1,000,000 micrograms (mcg) = 1 gram (g)
1000 micrograms (mcg) = 1 milligram (mg)
1000 milligrams (mg) = 1 gram (g)
1000 grams (g) = 1 kilogram (kg)

Volume
1000 milliliters (mL) = 1 liter (L)
1000 liters (L) = 1 kiloliter (kL)
1 cubic centimeter (cc) = 1 milliliter (mL)*

Metric Measure of Length
1 meter (m) = 1000 mm = 100 cm
1 centimeter (cm) = 10 mm = 0.01 m
1 millimeter (mm) = 0.1 cm = 0.001 m

*The abbreviations *cc* and *mL* should not be used interchangeably. Milliliters (mL) should be applied only to liquids, whereas cubic centimeters (cc) should be applied only to solids and gases.

✏ FYI A.2   CONVERSION OF METRIC MEASURES TO HOUSEHOLD MEASURES

METRIC MEASURE	HOUSEHOLD MEASURE
1 milliliter (mL)	15 drops (gtt)
5 milliliters (mL)	1 teaspoon (tsp)
15 milliliters (mL)	1 tablespoon (Tbsp)
180 milliliters (mL)	1 cup (c)
240 milliliters (mL)	1 glass
1 kilogram (kg), or 1000 grams (g)	2.2 pounds (lb)
2.5 cm	1 inch

METHODS OF DOSAGE CALCULATIONS

This section discusses the three methods of dosage calculations. All methods can help you correctly solve for accurate medication dosages.

Depending on the area in which you choose to work, you may need to use multiple methods to calculate medication dosages accurately. If you have previously learned a method that consistently gives correct answers, then stick with it. Practice problems and answers for all three methods of calculations are presented at the end of this appendix.

Ratio and Proportion Method

Nurses can use the ratio and proportion method (as just presented) to calculate dosages. You have already learned all the needed steps of this method. The following is an example of using the ratio and proportion method for dosage calculation.

Example	Prescribed: Codeine sulfate 15 mg PO q4h PRN pain Medication on hand: Codeine sulfate 10 mg/tablet How many tablets do you give?
Steps	Set up the proportion: The prescription and unknown is the first ratio (5 mg:*x*) The medication on hand is the second ratio (10 mg:1 tablet) The proportion is: 5 mg:*x*::10 mg:1 tablet Multiply the means by each other: 10 mg × *x* Multiply the extremes by each other: 15 mg × 1 tablet Place the product with the *x* on the left and the other product on the right for the new equation, separated by an equals (=) sign: 10x mg = 15 mg tablets Divide both sides of the equation by the number associated with *x*, which is also called isolating the *x*
Solve	This answer is: *x* = 1½ tablets

FORMULA METHOD

The formula method is another technique that RNs use to calculate medication dosages. If you have not previously tried using the formula method, you may find the following explanation helpful.

The following are two formulas that explain how to use this method of dosage calculation.

Formula 1: $D/A \times Q = x$ Use this formula for medications available as tablets or capsules

This formula is read as: "The desired, or ordered, *dose* (D) over the medication *available* (A) times the *quantity* (Q) of the available dose equals the amount to give, or *x*."

Formula 2: $D/H \times V = x$ Use this formula for medications available in liquid form

This formula is read as: "The desired *dose* (D) over the medication on *hand* (H) times the *volume* (V) of the available dose equals *x*."

To calculate a medication dosage, apply what you have learned about ratio and proportion, along with this formula method, to follow the steps in this example.

Example	*Prescribed:* amoxicillin 250 mg *Medication on hand:* 125 mg/capsule How many capsules do you give?
Steps	Using Formula 1 (medication available as capsule): Place the ordered dose over what is available, or on hand: 250 mg/125 mg Multiply 250 mg by how many capsules provide the amount (125 mg) or 1 capsule 250 mg × 1 capsule 125 mg
Solve	The answer is: *x* = 2 capsules

Many times it will be necessary to convert from household to metric measurement systems. Conversion needs to be done before using either of the formulas presented here. The units of the ordered dose and the on-hand or available dose must match before you try to calculate the dose; otherwise, you will make a critical calculation error. The formula method of dosage calculation will work with basic computations as long as you complete the appropriate conversions first.

DIMENSIONAL ANALYSIS (FACTOR LABELING) METHOD

As you advance in your nursing career, you will find it necessary to calculate dosages and IV rates in more advanced or specialty settings, such as intensive care or pediatrics. Nurses need to learn calculation methods specific to those areas. The third method of dosage calculation presented here can be used in both basic and advanced calculations.

Dimensional Analysis (DA) is especially useful for more complex calculations such as when conversions are required, when an IV-administered medication is ordered by weight, or when a pediatric dose must be verified. These are situations where errors can result because multiple factors are involved and some factors may be overlooked. In DA, you set up calculation problems with an easily mastered method that ensures a correct answer if all needed factors and labels are used.

Performing dosage calculations with DA is an organized method that works because all factors are labeled, and the factors involved are related to each other. It requires you to:

1. Identify the beginning point of the calculation (usually the prescriber's order);
2. Identify the ending point (the label for the specific dosage you seek); and
3. Include all other factors needed (conversion factors, strength/form of the medication that will be administered, patient weight, IV tubing drop factor, etc.) in your problem pathway.

When using the DA method, you build on what you already know about math and calculations (see the Basic Math Review at the start of this appendix). The DA method simplifies the process of converting between household and metric systems, as well as within the metric system, because all conversions are included in each problem pathway. DA works when all the labeled numeric factors and conversion factors are placed in the problem in a way that allows "unwanted" labels to be cancelled from the problem.

It is important not to take shortcuts, such as omitting a factor label, since that can lead to errors. The following examples show why labels must be used.

This math statement is **not true** : $\dfrac{1}{2} = \dfrac{2}{1}$
(no labels used)

This math statement is **true** : $\dfrac{1\ dose}{2\ tablets} = \dfrac{2\ tablets}{1\ dose}$
(read as: "1 dose per 2 tablets equals 2 tablets per 1 dose")

This math statement is **true** : $\dfrac{1\ mg}{2\ mL} = \dfrac{2\ mL}{1\ mg}$
(read as: "1 mg per 2 mL equals 2 mL per 1 mg")

The true statements are true because labels are attached to the numbers (factors). When you use DA, you decide how to express the strength of the medication or the needed conversion factor(s) so that you can cancel labels in the problem pathway. You decide to use "1 mg/2 mL" or "2 mL/1mg." You will see this in the examples that follow.

BASIC DOSAGE CALCULATIONS USING DIMENSIONAL ANALYSIS

Use Steps A through F found in Chart A.1.

I. Basic Calculations When No Conversion Factor Is Needed

Prescribed: Codeine sulfate 15 mg PO q4h PRN pain. *Available:* Codeine sulfate 10 mg/tablet. How much (how many tablets) do you give?

Step A: What did the prescriber order?

$$\frac{15 \text{ mg}}{1 \text{ dose}^*}$$

Step B. What is the available form of the medication to be given/the label of the final answer?

Tablet

Step C. What is the strength (concentration) of the medication on hand?

$$\frac{1 \text{ Tablet}^{**}}{10 \text{ mg}} \quad \text{or} \quad \frac{10 \text{ mg}}{1 \text{ Tablet}}$$

Step D. Conversion factor(s) needed:

No conversions needed

Step E. What is the problem pathway?

TABLE A.1		
STEP A	**STEP C**	**STEP B**
$\dfrac{15 \text{ mg}}{1 \text{ dose}^*}$ $\times$	$\dfrac{1 \text{ Tablet}}{10 \text{ mg}}$ $=$	$\dfrac{\_\_\_\_ \text{ Tablet}}{1 \text{ dose}^*}$

Step F. Solve:

$$\frac{15 \text{ mg}}{1 \text{ dose}^*} \times \frac{1 \text{ Tablet}}{10 \text{ mg}} = \frac{1\frac{1}{2} \text{ Tablet}}{1 \text{ dose}^*}$$

II. Basic Calculations When a Conversion Factor Is Needed

Prescribed for home use: Codeine sulfate 15 mg PO q4h PRN pain. *Available:* Codeine sulfate 10 mg/5 mL solution. How many teaspoons will be given in one dose?

---

*The label "dose" is given to the denominator of the first factor in this method of dosage calculations. It is understood that a "dose" is always what is being calculated, so this label for the first factor in the denominator can be omitted. The label of "dose" will be omitted in future examples.

**The medication strength (concentration) is written as 1 tablet/10 mg to allow you to cancel out the unwanted label (mg) in this denominator with the unwanted label (mg) in the numerator of the prescriber's order. This cancellation would not be possible if the strength was written as 10 mg/1 tablet. This lets you end up with the desired label (tablet/dose) as the only remaining labels on both the left side and right side of your problem pathway.

CHART A.1   BASIC STEPS TO CALCULATE DOSAGES USING DIMENSIONAL ANALYSIS

STEP	TASK	EXAMPLES/EXPLANATION
A	Identify what the prescriber ordered, express it as a whole number with a denominator of 1 (dose).	This is the first factor in calculation (e.g., prescribed: 20 mg PO daily). Write this as 20 mg/1 dose.
B	Identify the form of the dose to be given (the label for this dose) Write this label on the right side of problem pathway.	This is the label of the final answer (what form of medication is on hand/how medication will be administered) PO: mL or tablets or tsp or Tbsp IV: mL/hr or gtt/hr Pediatric dosages: mg/dose
C	Identify the strength of the medication on hand and where to place it in the problem pathway.	Include specifics about the actual medication that is on hand.
D	Include other needed factors for this pathway.	Include conversion factors specific to this problem for the pathway, PRN (e.g., 1 kilogram/2.2 lb) 1 tablet/2 mg 5 mL/1 tsp 1000 mcg/1 mg For IV rates in gtt/min, this includes the tubing drop factor.
E	Set up the problem pathway (make sure that "like"/ unwanted labels can be cancelled between a numerator and a denominator.	Correctly placed pathway will let you cancel out unwanted labels on the left side so that only the label(s) identified for Step B (for the right side of the problem pathway) remain.
F	Solve using basic math principles to perform calculations and reach the numeric value of the dose you seek.	Cancel "like"/unwanted labels between a numerator and a denominator; only the label identified in Step B should remain. Multiply all numerators together. Multiply all denominators together. Divide the product of all numerators by the product of all denominators. You can reduce numeric factors between any numerators and any denominators.

Step A. What did the prescriber order?

$$\frac{15\,mg}{1}$$

Step B. What is the available form of the medication to be given/the label of the final answer?

mL (of liquid medication)

Step C. What is the strength of the medication on hand?

$$\frac{5\ mL^*}{10\ mg} \quad \text{or} \quad \frac{10\ mg}{5\ mL}$$

Step D. Conversion factor(s) needed:

$$\frac{1\,tsp^*}{5\,mL} \quad \text{or} \quad \frac{5\,mL}{1\,tsp}$$

Step E. What is the problem pathway?

TABLE A.2

STEP A		STEP C		STEP D		STEP B
$\dfrac{15\ mg}{1}$	×	$\dfrac{5\ mL}{10\ mg}$	×	$\dfrac{1\ tsp}{5\ mL}$	=	_____ tsp

Step F. Solve:

$$\frac{15\ \cancel{mg}}{1} \times \frac{5\ \cancel{mL}}{10\ \cancel{mg}} \times \frac{1\,tsp}{5\ \cancel{mL}} = 1\tfrac{1}{2}\ tsp$$

III. Basic Calculations of IV Rates Using Dimensional Analysis

When IV therapy is ordered, the nurse must check to make sure all the necessary information is contained in the order, including the kind of fluid and the amount of fluid over a given amount of time. The RN is responsible for ensuring that IV fluid therapy is initiated and maintained in a safe and accurate manner. IV therapy may be delivered by a pump or by using gravity.

A. Calculating simple IV rates in mL/hr

Computerized IV pumps deliver IV fluids that can be set at rates in tenths of a mL/hr.

Format to set up the problem using DA:

Always divide volume in mL by the amount of time for the infusion

$$\frac{\text{Total volume to be infused (VTBI) in mL}}{\text{Total time for infusion in hours}} = \frac{mL}{hr}$$

Example of calculations when no conversion factor is required:

Prescribed : D$_5$½ NS 1000 mL over 10 hours

---

*Medication strength is written as 5 mL/10 mg and the conversion factor is written as 1 tsp/5 mL, to allow you to cancel out the unwanted labels (mg and mL) so that only the label identified in Step B (tsp) will remain.

$$\frac{1000\,mL}{10\,hr} = \frac{100\,mL}{1\,hr}$$

Example of calculations when a conversion factor is required for small volumes TBI in < 1 hr:

Prescribed : D₅½ NS 100 mL over 30 minutes

Steps A through D and Step E (problem pathway):

TABLE A.3

STEP A		STEP D		STEP B
$\dfrac{100\ mL}{30\ min}$	×	$\dfrac{60\ min}{1\ hr}$	=	$\dfrac{mL}{1\ hr}$

Step F. Solve:

$$\frac{100\ mL}{30\ \cancel{min}} \times \frac{60\ \cancel{min}}{1\ hr} = \frac{200\ mL}{1\ hr}$$

By using the following time equivalents (conversion factors) you can eliminate the required conversion (Step D).

$$15\,min = 0.25\ hr$$
$$20\,min = 0.33\ hr$$
$$30\,min = 0.50\ hr$$
$$40\,min = 0.67\ hr$$
$$45\,min = 0.75\ hr$$

Then Steps A through E result in this problem pathway and solution:

$$\frac{100\ mL}{0.5\ hr} = \frac{200\ mL}{1\ hr}$$

   B. Calculating simple IV rates in gtt/min

To initiate IV therapy by gravity you must know the **drop factor**, or established number of drops that the IV set provides to deliver 1 mL of fluid. This drop factor is usually found on the manufacturer's packaging. The two general types of IV sets are macrodrip and microdrip. The macrodrip delivers 10, 15, or 20 drops per mL (gtt/mL), and the microdrip delivers 60 gtt/mL of fluid. Blood administration tubing provides 10 gtt/mL.

The drop factor for the IV tubing must be included in the problem pathway as a conversion factor.

FORMAT TO SET UP THE IV RATE PROBLEM USING DA:

$$\frac{Total\ volume\ TBI\ (mL)}{Total\ time\ TBI\ (hours)} \times \frac{gtt}{mL} \times \frac{1\,hr}{60\,min} = \frac{gtt}{min}$$

EXAMPLE OF CALCULATIONS:

Prescribed: 1 L D$_5$NS with 20 mEq KCl over 10 hours. IV tubing package gives a drop factor of 15 gtt/mL. Steps A through D and Step E (problem pathway):

TABLE A.4

STEP A	STEP D	STEP C	STEP D	STEP B
1 L ×	1000 mL ×	15 gtt ×	1 hr =	_____ gtt
10 hrs	1 L	1 mL	60 min	min

Step F. Solve:

$$\frac{1000\ \text{mL}}{10\ \text{hr}} \times \frac{15\ \text{gtt}}{1\ \text{mL}} \times \frac{1\ \text{hr}}{60\ \text{min}} = \frac{15000}{600} = \frac{25\ \text{gtt}}{1\ \text{min}}$$

ADVANCED STEPS TO CALCULATE DOSAGES USING DIMENSIONAL ANALYSIS

"Advanced" dosages in this section refers to doses requiring more complex calculations. In addition to factors used in basic calculations, the problem pathways incorporate any or all of the following possible factors: patient's weight, time factor, drop factor of IV tubing, metric conversions, and strength/form of medication to administer.

For these calculations, use Steps A through F found in Chart A.2. Also, incorporate the following advanced steps as needed for complex calculations:
- Advanced Dosage Calculations Using Dimensional Analysis
- These steps are used with Steps A through F for Basic Calculations
I. Calculating IV Rates for Medications Ordered by Body Weight
Round final answer to the nearest tenth (0.1). IV pumps can be programmed to tenths, and potent medications must be delivered as exactly as possible.

EXAMPLE OF COMPLEX IV RATE CALCULATIONS:

Prescribed: Dobutrex at 5 mcg/kg/min. Patient weighs 182 lb. *Available:* dobutamine (Dobutrex) 500 mg in a 250 mL bag of D$_5$W. At what rate will you set the IV pump to deliver the medication as prescribed?

Step Pre-A. What is the patient's weight and needed conversion factor?

$$\frac{182\ \text{lb}}{1} \times \frac{1\ \text{kg}}{2.2\ \text{lb}}$$

Step A. What did the prescriber order?

$$\frac{5\ \text{mcg}}{\text{kg/min}}$$

Step B. What is the available form of the medication to be given/the label of the final answer?

$$\text{mL/hr}$$

CHART A.2 ADVANCED STEPS TO CALCULATE DOSAGES USING DIMENSIONAL ANALYSIS

STEP	TASK	EXAMPLE/EXPLANATION
Pre-A	Include weight conversion and/or weight in problem pathway at far left side.	Patient's weight is given in lbs but prescription is for a metric weight (kg). Include this conversion at the start of problem/place before Step A in problem pathway.
A (Use for *complex IV calculations*/ for any prescription with three labels)	Complex IV rate calculation Set up the problem pathway for a prescription labeled with three factors.	For example, prescription is for 5 mcg/kg/min. Place first factor label in numerator. Place second and third factor labels in denominator.
A (Use *to verify a prescribed pediatric dose* as appropriate)	Calculate the low, therapeutic dose and/or the high, safe dose for this medication for this patient Identify what has been determined to be appropriate for pediatric patients	Refer to an approved drug guide for this information—the prescribed dose is not used in these calculations. Once ordered dose has been verified as appropriate, use basic calculation Steps A-F to calculate amount for one dose.
B through F (Use to calculate the pediatric dose to administer)	See Chart 6.1 for tasks.	See Chart 6.1 for explanations.

Step C. What is the strength of the medication on hand?

$$\frac{250\,\text{mL}}{500\,\text{mg}}$$

Step D. Conversion factor(s) needed:

$$\frac{1\,\text{mg}}{1000\,\text{mcg}} \quad\text{and}\quad \frac{60\,\text{min}}{1\,\text{hr}}$$

Step E. What is the problem pathway?

TABLE A.5

STEP PRE-A	STEP A**		STEP C	STEP D	STEP C	STEP B
$\frac{182\,\text{lb} \times 1\,\text{kg}}{1\,2.2\,\text{lb}}$	$\times$	$\frac{5\,\text{mcg}}{\text{kg/min}}$ $\times$	$\frac{1\,\text{mg}}{1000\,\text{mcg}}$ $\times$	$\frac{250\,\text{mL}}{500\,\text{mg}}$ $\times$	$\frac{60\,\text{min}}{1\,\text{hr}}$	= ____ mL/hr

Step F. Solve:

$$\frac{182 \text{ lb}}{1} \times \frac{1 \text{ kg}}{2.2 \text{ lb kg/min}} \times \frac{5 \text{ mcg}}{1000 \text{ mcg}} \times$$

$$\frac{1 \text{ mg}}{500 \text{ mg}} \times \frac{250 \text{ mL}}{1 \text{ hr}} \times \frac{60 \text{ min}}{\text{hr}} = 12.4 \text{ mL}$$

II Verifying and Calculating Pediatric Dosages

The RN must determine that a dose ordered for a pediatric patient is within a safe and therapeutic range prior to giving that dose. A dose is safe and therapeutic if it lies within the range specified for that medication in the drug book used by the facility. The RN shares an equal responsibility with the prescribing health care provider for the administration of a dose which is too high to be safe or too low to be therapeutic.

Safe and therapeutic doses are based on the body weight of the child and are listed in drug guides as mg, mcg, or unit (per kg per day or per kg per dose). This calculation is done to verify appropriate dosing for medications for every pediatric patient. When a prescribed pediatric dose has been verified to be safe and therapeutic, the RN will then use DA to calculate the amount of medication to administer. Answers should be rounded to the nearest tenth (0.1).

EXAMPLE OF VERIFYING A PEDIATRIC MEDICATION ORDER:

Prescribed: Morphine sulfate 4.5 mg IV now. Child weighs 54 lb. Drug guide lists appropriate pediatric dose range: 0.1-0.2 mg/kg/dose.

A. Calculate the lowest/therapeutic (effective) dose for this patient

Step Pre-A. What is the patient's weight and needed conversion factor?

$$\frac{54 \text{ lb} \times 1 \text{ kg}}{1 \ 2.2 \text{ lb}}$$

Step A. What is the low end of the appropriate pediatric dosing range?

0.1 mg/kg/dose

Step B. What is the label of the final answer of this calculation?

mg/dose

Step C. What is the strength of the medication on hand?
This step is not needed for this calculation
Step D. Conversion factor(s) needed:
No conversions needed
Step E. What is the problem pathway?

TABLE A.6

STEP PRE-A		STEP A		STEP B
54 lb × 1 kg 1 2.2 lb	×	0.1 mg Kg/dose	=	_____ mg/dose

Step F. Solve for the lowest/therapeutic appropriate dose for this child:

$$\frac{54 \ \cancel{lb}}{1} \times \frac{1 \ \cancel{kg}}{2.2 \ \cancel{lb}} \times \frac{0.1 mg}{\cancel{kg}/dose} = \frac{5.2}{2.2} = \frac{2.4 \, mg}{dose}$$

B. Calculate the highest/safe dose for this patient

Step Pre-A. What is the patient's weight and needed conversion factor?

$$\frac{54 \, lb}{1} \times \frac{1 \, kg}{2.2 \, lb}$$

Step A. What is the high end of the appropriate pediatric dosing range?

0.2 mg/kg/dose

Step B. What is the label of the final answer of this calculation?

mg/dose

Step C. What is the strength of the medication on hand?
This step is not needed for this calculation
Step D. Conversion factor(s) needed:
No conversions needed
Step E. What is the problem pathway?

TABLE A.7				
STEP PRE-A		**STEP A**		**STEP B**
54 lb × 1 kg 1 2.2 lb	×	0.2 mg Kg/dose	=	_____ mg/dose

Step F. Solve for the highest/safe appropriate dose for this child:
C. Ask yourself: "Is the ordered dose within the safe and therapeutic pediatric dosing range of 2.4 mg to 4.7 mg?"

Lowest/therapeutic dose for this child   2.4 mg/dose
Prescribed dose   4.5 mg
Highest/safe dose for this child   4.7 mg/dose

In this case the answer is, "Yes, 4.5 mg falls between 2.4 mg and 4.7 mg." You can proceed to calculate the exact amount of medication to administer to this patient. If the prescribed dose did not fall within the drug guide's identified appropriate dosing range, the RN will hold the ordered dose and contact the prescribing health care provider.
D. Calculate the dose of medication to give and administer
Prescribed: Morphine sulfate 4.5 mg IV now
Medication available: Morphine sulfate 2 mg/mL
Steps A through F result in solving this problem as follows:

$$\frac{45 \ \cancel{mg}}{1} \times \frac{1 \, mL}{2 \ \cancel{mg}} = \frac{4.5}{2} = 2.3 \, mL$$

Accuracy when calculating dosages is critical. Once you have made your calculation, think about it. Does it make sense? If you are unsure, ask another nurse to check your math.

CRITICAL THINKING QUESTIONS

1. A patient receives a medication at 1 g intravenous piggyback (IVPB) every 12 hours (q12h). The medication comes in a unit dose of 1 g in 250 mL and, according to the manufacturer's recommendation, should be administered over 1 hour. The medication pumps are all in use, and you must use a primary tubing with a 15 gtt/mL factor. At what rate (in gtt/min) must the IV run?
   a. What interventions would you institute if your patient were at risk for pulmonary edema?
   b. The patient has one IV line, and the IVPB is incompatible with the continuous IV medication, which cannot be stopped for the duration of the IVPB. What needs to be done? What if the patient was a difficult IV start?
2. You have a 3-year-old pediatric patient who weighs 35 lb. You are to give a medication 30 mg/kg/24 hours in divided doses q8h. The unit dose medication comes in a 75 mg/mL of liquid. How many mL would you need to give your patient per dose?
   a. What would you do if your patient had a 22-gauge IV needle in the hand?
   b. The patient complains that the IV hurts. What is your intervention?
3. Your patient is to receive morphine sulfate 4 mg IVPB for breakthrough pain q2h PRN. The patient is on a continuous morphine drip at 4 mg/hr from a peripherally inserted central catheter (PICC) line, with a morphine sulfate concentration of 50 mg in 50 mL. Over an 8-hour shift the patient receives three PRN doses. What is the total mg of morphine sulfate the patient received for the shift?
   a. The patient has not had a bowel movement in the past 3 days. What interventions must be made?
   b. The prescriber has indicated that the patient is to have MS Content PO after the patient's first bowel movement. What is the equivalent dose of the MS Content PO to the IV dose the patient has been receiving?

WEB RESOURCES

http://mathforum.org/library/drmath/view/58519.html
http://www.hotmath.com/
http://www.dosagehelp.com/
http://www.tutor.com/subjects/math.aspx
https://www.youtube.com/watch?v=LRYAzR20cyw
https://www.youtube.com/watch?v=pd9girgZeY4
http://www.unc.edu/~bangel/quiz/quiz5.htm

Page numbers followed by *f* indicate figures, *t* indicate tables, and *b* indicate boxes.